Tucholsky Wagner Zola Scott Sydow Freud Schlegel
Turgenev Wallace Fonatne
Twain Walther von der Vogelweide Fouqué Friedrich II. von Preußen
Weber Freiligrath Frey
Fechner Fichte Weiße Rose von Fallersleben Kant Ernst Frommel
Richthofen
Engels Fielding Hölderlin
Fehrs Faber Flaubert Eichendorff Tacitus Dumas
Eliasberg Ebner Eschenbach
Feuerbach Maximilian I. von Habsburg Fock Eliot Zweig
Ewald Vergil
Goethe Elisabeth von Österreich London
Mendelssohn Balzac Shakespeare Dostojewski Ganghofer
Lichtenberg Rathenau
Trackl Stevenson Doyle Gjellerup
Tolstoi Hambruch
Mommsen Lenz Droste-Hülshoff
Thoma Hanrieder
Dach Verne von Arnim Hägele Hauff Humboldt
Reuter Rousseau Hagen Hauptmann Gautier
Karrillon Garschin
Defoe Baudelaire
Damaschke Hebbel
Descartes Hegel Kussmaul Herder
Wolfram von Eschenbach Dickens Schopenhauer Rilke George
Darwin Melville Grimm Jerome Bebel Proust
Bronner Campe Horváth Aristoteles Federer
Bismarck Vigny Barlach Voltaire Herodot
Gengenbach Heine
Storm Casanova Tersteegen Grillparzer Georgy
Chamberlain Lessing Langbein Gryphius
Brentano Lafontaine
Strachwitz Claudius Schiller Kralik Iffland Sokrates
Katharina II. von Rußland Bellamy Schilling
Gerstäcker Raabe Gibbon Tschechow
Löns Hesse Hoffmann Gogol Wilde Gleim Vulpius
Luther Heym Hofmannsthal Klee Hölty Morgenstern
Roth Heyse Klopstock Kleist Goedicke
Luxemburg Puschkin Homer Mörike
La Roche Horaz Musil
Machiavelli Kierkegaard Kraft Kraus
Navarra Aurel Musset Moltke
Nestroy Marie de France Lamprecht Kind Kirchhoff Hugo
Laotse Ipsen Liebknecht
Nietzsche Nansen Ringelnatz
Marx Lassalle Gorki Klett Leibniz
von Ossietzky May Irving
vom Stein Lawrence
Petalozzi Platon Knigge
Pückler Michelangelo Kock Kafka
Sachs Poe Liebermann Korolenko
de Sade Praetorius Mistral Zetkin

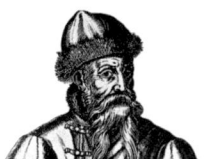

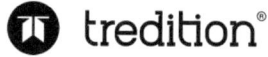

tredition was established in 2006 by Sandra Latusseck and Soenke Schulz. Based in Hamburg, Germany, tredition offers publishing solutions to authors and publishing houses, combined with worldwide distribution of printed and digital book content. tredition is uniquely positioned to enable authors and publishing houses to create books on their own terms and without conventional manufacturing risks.

For more information please visit: www.tredition.com

Civics and Health

William H. Allen

Imprint

This book is part of the TREDITION CLASSICS series.

Author: William H. Allen
Cover design: toepferschumann, Berlin (Germany)

Publisher: tredition GmbH, Hamburg (Germany)
ISBN: 978-3-8491-7404-0

www.tredition.com
www.tredition.de

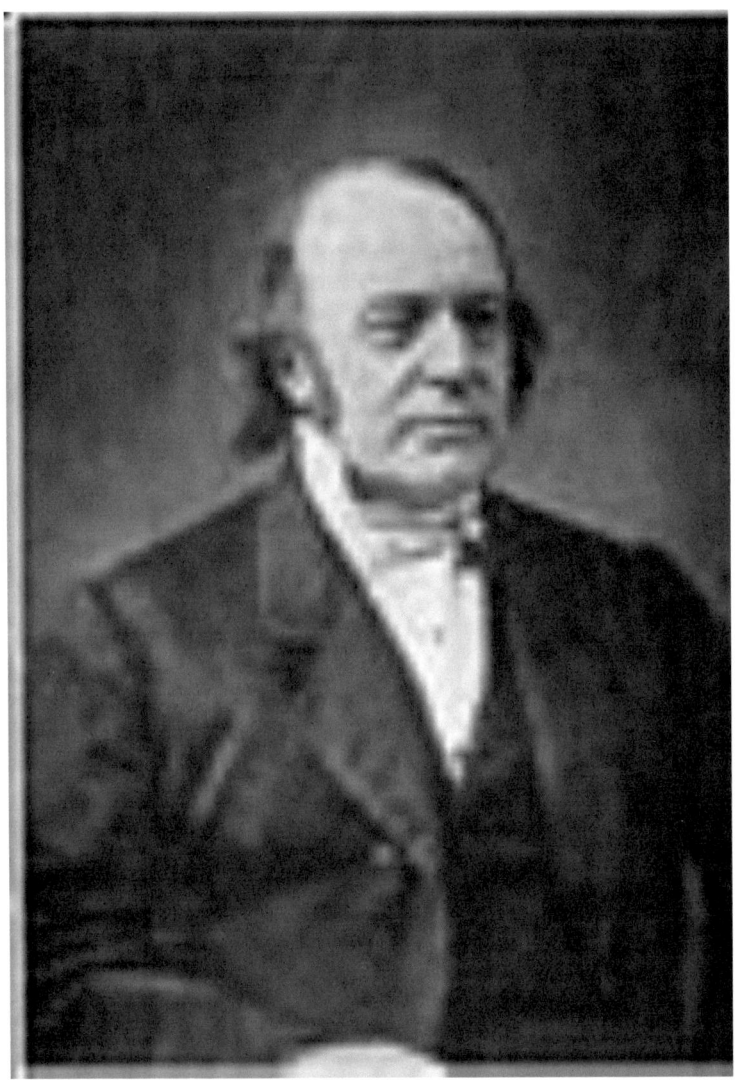

LOUIS AGASSIZ
"A natural law is as sacred as a moral principle"

INTRODUCTION

It is a common weakness of mankind to be caught by an idea and captivated by a phrase. To rest therewith content and to neglect the carrying of the idea into practice is a weakness still more common. It is this frequent failure of reformers to reduce their theories to practice, their tendency to dwell in the cloudland of the ideal rather than to test it in action, that has often made them distrusted and unpopular.

With our forefathers the phrase *mens sana in corpore sano* was a high favorite. It was constantly quoted with approval by writers on hygiene and sanitation, and used as the text or the finale of hundreds of popular lectures. And yet we shall seek in vain for any evidence of its practical usefulness. Its words are good and true, but passive and actionless, not of that dynamic type where words are "words indeed, but words that draw armed men behind them."

Our age is of another temper. It yearns for reality. It no longer rests satisfied with mere ideas, or words, or phrases. The modern Ulysses would drink life to the dregs. The present age is dissatisfied with the vague assurance that the Lord will provide, and, rightly or wrongly, is beginning to expect the state to provide. And while this desire for reality has its drawbacks, it has also its advantages. Our age doubts absolutely the virtues of blind submission and resignation, and cries out instead for prevention and amelioration. Disease is no longer regarded, as Cruden regarded [vi]it, as the penalty and the consequence of sin. Nature herself is now perceived to be capable of imperfect work. Time was when the human eye was referred to as a perfect apparatus, but the number of young children wearing spectacles renders that idea untenable to-day.

Meanwhile the multiplication of state asylums and municipal hospitals, and special schools for deaf or blind children and for cripples, speaks eloquently and irresistibly of an intimate connection between civics and health. There is a physical basis of citizenship, as there is a physical basis of life and of health; and any one who will take the trouble to read even the Table of Contents of this book will see that for Dr. Allen prevention is a text and the making of sound citizens a sermon. Given the sound body, we have nowadays small fear for the sound mind. The rigid physiological dualism implied in the phrase *mens sana in corpore sano* is no longer allowed. To-day the sound body generally includes the sound mind, and vice versa. If mental dullness be due to imperfect ears, the remedy lies in medical treatment of those organs, — not in education of the brain. If lack of initiative or energy proceeds from defective aëration of the blood due to adenoids blocking the air tides in the windpipe, then the remedy lies not in better teaching but in a simple surgical operation.

Shakespeare, in his wildwood play, saw sermons in stones and books in the running brooks. We moderns find a drama in the fateful lives of ordinary mortals, sermons in their physical salvation from some of the ills that flesh is heir to, and books — like this of Dr. Allen's — in striving to teach mankind how to become happier, and healthier, and more useful members of society.

Dr. Allen is undoubtedly a reformer, but of the modern, not the ancient, type. He is a prophet crying in our present [vii]wilderness; but he is more than a prophet, for he is always intensely practical, insisting, as he does, on getting things done, and done soon, and done right.

No one can read this volume, or even its chapter-headings, without surprise and rejoicing: surprise, that the physical basis of effective citizenship has hitherto been so utterly neglected in America; rejoicing, that so much in the way of the prevention of incapacity and unhappiness can be so easily done, and is actually beginning to be done.

The gratitude of every lover of his country and his kind is due to the author for his interesting and vivid presentation of the outlines of a subject fundamental to the health, the happiness, and the well-being of the people, and hence of the first importance to every American community, every American citizen.

WILLIAM T. SEDGWICK

Massachusetts Institute of Technology

CONTENTS

PART IV. OFFICIAL MACHINERY FOR ENFORCING HEALTH RIGHTS

PART V. ALLIANCE OF HYGIENE, PATRIOTISM, AND RELIGION

[3]

PART I. HEALTH RIGHTS

CHAPTER IToC

HEALTH A CIVIC OBLIGATION

In forty-five states and territories the teaching of hygiene with special reference to alcohol and tobacco is made compulsory. To hygiene alone, of the score of subjects found in our modern grammar-school curriculum, is given statutory right of way for so many minutes per week, so many pages per text-book, or so many pages per chapter. For the neglect of no other study may teachers be removed from office and fined. Yet school garrets and closets are full of hygiene text-books unopened or little used, while of all subjects taught by five hundred thousand American teachers and studied by twenty million American pupils the least interesting to both teacher and pupil is that forced upon both by state legislation. To complete the paradox, this least interesting subject happens also to be the most vital to the child, to the home, to industry, to social welfare, and to education itself.

Whether the subject of hygiene is necessarily dull, whether the statutes requiring regular instruction in the laws of health are violated with impunity, whether health principles are flaunted by health practice at school, — these are questions of immediate concern to parents as a class, to employers as a class, to every pastor, every civic leader, every health officer, every taxpayer.

Interviews with teachers and principals regarding the present apathy to formal hygiene instruction have brought [4]out the following points that merit the serious consideration of those who are struggling for higher health standards.

1. *There is many a slip 'twixt the making of a law and its enforcement.* If laws regarding hygiene instruction are not enforced, we should not be surprised. It has been nobody's business to see whether and how hygiene is being taught. The moral crusade spent itself in forcing compulsory laws upon the statute books of every state and territory. Making a fetish of *Legislation*, the advocates of anti-alcohol and anti-tobacco instruction failed to see the truth that experienced political reformers are but slowly coming to see — *Legislation which does not provide machinery for its own enforcement is apt to do little good and frequently will do much harm.* Machinery, however admirably adapted to the work to be done, will get out of order and become useless, or even harmful, unless constantly watched and efficiently directed. Of what possible use is it to say that state money may be withheld from any school board which fails to enforce the law regarding instruction in hygiene, if state officials never enforce the penalty? So long as the penalty is not enforced for flagrant violation, what difference does it make whether the reason is indifference, ignorance, or desire to thwart the law? Fortunately, it is easy for each one of us to learn how often and in what way the children in our community are being taught hygiene, and how the schools of our state teach and practice the laws of health. If either the spirit or the letter of the law regarding instruction in hygiene is being violated, we can measure the penalty paid in health and morals by our children and our community. We can learn whether law, text-book, curriculum, or teacher should be changed. We can insist upon discussion of the facts and upon remedies suggested by the facts.

2. *Teachers give as one reason for neglecting hygiene, that they are often compelled to struggle with a curriculum which [5]requires more than they are able to teach and more than pupils are able to learn in the time allowed.* While an overcharged curriculum may explain, it surely does not justify, the violation of law and the dropping of hygiene from our school curriculum. If there is any class of citizen who should teach

and practice respect for law as law, it is the teacher. Parents, school directors, county and state superintendents, university presidents, social workers, owe it not only to themselves, but to the American school-teacher, either to repeal the laws that enjoin instruction in hygiene or else so to adjust the curriculum that teachers can comply with those laws. The present situation that discredits both law and hygiene is most demoralizing to teacher, pupil, and community. Many of us might admire the man teacher who frankly says he never explains the evils of cigarettes because he himself is an inveterate smoker of cigarettes. But what must we think of the school system that shifts to such a man the right and the responsibility of deciding whether or not to explain to underfed and overstimulated children of the slums the truth regarding cigarettes? If practice and precept must be consistent, shall the man be removed, shall he change his habits, shall the law regarding instruction in hygiene be changed, or shall other provision be made for bringing child and essential facts together in a way that will not dull the child's receptivity?

3. *Teachers are made to feel that while arithmetic and reading are essential, hygiene is not essential.* Whatever may be the facts regarding the relative value of arithmetic and hygiene, whether or not our state legislators have made a mistake in declaring hygiene to be essential, are questions altogether too important for child and state to be left to the discretion of the individual teacher or superintendent. It is fair to the teachers who say they cannot afford to turn aside from the three R's to teach hygiene, to admit [6]that they have not hitherto identified the teaching of hygiene with the promotion of the physical welfare of children. Teachers awake to the opportunity will sacrifice not only hygiene but any other subject for the sake of promoting children's health. They do not really believe that arithmetic is more important than health. What they mean to say is that hygiene, as taught by them, has not heretofore had an appreciable effect upon their pupils' health; that other agencies exist, outside of the school, to teach the child how to avoid certain diseases and how to observe the fundamental laws of health, whereas no other agencies exist to give the child the essentials of arithmetic, reading, and geography. "We teach (or try to teach) what our classes are examined in. If you want a subject taught, you must test a class in it and

hold a teacher responsible for results, and examinations are mercilessly unhygienic, you know."

4. *Teachers believe that they get better results for their children from teaching hygiene informally and indirectly than from stated formal lessons.* Whether instruction should be informal or formal is merely a question of method to be determined by results. What the results are, can be determined by principals, superintendents, and students of education. It is easy to understand how at the time of a fever epidemic children could be taught as much in one week about infection, disease germs, antiseptics, value of cleanliness, etc., as in five or ten months when vivid illustration is lacking. Physicians themselves learn more from one epidemic of smallpox than from four years of book study. To make possible and to require a daily shower bath will undoubtedly do more to inculcate habits of health than repeated lessons about the skin, pores, evaporation, and discharge of impurities.

If one illustration is better than ten lessons, if an open window is worth more than all that text-books have to say [7]about ventilation, if a seat adjusted to the child is better than an anatomical chart, this does not mean that instruction in hygiene should cease. On the contrary, it means that provision should be made for every teacher to open windows, to adjust desks, to use the experience of individual children for the education of the class. If the rank and file of teachers have not hitherto been sufficiently observant of physiological and hygienic facts, if they are unprepared from their own lives to detect or to furnish illustrations for the child, this again does not mean that the child should be denied the illustrations, but that the teacher should either have instruction and experience to incite interest and to stimulate powers of observation, or else be asked to give place to another teacher who is able to furnish such qualifications.

5. *Children, like adults, can be interested in other people, in rules of conduct, in social conditions, in living and working relations more easily than in their own bodies.* The normal, healthy child thinks very little of himself apart from the other boys and girls, the games, the studies, the animals, the nature wonders, the hardships that come to him from the outside. So true is this that one of the best means of mitigating or curing many ailments is to divert the child's attention

from himself to things outside of himself that he can look at, hear, enjoy. The power to concentrate attention upon oneself is a sign either of a diseased body, a diseased mind, or a highly trained mind. To study others and to recognize the similarity between others and oneself is as natural as the body itself. Teachers are consulting this line of easiest access to children's attention when they honor children according to cleanliness of hands, of teeth, of shoes. Human interest attaches to what parks or excursions are doing for sickly children, how welfare work is improving factory employees, how smallpox is conquered by vaccination, how insurance companies [8]refuse to take risks upon the lives of men or women addicted to the excessive use of alcohol or tobacco.

Other people's interests—tenement conditions, factory rules—can be described in figures and actions that appeal to the imagination and impress upon the mind pictures that are repeatedly reawakened by experience and observation on the playground, at home, on the way to school or to work. "Once upon a time—" will always arrest attention more quickly than "The human frame consists—." What others think of me helps me to obey law—statutory, moral, or hygienic—more than what I know of law itself. How social instincts dominate may be illustrated by an experience in advertising a public bath near a thoroughfare traveled daily by thousands of working girls. I prepared a card to be distributed among these girls that began: "A cool, refreshing bath, etc." This card was criticised by one who knows the ways of girls and women, as follows: "Of course you get no success when you have a man stand on the street corner and pass out cards telling girls to get clean. Every girl that is worth while is affronted by the insinuation." Acting upon this expert advice, we then got out a neatly printed card reading as follows: "For a clear complexion, sprightly step, and bounding vitality, visit the Center Market Baths, open from 6 A.M. to 9 P.M. daily." The board of managers shook their sage masculine heads and reluctantly gave permission to issue these appeals. Woman's judgment was vindicated, however, and the advantage was proved of urging health for "society's" sake rather than for health's sake, when the patronage of the bath jumped at once to considerable proportions.

6. *Other people's habits of health influence our well-being quite as much, if not more, than our own.* Because we are social beings, ability

to get along with our families, our friends, our employers, is—at least so it seems to most of us—quite as important as individual health. For too [9]many of us, living hygienically is absolutely impossible without inconveniencing and bothering the majority of persons with whom we live. I remember a girl in college,—a fresh-air fiend,—who every morning, no matter how cold, threw the windows wide open. Then, with forty others, I thought this girl a nuisance as well as a menace to health, but now, twenty years afterwards, I find myself wanting to do the same thing. Professor Patten, the economist, whom I shall quote many times because he is particularly interested in the purpose of this book, was recently dining at my house and illustrated from his own health the importance of teaching hygiene so as to affect social as well as personal standards. "To be true to my own health needs, I ought to have declined nearly everything that has been offered me for dinner, but in the long run, if I am going to visit, my eating what is placed before me is better for society than making those who entertain me feel uncomfortable."

Most of us know what uphill work it is to live hygienically in an unhygienic environment. I remember how hard it was to eat happily when sitting beside a college professor who took brown pills before each meal, yellow pills between each course, and a dose of black medicine after the meal was over. Mariano, an Italian lad cured of bone tuberculosis by out-of-door salt air at Sea Breeze, returned to his tenement home an ardent apostle of fresh air day and night, winter and summer. His family allowed him to open the window before going to bed, but closed it as soon as he was asleep. Lawrence Veiller, our greatest expert on tenement conditions, says: "To bathe in a tenement where a family of six occupy three rooms often involves the sacrifice of privacy and decency, which are quite as important to social betterment as cleanliness."

To live unhygienically where others live hygienically is quite as difficult. Witness the speedy improvement of dissipated men when boarding with country friends who eat [10]rationally and retire early. It must have been knowledge of this fact that prompted the tramways of Belfast to post conspicuous notices: "Spitting is a vile and filthy habit, and those who practice it subject themselves to the disgust and loathing of their fellow-passengers." It is almost impossible to have indigestion, blues, and headache when one is camping, particularly where action and enjoyment fill the day. Our practical question is, therefore, not "What shall I eat, how many hours shall I sleep, what shall I wear," but "How can I manage to get into an environment among living and working conditions where the people I live with and want to please, those who influence me and are influenced by me, make healthy living easy and natural?"

7. *Because the problems of health have to do principally with environment, — home, street, school, business, — it is worth while trying to relate hygiene instruction to industry and government, to preach health from the standpoint of industrial and national efficiency rather than of individual well-being.* Since healthful living requires the coöperation of all persons in a household, in a group, or in a community, we must find some working programme that will make it easy for all the members of the group to observe health standards. A city government that spends taxes inefficiently can produce more sickness, wretchedness, incapacity in one year than pamphlets on health can offset in a generation. Failure to enforce health laws is a more serious menace to health and morals than drunkenness or tobacco cancer. Unclean streets, unclean dairies, unclean, overcrowded tenements can do more harm than alcohol and tobacco because they can breed an appetite that craves stimulants and drugs. Others have taught how the body acts, what we ought to eat, how we should live. We are concerned here not with repeating the laws of health, but with a consideration of the mechanism that will make it possible for us so to work together that we can observe those laws.

[11]

SEVEN HEALTH MOTIVES AND SEVEN CATCHWORDS

In making a health programme as in making a boat, a garden, or a baseball team, the first step is to look about and see what material there is to work with. A baseball team will fail miserably unless the captain places each man where he can play best. Gardening is profitless when the gardener does not know the habits of plants and the possibilities of different kinds of soil. So in planning a health programme we must study our materials and use each where it will fit best. The materials of first importance to a health programme in civilized countries are men; for men working together can control water sources, drainage, and ventilation, or else move away to surroundings better suited to healthful living. Therefore the first concern of the leader in a health crusade is the human kind he has to work for and work with.

Seven kinds of man are to be found in every community, seven different points of view with regard to health administration. Each individual, likewise, may have seven attitudes toward health laws, seven reasons for demanding health protection. These seven points of view, seven stages of development, are clearly marked in the evolution of sanitary administration throughout the civilized world. With few exceptions, it is possible, by examining ourselves, our friends, and our communities, to see where one motive begins and leaves off, giving way to or mixing with one or more other motives. A friend once asked me if I could keep this number seven from growing to eight or nine. Perhaps not. Perhaps there are more kinds of people, [12]more health motives, more stages in health progress; but I am sure of these seven, and certain that they have been of great help to me in planning health crusades for the state of New Jersey and for New York City. The number seven was not reached hit-or-miss fashion, nor was it chosen for its biblical prestige. On the contrary, it came as the result of studying health administration in twoscore British and American cities, and of reading scores of books on sanitary evolution.

Seven catchwords make it easy to remember the characteristics and the source of every motive, every kind of person, and every stage in the evolution of sanitary standards. These seven catchwords are: *Instinct, Display, Commerce, Anti-nuisance, Anti-slum, Pro-slum, Rights*. By the use of these catchwords any teacher, parent, public official, educator, or social worker should be able to size up the situation, the needs, and the opportunity of the individuals or the communities for whom a health crusade is planned.

Instinct was the first health officer and made the first health laws. Instinct warns us against unusual and offensive odors, sights, and noises, just as it causes us to seek that which is agreeable. Primitive man in common with other animals learned by sad experience to avoid certain herbs as poisons; to bury or to move away from the dead; to shun discolored drinking water. During the roaming period sun and air and water acted as scavengers. When tribes settled down in one spot for long periods, habits that had hitherto been inoffensive and safe became noticeably injurious and unpleasant. Heads of tribes gave orders prohibiting such habits and restricting disagreeable acts and objects to certain portions of the camp. Instinct places outhouses on our farms and then gradually removes them farther and farther from dwellings. In many school yards, more particularly in country districts and small towns, [13]outhouses are a crying offense against animal instinct. In visiting slum districts in Irish and Scotch cities, and in London, Paris, Berlin, and New York, I never found conditions so offensive to crude animal instinct as those I knew when a boy in Minnesota school yards, or those I have since seen in a Boy Republic. But the evil is not corrected because it is not made anybody's business to execute instinct's mandates. In the Boy Republic the leaders were waiting for the children themselves to revolt, as does primitive man.

Table I

Typhoid a Rural Disease[1]

	Average Per Cent of Rural Population	Average Typhoid Fever Death Rate per 100,000
Five states in which the urban population was more than 60% of the total	30	25
Six states in which the urban population was between 40% and 60%	49	42
Seven states in which the urban population was between 30% and 40%	67	38
Eight states in which the urban population was between 20% and 30%	75	46
Twelve states in which the urban population was between 10% and 20%	87	62
Twelve states in which the urban population was between 0 and 10%	95	67

Among large numbers of persons, in city as well as country, washing the body is still a matter of instinct, a bath not being taken until the body is offensive, the hands not being washed until their condition interferes with the enjoyment of food or with one's treatment by others. There is a point of neglect beyond which instinct will not [14]permit even a tramp to go. If cleanliness is next to godliness, the average child is most ungodly by nature, for it loathes the means of cleanliness and otherwise observes instinct's health warnings only after experience has punished or after other motives from the outside have prompted action. The chief form of legislation of the instinct age is provision of penalties for those who poison food, water, or fellow-man. There are districts in America where hygiene is supposed to be taught to children that are conscious of no other sanitary legislation but that which punishes the poisoner.

Display has always been an active health crusader. Professor Patten says the best thing that could happen to the slums of every city would be for every girl and woman to be given white slippers, white stockings, a white dress, and white hat. Why? Because they would at once notice and resent the dirt on the street, in their hallways, and in their own homes. People that have nothing to "spoil" really do not see dirt, for it interferes in no way with their comfort so far as they can see. Their windows are crusted with dust, their babies' milk bottles are yellow with germs. Who cares? Similar conditions exist among well-to-do women who live on isolated farms with no one to notice their personal appearance except others of the family who prefer rest to cleanliness. But let the tenement mother or the isolated farmer's wife entertain the minister or the schoolteacher, the candidate for sheriff or the ward boss, let her go to Coney Island or to the county fair, and at once an outside standard is set up that requires greater regard for personal appearance and leads to "cleaning up."

Elbow sleeves and light summer waists have led many a girl to daily bathing of at least those parts of the body that other people see. Entertainments and sociables, Saturday choir practice and church have led many a young man to bathe for others' sake when quite satisfied [15]to forego the ordeal so far as his own comfort and health were concerned. Streets on which the well-to-do live are kept clean. Why? Not because Madam Well-to-do cares so much for health, but because she associates cleanliness with social prestige. It is necessary for the display of her carriages and dresses, just as paved streets and a plentiful supply of water for public baths and private homes were essential to the display of Rome's luxury. Generally speaking, residence streets are cleaned in small towns just as waterworks are introduced, to gratify the display motive of those who have lawns to water and clothes to show.

Instinct strengthens the display motive. As every one can be interested in instinct hygiene, so every one is capable of this display motive to the extent that his position is affected by other people's opinion. It was love of display quite as much as love of beauty that gave Greece the goddess Hygeia, the worship of whom expressed secondarily a desire for universal health, and primarily a love of the beautiful among those who had leisure to enjoy it.

Commerce brooks no preventable interference with profits, whether by disease, death, impassable streets, or disabled men. The age of chivalry was also the age of indescribable filth, plague, Black Death, and spotted fever that cost the lives of millions. It would be impossible in the civilized world to duplicate the combination of luxury and filthy, disease-breeding conditions in the midst of which Queen Bess and her courtiers held their revels. The first protest was made, not by the church, not by sanitarians, but by the great merchants who were unable to insure against loss and ruin from the plagues that thrived on filth and overcrowding. By an interesting coincidence the first systematic street cleaning and the first systematic ship cleaning—maritime quarantine—date from the same year, 1348 A.D.; the former in the foremost German [16]trading town, Cologne, and the latter in Venice, the foremost trading town of Italy. The merchants of Philadelphia and New York started the first boards of health in the United States. For what purpose? To prevent business losses from yellow fever. Desire for passable streets, drains, waterworks, and strong boards of health has generally started with merchants. For commercial reasons many of our states vote more money for the protection of cattle than for the protection of human life, and the United States votes millions for the study of hog cholera, chicken pip, and animal tuberculosis, while neglecting communicable diseases of men. No class in a community will respond more quickly to an appeal for the rigid enforcement of health laws than the merchant class; none will oppose so bitterly as that which makes profits out of the violation of health laws.

Table II

Cost in Life Capital of Preventable Diseases[2]

Age	Estimated Value of Human Life	Multiply by the number of deaths for each age group to learn the cost in life capital to your community in loss of life from one or all preventable diseases.
0- 5 years	$1,500	
5-10 years	2,300	

10-15 years	2,500
15-20 years	3,000
20-25 years	5,000
25-30 years	7,500
30-35 years	7,000
35-40 years	6,000
40-45 years	5,500
45-50 years	5,000
50-55 years	4,500
55-60 years	4,500
60-65 years	2,000
65-70 years	1,000
70- years	1,000

[17]*Anti-nuisance* motives do not affect health laws until people with different incomes and different tastes try to live together. In a small town where everybody keeps a cow and a pig, piggeries and stables offend no one; but when the doctor, the preacher, the dressmaker, the lawyer, and the leading merchant stop keeping pigs and cows, they begin to find other people's stables and piggeries offensive. The early laws against throwing garbage, fish heads, household refuse, offal, etc., on the main street were made by kings and princes offended by such practices. The word "nuisance" was coined in days when neighbors lived the same kind of life and were not sensitive to things like house slops, ash piles, etc. The first nuisances were things that neighbors stumbled over or ran into while using the public highway. Next, goats and other animals interfering with safety were described as nuisances, and legal protection against them was worked out. It has never been necessary to change the maxim which originally defined a nuisance: "So use your own property that you will not injure another in the use of his property." The thing that has changed and grown has been society's knowledge of acts and objects that prevent a man from enjoying his own property. To-day the number of things that the law calls nui-

sances is so great that it takes hundreds of pages to describe them. Stables and outhouses must be set back from the street. Every man must dispose of garbage and drainage on his own property. Stables and privies must be at least a hundred feet from water reservoirs. Factories may not pollute streams that furnish drinking water. Merchants may be punished if they put banana skins in milk cans, or if they fail to scald and cleanse all milk receptacles before returning them to wholesalers. Automobile drivers may be punished for disturbing sleep. Anything that injures my health will be declared a nuisance and abolished, if I can prove that my health is being injured and that I am doing all I can to [18]avoid that injury. No educational work will accomplish more for any community than to make rich and poor alike conscious of nuisances that are being committed against themselves and their neighbors. The rich are able to run away from nuisances that they cannot have abated. If proper publicity is given to living conditions among those who do not resist nuisances, the presence of such conditions will itself become offensive to the well-to-do, who will take steps to remove the nuisance. Jacob Riis in this way made the slums a nuisance to rich residents in New York City and stimulated tenement reform, building of parks, etc.

Anti-slum motives originated in cities where there is a clear dividing line between the clean and the unclean, the infected and the uninfected, the orderly and the disorderly, high and low vitality. As soon as one district becomes definitely known as a source of nuisance, infection, and disease, better situated districts begin to make laws to protect themselves. A great part of our existing health codes and a very large part of the funds spent on health administration are designed to protect those of high income against disease incident to those of low income, high vitality against low vitality, houses with rooms to spare against houses that are overcrowded. To the small town and the country the slum means generally the near-by city whose papers talk of epidemic scarlet fever, diphtheria, or smallpox. Cities have only recently begun to experience anti-slum aversion to country dairies whose uncleanliness brings infected milk to city babies, or to filthy factories and farms that pollute water reservoirs and cause typhoid. The last serious smallpox epidemic in the East came from the South by way of rural districts that failed to notify the Pennsylvania state board of health of the outbreak until the disease was scattered broadcast. Every individual knows of some family or some district that is immediately pictured when terms like "disease," "epidemic," "slum," are [19]pronounced. The steps worked out by the anti-slum motive to protect "those who have" from disease arising from "those who have not" are given on page 31.

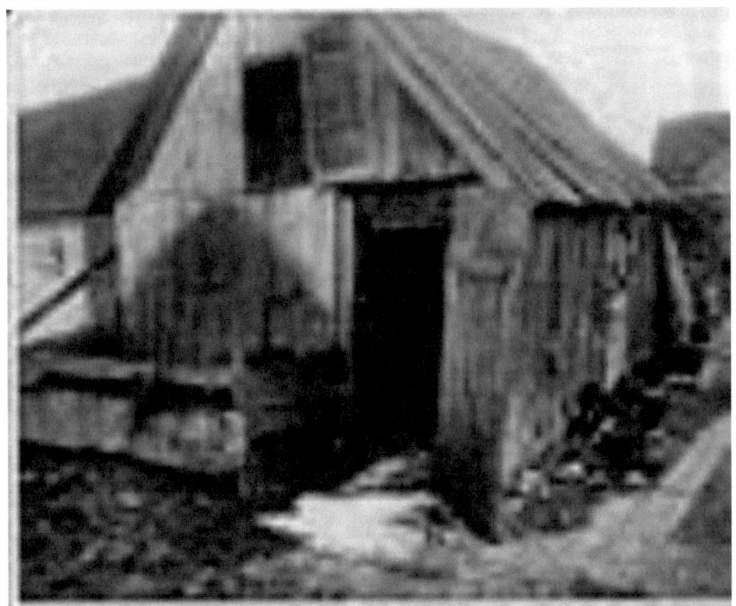

A COUNTRY MENACE TO CITY HEALTH

Pro-slum motives are not exactly born of anti-slum motives, but, thanks to the instinctive kindness of the human heart, follow promptly after the dangers of the slum have been described. You and I work together to protect ourselves against neglect, nuisance, and disease. In a district by which we must pass and with which we must deal, one of us or a neighbor or friend will turn our attention from our danger to the suffering of those against whom we wish to protect ourselves. Charles Dickens so described Oliver Twist and David Copperfield that Great Britain organized societies and secured legislation to improve the almshouse, school, and working and living conditions. When health reports, newspapers, and charitable societies [20]make us see that the slum menaces our health and our happiness, we become interested in the slum for its own sake. We then start children's aid societies, consumer's leagues, sanitary and prison associations, child-labor committees, and "efficient government" clubs.

Rights motives are the last to be evolved in individuals or communities. The well-to-do protect their instinct, their comfort, their commerce, but run away from the slums and build in the secluded spots or on the well-policed and well-cleaned avenues and boulevards. Uptown is often satisfied with putting health officials to work to protect it against downtown. Pro-slum motives are shared by too few and are expressed too irregularly to help all of those who suffer from crowded tenements, impure milk, unclean streets, inadequate schooling. So long as those who suffer have no other protection than the self-interest or the benevolence of those better situated, disease and hardship inevitably persist. Health administration is incomplete until its blessings are given to men, women, and children as rights that can be enforced through courts, as can the right to free speech, the freedom of the press, and trial by jury. There is all the difference in the world between having one's street clean because it is a danger to some distant neighbor, or because that neighbor takes some philanthropic interest in its residents, and because one has a right to clean streets, regardless of the distant neighbor's welfare or interest. When the right to health is granted health laws are made, and all men within the jurisdiction of the lawmaking power own health machinery that provides for the administration of those laws. A system of public baths takes the place of a bathhouse supported by charity; a law restricting the construction and management of all tenements takes the place of a block of model tenements, financed by some wealthy man; medical examination of all school children takes the place of a private dispensary; [21]a probation law takes the place of the friendly visitor to the county jail.

Most of the rights we call inalienable are political rights no longer questioned by anybody and no longer thought of in connection with our everyday acts, pleasures, and necessities. When our political rights were formulated in maxims, living was relatively simple. There was no factory problem, no transportation problem, no exploitation of women and children in industry. Our ancestors firmly believed that if the strong could be prevented from interfering with the political rights of the weak, all would have an equal chance. The reason that our political maxims mean less to-day than two hundred years ago is that nobody is challenging our right to move from place to place if we can afford it, to trial by jury if charged with crime, to speak or print the truth about men or governments. If, however, anybody should interfere with our freedom in this respect, it would be of tremendous help that everybody we know would resent such interference and would point to maxims handed down by our ancestors and incorporated in our national and state constitutions as formal expressions of unanimous public opinion.

The time is past when any one seriously believes that political freedom or personal liberty will be universal, just because everybody has a right to talk, to move from place to place, to print stories in the newspapers. The relation of man to man to-day requires that we formulate rules of action that prevent one man's taking from another those rights, economic and industrial, that are as essential to twentieth-century happiness as were political rights to eighteenth-century happiness. Political maxims showed how, through common desire and common action, steps could be taken by the individual and by the whole of society for the protection of all. Health rights, likewise, are to be obtained through common action. A modern city must [22]know who is accountable when an automobile runs over a pedestrian, when a train load of passengers lose their lives because of an engineer's carelessness, when an employee is incapacitated for work by an accident for which he is not responsible, or when fever epidemics threaten life and liberty without check. How can a child who is prevented by removable physical defects from breathing through his nose be enthusiastic over free speech? Of what use is freedom of the press to those who find reading harder than factory toil? How futile the right to trial by jury if removable physical defects make children unable to do what the law expects! Who would not exchange rights of petition for ability to earn a living? Children permanently incapacitated to share the law's benefits cannot appreciate the privilege of pursuing happiness.

Succeeding chapters will enumerate a number of health rights and will show through what means we can work together to guarantee that we shall not injure the health of our neighbor and that our neighbor shall not injure our health. The truest index to economic status and to standards of living is health environment. The best criterion of opportunity for industrial and political efficiency is the conditions affecting health. The seven catchwords that describe seven motives to health legislation and health administration, seven ways of approaching health needs, and seven reasons for meeting them, should be found helpful in analyzing the problem confronting the individual leader. Generally speaking, we cannot watch political rights grow, but health rights are evolved before our eyes all the time. If we wish, we can see in our own city or township the steps taken, one by one, that have slowly led to granting a large number of health rights to every American.

FOOTNOTES:

[1] Prepared by Dr. John S. Fulton, secretary of the state board of health, Maryland, and quoted by Dr. George C. Whipple in *Typhoid Fever*.

[2] Marshall O. Leighton, quoted in Whipple's *Typhoid Fever*.

[23]

CHAPTER IIIToC

WHAT HEALTH RIGHTS ARE NOT ENFORCED IN YOUR COMMUNITY?

Laws define rights. Men enforce them. For definitions we go to books. For record of enforcement we go to acts and to conditions.[3] What health rights a community pretends to enforce will, as a rule, be found in its health code. What health rights are actually enforced can be learned only by studying both the people who are to be protected and the conditions in which these people live. A street, a cellar, a milk shop, a sick baby, or an adult consumptive tells more honestly the story of health rights enforced and health rights unenforced than either sanitary code or sanitary squad. Not until we turn our attention from definition and official to things done and dangers remaining can we learn the health progress and health needs of any city or state.

The health code of one city looks very much like the health code of every other city. This is natural because those who write health codes generally copy other codes. Even small cities are given complicated sanitary legislative powers by state legislatures. Therefore those who judge a community's health rights by its health laws will get as erroneous an impression as those who judge hygiene instruction in our public schools from printed statements about the frequency and character of such instruction. Advocates of health codes have thought the battle won when boards of health were given almost unlimited power to abate nuisances and told how to exercise those powers.

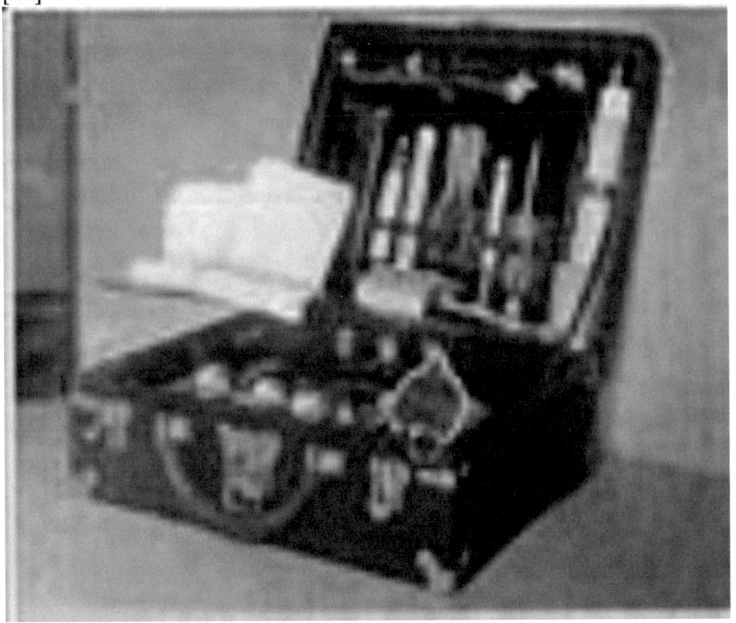

A DAIRY INSPECTOR'S OUTFIT

The slip 'twixt law making and law enforcement is everywhere found. In 1864 New York state prohibited the sale of adulterated milk. Law after law has been made since that time, giving health officials power to revoke licenses of milk dealers and to send men to jail who violated milk laws. We now know that no law will ever stop the present frightful waste of infant lives, counted in thousands annually, unless dairies are frequently inspected and forced to be clean; unless milk is kept at a temperature of about fifty degrees on the train, in the creamery, at the receiving station, and in the milk shop; unless dealers scald and thoroughly cleanse cans in which milk is shipped; unless licenses are taken from farmers, creameries, and retailers who violate the law; unless magistrates use their power to fine or imprison those who poison helpless babies by violating milk laws; and unless mothers are taught to scald [25]and thoroughly cleanse bottles, nipples, cups, and dishes from which milk is fed to the baby. We know that these things are not being done except where men or women make it their business to see that they are done. Experience tells us that inspectors will not consistently do their duty unless those who direct them have regular records of their inspections, study those records, find out work not done properly or promptly, and insist upon thorough inspection.

Whether work is done right, whether inspectors do their full duty, whether babies are protected, can be learned only from statements in black and white that show accurately the conditions of dairies and milk shops, the character of milk found and tested by inspectors, and the number of babies known to have been sick or known to have died from intestinal diseases chiefly due to unsafe milk. Any teacher or parent can learn for himself, or can teach children to learn, what steps are taken to guarantee the right to pure milk by using a table such as Table III. Whether conditions at the dairy make pure milk impossible can be told by any one who can read the score card used by New York City (Table IV).

Table III[26]

MILK INSPECTION WITHIN NEW YORK CITY, 1906

	New York		Each borough	
	Stores	Wagons	Stores	Wagons
FIELD				
Permits issued during 1906				
Permits revoked during 1906				
For discontinuance of selling				
For violation of law				
Average permits in force in 1906				
INSPECTION				
Regular inspections				
Inspections at receiving stations				
Total				
Average inspections per permit per year				
Specimens examined				
Samples taken				

CONDITIONS FOUND

Inspections finding milk above 50°

% of such discoveries to total inspections

Inspections finding adulteration

  Warning given

  Prosecuted

% of adulterations found to inspections

Rooms connected contrary to sanitary code

Ice box badly drained

Ice box unclean

Store unclean

Utensils unclean

Milk not properly cooled

Infectious disease

Persons found selling without permit

ACTION TAKEN

DESTRUCTION OF MILK

  Lots of milk destroyed for being over 50°

  Quarts so destroyed

  Lots of milk destroyed for being sour

  Quarts so destroyed

  Lots of milk destroyed for being otherwise adulterated

  Quarts so destroyed

  Total quarts destroyed

NOTICES ISSUED

  To drain and clean ice box

  To clean store

CRIMINAL ACTIONS BEGUN
    For selling adulterated milk
    For selling without permit
    For interference with inspector
    Total

[27]

Table IV

Perfect Score 100%
Score allowed ...%

File No............

DEPARTMENT OF HEALTH

(Thirteen items are here omitted)

Dairy InspectionDivision of Inspections

1 Inspection No. ....   Time .... A. P. M.   Date 190

2 All persons in the households of those engaged in producing or handling milk are .... free from all infectious disease ....

3 Date and nature of last case on farm ....

4 A sample of the water supply on this farm taken for analysis .... 190... and found to be ....

STABLE   Perfect Allow

	Perfect	Allow
5 **COW STABLE** is ...... located on elevated ground with no stagnant water, hog pen, or privy within 100 feet	1	...
6 **FLOORS** are ...... constructed of concrete or some nonabsorbent material	1	...
7 Floors are ...... properly graded and water-tight	2	...
8 **DROPS** are ...... constructed of concrete, stone, or	2	...

some nonabsorbent material		
9 Drops are ...... water-tight	2	...
10 **FEEDING TROUGHS**, platforms, or cribs are ...... well lighted and clean	1	...
11 **CEILING** is constructed of ...... and is ...... tight and dust proof	2	...
12 Ceiling is ...... free from hanging straw, dirt, or cobwebs	1	...
13 **NUMBER OF WINDOWS**...... total square feet ... which is ...... sufficient	2	...
14 Window panes are ...... washed and kept clean	1	...
15 **VENTILATION** consists of ...... which is sufficient 3, fair 1, insufficient 0	3	...
16 **AIR SPACE** is ...... cubic feet per cow which is ...... sufficient (600 and over − 3) (500 to 600 − 2) (400 to 500 − 1) (under 400 − 0)	3	...
17 **INTERIOR** of stable painted or whitewashed on ...... which is satisfactory 2, fair 1, never 0	2	...
18 **WALLS AND LEDGES** are ...... free from dirt, dust, manure, or cobwebs	2	...
19 **FLOORS AND PREMISES** are ...... free from dirt, rubbish, or decayed animal or vegetable matter	1	...
20 **COW BEDS** are ...... clean	1	...
21 **LIVE STOCK**, other than cows, are ...... excluded from rooms in which milch cows are kept	2	...
22 There is ...... direct opening from barn into silo or grain pit	1	...
23 **BEDDING** used is ...... clean, dry, and absorbent	1	...
24 **SEPARATE BUILDING** is ...... provided for cows when sick	1	...
25 Separate quarters are ...... provided for cows when calving	1	...
26 **MANURE** is ...... removed daily to at least 200 feet from the barn (... ft.)	2	...

27 Manure pile is ...... so located that the cows cannot get at it | 1 | ...

28 **LIQUID MATTER** is ...... absorbed and removed daily and ...... allowed to overflow and saturate ground under or around cow barn | 2 | ...

29 **RUNNING WATER** supply for washing stables is ...... located within building | 1 | ...

30 **DAIRY RULES** of the Department of Health are ...... posted | 1 | ...

COW YARD

31 **COW YARD** is ...... properly graded and drained | 1 | ...

32 Cow yard is ...... clean, dry, and free from manure | 2 | ...

[28]COWS

33 **COWS** have ...... been examined by veterinarian ... Date ...... 190 Report was | 3 | ...

34 Cows have ...... been tested by tuberculin, and all tuberculous cows removed | 5 | ...

35 Cows are ...... all in good flesh and condition at time of inspection | 2 | ...

36 Cows are ...... all free from clinging manure and dirt. (No. dirty ...) | 4 | ...

37 **LONG HAIRS** are ...... kept short on belly, flanks, udder, and tail | 1 | ...

38 **UDDER AND TEATS** of cows are ...... thoroughly cleaned before milking | 2 | ...

39 **ALL FEED** is ...... of good quality and all grain and coarse fodders are ...... free from dirt and mold | 1 | ...

40 **DISTILLERY** waste or any substance in a state of fermentation or putrefaction is ...... fed | 1 | ...

41 **WATER SUPPLY** for cows is ...... unpolluted and plentiful | 2 | ...

MILKERS AND MILKING

42 **ATTENDANTS** are ...... in good physical condition	1	...
43 Special Milking Suits are ...... used	1	...
44 Clothing of milkers is ...... clean	1	...
45 Hands of milkers are ...... washed clean before milking	1	...
46 **MILKING** is ...... done with dry hands	2	...
47 **FORE MILK** or first few streams from each teat is ...... discarded	2	...
48 Milk is strained at ...... and ...... in clean atmosphere	1	...
49 Milk strainer is ...... clean	1	...
50 **MILK** is ...... cooled to below 50° F. within two hours after milking and kept below 50° F. until delivered to the creamery ...... °	2	...
51 Milk from cows within 15 days before or 5 days after parturition is ...... discarded	1	...

UTENSILS

52 **MILK PAILS** have ...... all seams soldered flush	1	...
53 Milk pails are ...... of the small-mouthed design, top opening not exceeding 8 inches in diameter. Diameter	2	...
54 Milk pails are ...... rinsed with cold water immediately after using and washed clean with hot water and washing solution	2	...
55 Drying racks are ...... provided to expose milk pails to the sun	1	...

MILK HOUSE

56 **MILK HOUSE** is ...... located on elevated ground	1	...

with no hog pen, manure pile, or privy within 100 feet		
57 Milk house has ...... direct communication with ...... building	1	...
58 Milk house has ...... sufficient light and ventilation	1	...
59 Floor is ...... properly graded and water-tight	1	...
60 Milk house is ...... free from dirt, rubbish, and all material not used in the handling and storage of milk	1	...
61 Milk house has ...... running or still supply of pure clean water	1	...
62 Ice is ...... used for cooling milk and is cut from ...	1	...

WATER

63 **WATER SUPPLY** for utensils is from a ...... located ...... feet deep and apparently is ...... pure, wholesome, and uncontaminated	5	...
64 Is ...... protected against flood or surface drainage	2	...
65 There is ...... privy or cesspool within 250 feet (... feet) of source of water supply	2	...
66 There is ...... stable, barnyard, or pile of manure or other source of contamination within 200 feet (... feet) of source of water supply	1	...
	100	

[29]It is a great pity that we Americans have taken so long to learn that laws do not enforce themselves, that even good motives and good intentions in the best of officials do not insure good deeds. Thousands of lives are being lost every year, millions of days taken from industry and wasted by unnecessary sickness, millions of dollars spent on curing disease, the working life of the nation shortened, the hours of enjoyment curtailed, because we have not seen the great gap between health laws and health-law enforcement. In our municipal, state, and national politics we have made the same mistake of concentrating our attention upon the morals

and pretensions of candidates and officials instead of judging government by what government does. Gains of men and progress of law are useful to mankind only when converted into deeds that make men freer in the enjoyment of health and earning power. In protecting health, as in reforming government, an ounce of efficient achievement is worth infinitely more than a moral explosion. One month of routine — unpicturesque, unexciting efficiency — will accomplish more than a scandal or catastrophe. Such routine is possible only when special machinery is constantly at work, comparing work done with work expected, health practice with health ideals. Where such machinery does not yet exist, volunteers, civic leagues, boys' brigades, etc., can easily prove the need for it by filling out an improvised score card for the school building, railroad station, business streets, "well-to-do" and poor resident streets, such as follows:

Table V

Score Card for Citizen Use

	Perfect	Allow
Schoolhouse		
Well ventilated, 20; badly, 0-10	20	...
Cleaned regularly, 20; irregularly, 0-10	20	...
Feather duster prohibited, 10	10	...
No dry sweeping, 10	10	...
Has adequate play space, 10; inadequate, 0-5	10	...
Has clean drinking water, 10	10	...
Has clean outbuildings and toilet, 20: unclean, 0-10	20	...
	100	
Church and Sunday School		
Well ventilated, 20; badly, 0-10	20	...
Heat evenly distributed, 20; unevenly, 0-10	20	...
Cleaned regularly, 20; irregularly, 0-10	20	...
Without carpets, 20	20	...

Without plush seats, 20	20	...
	100	

Streets

Sewerage underground, 20; surface, 0-10	20	...
No pools neglected, 10	10	...
No garbage piled up, 10	10	...
Swept regularly, 20; irregularly, 0-10	20	...
Sprinkled and flushed, 10	10	...
Has baskets for refuse, 10	10	...
All districts equally cleaned, 20; unequally, 0-10	20	...
	100	

[30]Until recently the most reliable test of health rights not enforced was the number of cases of preventable, communicable, contagious, infectious, transmissible diseases, such as smallpox, typhoid fever, yellow fever, scarlet fever, diphtheria, measles, whooping cough. By noticing streets and houses where these diseases occurred, students learned a century ago that the darker and more congested the street the greater the prevalence of fevers and the greater the chance that one attacked would die. The well-to-do remove from their houses and their streets the dirt, the decomposed garbage, and stagnant pools from which fevers seem to spring. It was because fevers and congestion go together that laws were made to protect the well-to-do, the comfortable, and the clean against the slum. It is true to-day that if you study your city and stick a pin in the map, street for street, where infection is known to exist, you will find the number steadily increase as you go from uncongested to congested streets and houses, from districts of high rent to districts of low rent. Because it is easier to learn the number of persons who have measles and diphtheria and smallpox than it is to learn the incomes and living conditions prejudicial to health, and because our laws grant protection against communicable diseases to a child in whatever district he may be born, the record of cases of communicable diseases has heretofore been the best test of health rights unenforced. Even in country schools it would make a good lesson in hygiene and civics to have the children keep a record of absences on

account of transmissible disease, and then follow up the record with a search for conditions that gave the disease a good chance.

But to wait for contagion before taking action has been found an expensive way of learning where health protection is needed. Even when infected persons and physicians are prompt in reporting the presence of disease it is often [31]found that conditions that produced the disease have been overlooked and neglected.

For example, smallpox comes very rarely to our cities to-day. Wherever boards of health are not worried by "children's diseases," as is often the case, and wait for some more fearful disease such as smallpox, there you will find that garbage in the streets, accumulated filth, surface sewers, congested houses, badly ventilated, unsanitary school buildings and churches are furnishing a soil to breed an epidemic in a surprisingly short time. Where, on the other hand, boards of health regard every communicable disease as a menace to health rights, you will find that health officials take certain steps in a certain order to remove the soil in which preventable diseases grow. These steps, worked out by the sanitarians of Europe and America after a century of experiment, are seen to be very simple and are applicable by the average layman and average physician to the simplest village or rural community. How many of these steps are taken by your city? by your county? by your state?

1. Notification of danger when it is first recognized.

2. Registration at a central office of facts as to each dangerous thing or person.

3. Examination of the seat of danger to discover its extent, its cost, and new seats of danger created by it.

4. Isolation of the dangerous thing or person.

5. Constant attention to prevent extension to other persons or things.

6. Destruction or removal of disease germs or other causes of danger.

7. Analysis and record, for future use, of lessons learned by experience.

8. Education of the public to understand its relation to danger checked or removed, its responsibility for preventing a recurrence of the same danger, and the importance of promptly recognizing and checking similar danger elsewhere.

[32]With a chart showing what districts have the greatest number of children and adults suffering from measles, typhoid fever, scarlet fever, consumption, one can go within his own city or to a strange city and in a surprisingly short time locate the nuisances, the dangerous buildings, the open sewers, the cesspools, the houses without bathing facilities, the dark rooms, the narrow streets, the houses without play space and breathing space, the districts without parks, the polluted water sources, the unsanitary groceries and milk shops. In country districts a comparison of town with town as to the prevalence of infection will enable one easily to learn where slop water is thrown from the back stoop, whether the well, the barn, and the privy are near together.

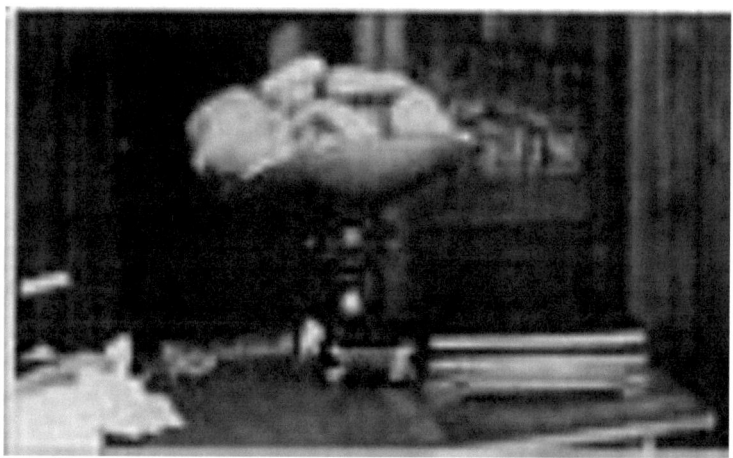

THE BABY, NOT THE LAW, IS THE TEST OF INFANT PROTECTION IN COUNTRY AND IN CITY

Testing health rights requires not only that there be a board of health keeping track of and publishing every case of infection, but it requires further that one community be compared with other communities of similar size, and that each community be compared with itself year for year. These comparisons have not been made and records do not exist in many states.

FOOTNOTES:

[3] A striking demonstration of law enforcement that followed lawmaking is given in *The Real Triumph of Japan*, L.L. Seaman, M.D.

[33]

THE BEST INDEX TO COMMUNITY HEALTH IS THE PHYSICAL WELFARE OF SCHOOL CHILDREN

Compulsory education laws, the gregarious instinct of children, the ambition of parents, their self-interest, and the activities of child-labor committees combine to-day to insure that one or more representatives of practically every family in the United States will be in public, parochial, or private schools for some part of the year. The purpose of having these families represented in school is not only to give the children themselves the education which is regarded as a fundamental right of the American child, but to protect the community against the social and industrial evils and the dangers that result from ignorance. Great sacrifices are made by state, individual taxpayer, and individual parent in order that children and state may be benefited by education. Almost no resistance is found to any demand made upon parent or taxpayer, if it can be shown that compliance will remove obstructions to school progress. If, therefore, by any chance, we can find at school a test of home conditions affecting both the child's health and his progress at school, it will be easy, in the name of the school, to correct those conditions, just as it will be easy to read the index, because the child is under state control for six hours a day for the greater part of the years from six to fourteen.[4]

[34]

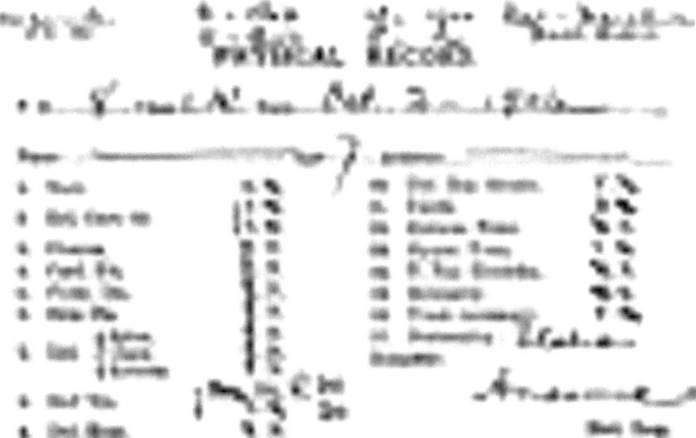

What, then, is this test of home conditions prejudicial to health that will register the fact as a thermometer tells us the temperature, or as a barometer shows moisture and air pressure? The house address alone is not enough, for many children surrounded by wealth are denied health rights, such as the right to play, to breathe pure air, to eat wholesome food, to live sanely. Scholarship will not help, because the frailest child is often the most proficient. Manners mislead, for, like dress, they are but externals, the product of emulation, of other people's influence upon us rather than of our living conditions. Nationality is an index to nothing significant in America, where all race and nationality differences melt into Americanisms, all responding in about the same way to American opportunity. No, our test must be something that cannot be put on and off, cannot be left at home, cannot be concealed or pretended, something inseparable from the child and beyond his control. This test it has been conclusively proved in Chicago, Boston, Brookline, Philadelphia, and particularly in New York City, is the physical condition of the school child. To learn this condition the child must be examined and reëxamined for [35]the physical signs called for by the card on page 34. Weight, height, and measurements are needed to tell the whole story.

When this card is filled out for every child in a class or school or city, the story told points directly to physical, mental, or health rights neglected. If for every child there is begun a special card, that will tell his story over and over again during his school life, noting every time he is sick and every time he is examined, the progress of the community as well as of the child will be clearly shown. Such a history card (p. 314) is now in use in certain New York schools, as well as in several private schools and colleges.

Have you ever watched such an examination? By copying this card your family physician can give you a demonstration in a very short time as to the method and advantage of examination at school. The school physician goes at nine o'clock to the doctor's room in the public school, or, if there is no doctor's room, to that portion of the hall or principal's office where the doctor does his work. The teacher or the nurse stands near to write the physician's decision. The doctor looks the child over, glances at his eyes, his color, the fullness of his cheeks, the soundness of his flesh, etc. If the physician says "B," the principal or nurse marks out the other letter opposite to number 1, so that the card shows that there is bad nutrition.

In looking at the teeth and throat a little wooden stick is used to push down the tongue. There should be a stick for every child, so that infection cannot possibly be carried from one to the other. If this is impossible, the stick should be dipped in an antiseptic such as boric acid or listerine. If, because of swollen tonsils, there is but a little slit open in the throat, or if teeth are decayed, the mark is Y or B. The whole examination takes only a couple of minutes, but the physician often finds out in this short time facts that will save a boy and his parents a great deal of trouble. Very often this examination tells a story that overworked [36]mothers have studiously concealed by bright ribbons and clean clothes. I remember one little girl of fourteen who looked very prosperous, but the physician found her so thin that he was sure that for some time she had eaten too little, and called her anæmic. He later found that the mother had seven children whom she was trying to clothe and shelter and feed with only ten dollars a week. A way was found to increase her earnings and to give all the children better living conditions,—all because of the short story told by the examination card. In another instance the card's story led to the discovery of recent immigrant parents earning enough, but, because unacquainted with American ways and with their new home, unable to give their children proper care.

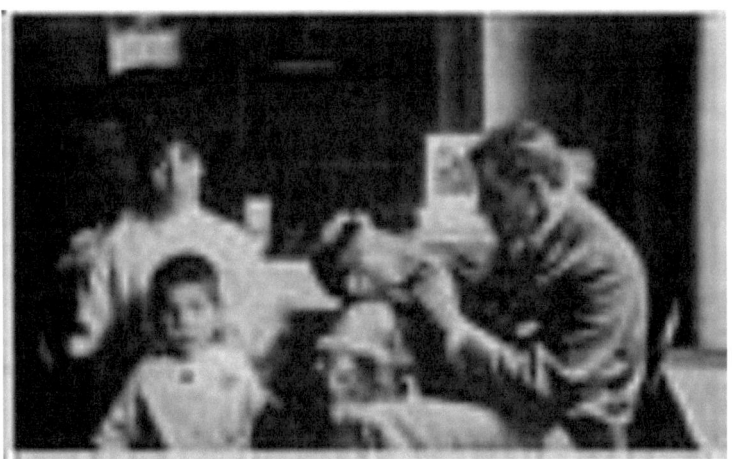

LOOKING FOR ENLARGED TONSILS AND BAD TEETH
Note the mouth breather waiting

The most extensive inquiry yet made in the United States as to the physical condition of school children is that conducted by the board of health in New York City since 1905. From March, 1905, to January 1, 1908, 275,641 children have been examined, and 198,139 or 71.9 per cent have been found to have defects, as shown in Table VI.

Table VI[37]

Physical Examination of School Children — performed by the Department of Health in the Borough of Manhattan, 1905-1907

	Total	Percentage
Number of children examined	275,641	100
Number of children needing treatment	198,139	71.9
Defects found:		
Malnutrition	16,021	5.8
Diseased anterior or posterior cervical glands	125,555	45.5

Chorea	3,776	1.3
Cardiac disease	3,385	1.2
Pulmonary disease	2,841	1.0
Skin disease	4,557	1.6
Deformity of spine, chest, or extremities	4,892	1.7
Defective vision	58,494	21.2
Defective hearing	3,540	1.2
Obstructed nasal breathing	43,613	15.8
Defective teeth	136,146	49.0
Deformed palate	3,625	1.3
Hypertrophied tonsils	75,431	27.4
Posterior nasal growths	46,631	16.9
Defective mentality	7,090	2.5

It is generally believed that New York children must have more defects than children elsewhere. If this assumption is wrong, if children in other parts of the United States are as apt to have eye defects, enlarged tonsils, and bad teeth as the children of the great metropolis, then the army of children needing attention would be seven out of ten, or over 14,000,000.

Whether these figures overstate or understate the truth, the school authorities of the country should find out. The chances are that the school in which you are particularly interested is no exception. To learn what the probable number needing attention is, divide your total by ten and multiply the result by seven.

[38]The seriousness of every trouble and its particular relation to school progress and to the general public health will be explained in succeeding chapters. The point to be made here is that the examination of the school child discloses in advance of epidemics and breakdowns the children whose physical condition makes them most likely to "come down" with "catching diseases," least able to withstand an attack, less fitted to profit fully from educational and industrial opportunity.

The only index to community conditions prejudicial to health that will make known the child of the well-to-do who needs attention is the record of physical examination. No other means to-day exists by which the state can, in a recognized and acceptable way, discover the failure of these well-to-do parents to protect their children's health and take steps to teach and, if necessary, to compel the parents to substitute living conditions that benefit for conditions that injure the child.

Among the important health rights that deserve more emphasis is the right to be healthy though not "poor." A child's lungs may be weak, breathing capacity one third below normal, weight and nutrition deficient, and yet that child cannot contract tuberculosis unless directly exposed to the germs of that disease. But such a child can contract chronic hunger, can in a hundred ways pay the penalty for being pampered or otherwise neglected. Physical examination is needed to find every child that has too little vitality, no zest for play, little resistance, even though sent to a private school and kept away from dirt and contagion.

The New York Committee on the Physical Welfare of School Children visited fourteen hundred homes of children found to have one or more of the physical defects shown on the above card. While they found that low incomes have more than their proper share of defects and of unsanitary living conditions, yet they saw emphatically [39]also that low incomes do not monopolize physical defects and unsanitary living conditions. Many families having $20, $30, $40 a week gave their children neither medical nor dental care. The share each income had in unfavorable conditions is shown by the summary in the following table.

Table VII

Showing Per Cent Share of Physical Defects of Children, Unfavorable Housing Conditions, and Child Mortality found among each Family-income Group

Weekly Family Income						
$0-	$10-	$16-	$20-	$25-	$30	$100

	10	15	19	25	29	and over	
	%	%	%	%	%	%	%
Proportion to total families	8.4	32.7	15.2	23.8	3.9	15.6	100
Physical defects:							
Malnutrition	13.8	43.4	12.4	17.9	3.4	9.	"
Enlarged glands	8.6	37.4	14.6	22.6	3.6	13.2	"
Defective breathing	9.6	32.3	15.5	24.4	2.8	15.4	"
Bad teeth	8.1	32.2	15.3	24.5	4.8	15.1	"
Defective vision	8.2	34.6	16.5	22.1	1.4	17.3	"
Unfavorable housing conditions:							
Dark rooms	8.2	35.4	18.1	18.4	3.8	15.9	"
Closed air shaft	6.9	30.2	18.9	26.4	3.2	19.6	"
No baths	10.1	38.5	16.5	19.7	4.4	10.8	"
Paying over 25% rent	8.6	27.6	21.7	14.7	...	27.6	"
Child Mortality:							
Families losing children	10.3	35.5	14.7	20.5	5.4	13.6	"
Families losing no children	6.4	30.1	15.7	26.9	2.4	18.6	"
Children dead	11.7	36.2	13.1	20.8	6.1	12.1	"
Infants dying from intestinal diseases	8.9	37.6	18.3	18.8	4.	12.4	"
Children working	4.2	19.5	13.2	30.3	11.5	21.3	"

The index should be read in all grades from kindergarten to high school and college.

[40]Last winter the chairman of the Committee on the Physical Welfare of School Children was invited to speak of physical examination before an association of high-school principals. He began by saying, "This question does not concern you as directly as it does

the grammar-school principals, but you can help secure funds to help their pupils." One after another the high-school principals present told—one of his own daughter, another of his honor girls, a third of his honor boys—the same story of neglected headaches due to eye strain, breakdowns due to undiscovered underfeeding, underexercise, or overwork. Are we coming to the time when the state will step in to prevent any boy or girl in high school, college, or professional school from earning academic honors at the expense of health? Harmful conditions within schoolrooms and on school grounds will not be neglected where pupils, teachers, school and family physicians, and parents set about to find and to remove the causes of physical defects.

Disease centers outside of school buildings quickly register themselves in the schoolroom and in the person of a child who is paying the penalty for living in contact with a disease center. If a child sleeps in a dark, ill-ventilated, crowded room, the result will show in his eyes and complexion; if he has too little to eat or the wrong thing to eat, he will be underweight and undersized; if his nutrition is inadequate and his food improper, he is apt to have eye trouble, adenoids, and enlarged tonsils. He may have defective lung capacity, due to improper breathing, too little exercise in the fresh air, too little food. Existence of physical defects throws little light on income at home, but conclusively shows lack of attention or of understanding. Several days' absence of a child from school leads, in every well-regulated school, to a visit to the child's home or to a letter or card asking that the absence be explained. Even newly arrived immigrants have learned the necessity and [41]the advantage of writing the teacher an "excuse" when their children are absent. Furthermore, neighbors' children are apt to learn by friendly inquiry what the teacher may not have learned by official inquiry, why their playmate is no longer on the street or at the school desk. While physicians are sometimes willing to violate the law that compels notification of infection, rarely would a physician fail to caution an infected family against an indiscriminate mingling with neighbors. Whether the family physician is careless or not, the explanation of the absence which is demanded by the school would give also announcement of any danger that might exist in the home where the child is ill.

If it be said that in hundreds of thousands of cases the child labor law is violated and that therefore school examination is not an index to the poverty or neglect occasioning such child labor, it should be remembered that the best physical test is the child's presence at school. The first step in thorough physical examination is a thorough school census, — the counting of every child of school age. Moreover, a relatively small number of children who violate the child labor law are the only members of the family who ought to be in school. Younger children furnish the index and occasion the visit that should discover the violation of law.

Appreciation of health, as well as its neglect, is indexed by the physical condition of school children. Habits of health are the other side of the shield of health rights unprotected. Physical examination will discover what parents are trying to do as well as what they fail to do because of their ignorance, indifference, or poverty. In so far as parents are alive to the importance of health, the school examination furnishes the occasion of enlisting them in crusades to protect the public health and to enforce health rights. The Committee on the Physical Welfare of School Children found many parents unwilling to answer [42]questions as to their own living conditions until told that the answers would make it easier to get better health environment not only for their own children but for their neighbors' children. Generally speaking, fathers and mothers can easily be interested in any kind of campaign in the name of health and in behalf of children. The advantage of starting this health crusade from the most popular American institution, the public school, — the advantage of instituting corrective work through democratic machinery such as the public school, — is incalculable. To any teacher, pastor, civic leader, health official, or taxpayer wanting to take the necessary steps for the removal of conditions prejudicial to health and for the enforcement of health rights of child and adult, the best possible advice is to learn the facts disclosed by the physical examination of your school children. See that those facts are used first for the benefit of the children themselves, secondly for the benefit of the community as a whole. If your school has not yet introduced the thorough physical examination of school children, take steps at once to secure such examination. If necessary, volunteer to test the eyes and the breathing of one class, persuade one or two physicians to coöperate until you have proved to parent, taxpayer, health official, and teacher that such an examination is both a money-saving, energy-saving step and an act of justice.

We shall have occasion to emphasize over and over again the fact that it is the use of information and not the gathering of information that improves the health. The United States Weather Bureau saves millions of dollars annually, not because flags are raised and bulletins issued foretelling the weather, but because shipowners, sailors, farmers, and fruit growers obey the warnings. Mere examination of school children does little good. The child does not breathe better or see better because the school physician fills out a card stating that there is [43]something wrong with his eyes, nose, and tonsils. The examination tells where the need is, what children should have special attention, what parents need to be warned as to the condition of the child, what home conditions need to be corrected. If the facts are not used, that is an argument not against obtaining facts but against disregarding them.

In understanding medical examination we should keep clearly in mind the distinction between medical school inspection, medical school examination, and medical treatment at school. Medical inspection is the search for communicable disease. The results of medical inspection, therefore, furnish an index to the presence of communicable diseases in the community. Medical examination is the search for physical defects, some of which furnish the soil for contagion. Its results are an index not only to contagion but to conditions that favor contagion by producing or aggravating physical defects and by reducing vitality. Medical treatment at school refers to steps taken under the school roof, or by school funds, to remove the defects or check the infection brought to light by medical inspection and medical examination. Treatment is not an index. In separate chapters are given the reasons for and against trying to treat at school symptoms of causes that exist outside of school. When, how often, and by whom inspection and examination should be made is also discussed later. The one point of this chapter is this: if we really want to know where in our community health rights are endangered, the shortest cut to the largest number of dangers is the physical examination of children at school, — private, parochial, reformatory, public, high, college.

Apart from the advantage to the community of locating its health problems, physical examination is due every child. No matter where his schooling or at whose expense, every child has the right to advance as fast as his own powers [44]will permit without hindrance from his own or his playmates' removable defects. He has the right to learn that simplified breathing is more necessary than simplified spelling, that nose plus adenoids makes backwardness, that a decayed tooth multiplied by ten gives malnutrition, and that hypertrophied tonsils are even more menacing than hypertrophied playfulness. He has the right to learn that his own mother in his own home, with the aid of his own family physician, can remove his physical defects so that it will be unnecessary for outsiders to give him a palliative free lunch at school, thus neglecting the cause of his defects and those of fellow-pupils.

FOOTNOTES:

[4] Sir John E. Gorst in *The Children of the Nation* reads the index of the health of school children in the United Kingdom; John Spargo, in *The Bitter Cry of the Children*, and Simon N. Patten in *The New Basis of Civilization*, suggest the necessity for reading the index in the United States and for heeding it.

[45]

CHAPTER VToC

MOUTH BREATHING

If the physical condition of school children is our best index to community health, who is to read the index? Unless the story is told in a language that does not require a secret code or cipher, unless some one besides the physician can read it, we shall be a very long time learning the health needs of even our largest cities, and until doomsday learning the health needs of small towns and rural districts. Fortunately the more important signs can be easily read by the average parent or teacher. Fortunately, too, it is easy to persuade mothers and teachers that they can lighten their own labors, add to their efficiency, and help their children by being on the watch for mouth breathing, for strained, crossed, or inflamed eyes, for decaying teeth, for nervousness and sluggishness. Years ago, when I taught school in a Minnesota village, I had never heard of adenoids, hypertrophied tonsils, myopia, hypermetropia, or the relation of these defects and of neglected teeth to malnutrition, truancy, sickness, and dullness. I now see how I could have saved myself several failures, the taxpayers a great deal of money, the parents a great deal of disappointment, and many children a life of inefficiency, had I known what it is easy for all teachers and parents to learn today.

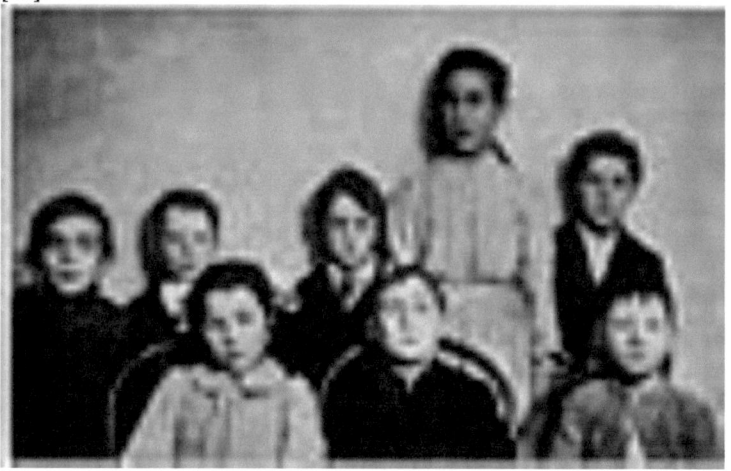

MOUTH BREATHERS BEFORE "ADENOID PARTY"

The features in the following cut are familiar to teachers the world over. Parents may reconcile themselves to such lips, eyes, and mouths, but seldom do even neglectful parents fail to notice "mouth breathing." Children afflicted by such features suffer torment from playfellows whose scornful epithets are echoed by the looking-glass. No fashion plate ever portrays such faces. No athlete, thinker, or hero looks out from printed page with such clouded, listless eyes. The more wonder, therefore, that the meaning of these outward signs has not been appreciated and their causes removed; conclusive reason, also, for not being misled by recent talk of mouth breathing, adenoids, and enlarged tonsils, into the belief that the race is physically deteriorating. Three generations ago Charles Dickens in his *Uncommercial Traveller* pointed out a relation between open mouths and backwardness and delinquency that would have saved millions of dollars and millions of life failures had the civilized world listened. He was speaking of delinquent girls from seventeen to twenty years old in Wapping Workhouse: "I have never [47]yet ascertained why a refractory habit should affect the tonsils and the uvula; but I have always observed that refractories of both sexes and every grade, between a Ragged School and the Old Bailey, have one voice, in which the tonsils and uvula gain a diseased ascendency."

To-day we are just beginning to see over again the connection between inability to breathe through the nose and inability to see clearly right from wrong and inability to want to do what teachers and parents wish. Physical examinations show now, and might just as well have shown fifty years ago, that the great majority of truants and juvenile offenders have adenoids and enlarged tonsils. A recent examination made by the New York board of health on 150 children in one school made up from the truant school, the juvenile court, and Randall's Island, showed that only three were without some physical defect and that 137 had adenoids and large tonsils. Dickens wrote his observations in 1860; in 1854 the New York Juvenile Asylum was started, and up to 1908 cared for 40,000 children; in 1860 William Meyer pointed out, so that no one need misunderstand, the harmful effects of adenoids. What would have been the story of juvenile waywardness, of sickness, of educational advancement, had examinations for defective breathing been started in 1853 or 1860 instead of 1905; if one per cent of the attention that has been given to teaching mouth breathers the ten commandments had been spent on removing the nasal obstructions to intelligence?

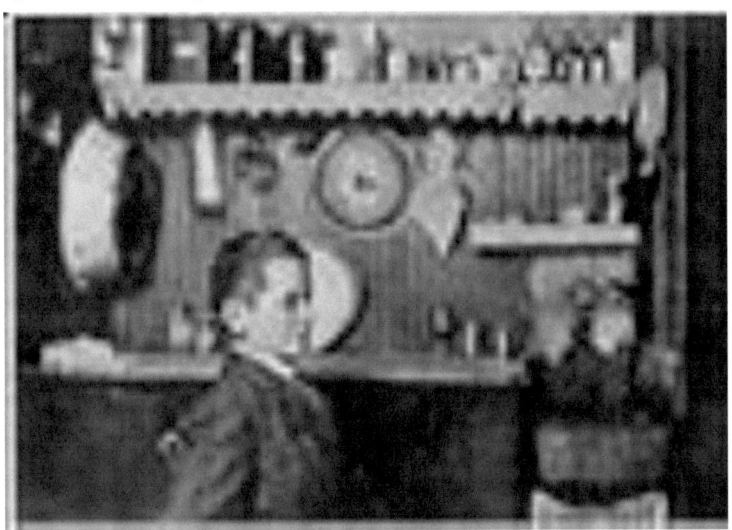

A "DEGENERATE" MADE NORMAL BY REMOVAL OF ADE-NOIDS

William Hegel, who is pictured on page 48, before his tonsils and adenoids were removed was described by his father in this way: "When playing with other boys on the street he seems dazed, and sluggish to grasp the various situations occurring in the course of the game. When he decides to do something he runs in a heedless, senseless way, as if running away,—will bump against something, [48]pedestrian or building, before he comes to himself; seems dazed all the time. When told something by his mother he giggles in the most exasperating way, for which he receives a whipping quite often." The father said the whipping was of no avail. The child was restless, talkative, and snored during sleep. He had an insatiable appetite. He was removed or transferred from five different schools in New York City. To get redress the father took him to the board of education, whence he was referred to the assistant chief medical inspector of the department of health, whose examination revealed immensely large fungous-looking tonsils and excessive pharyngeal granulations (adenoids). He was operated on at a clinic. The tonsils and adenoids removed are pictured on the opposite page, reduced one third. After the operation the child was visited by the assistant medical inspector. There was a marked improvement in his facial expression,—he looked intelligent, was alert and interested. When [49]asked how he felt, he answered, "I feel fine now." It required about fifteen minutes to get his history, during all of which time he was responsive and interested, constantly correcting statements of his father and volunteering other information. Eleven days after the operation he was reported to have had no more epileptic seizures. "Doesn't talk in sleep. Doesn't snore. Doesn't toss about the bed. Has more self-control. Tries to read the paper. His immoderate appetite is not present."

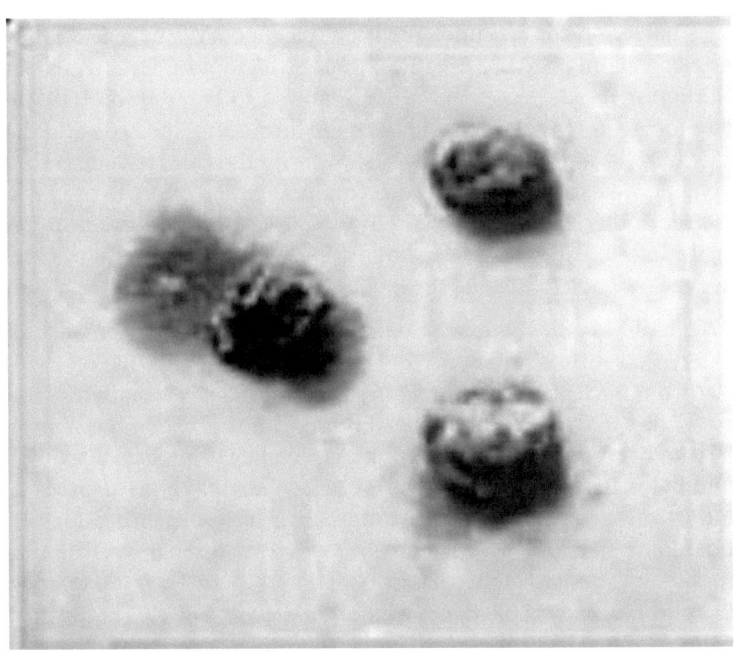

REASON ENOUGH FOR MOUTH BREATHING
Adenoid and tonsils reduced one third

While the open mouth is a sure sign of defects of breathing, it is not true that the closed mouth, when awake and with other people, is proof that there are no such defects. Children breathe through the mouth not because they like to, not because they have drifted into bad habits, not [50]because their parents did, not because the human race is deteriorating, but because their noses are stopped up, — because they must. A mouth breather is not only always taking unfiltered dirt germs into his system but is always in the condition of a person who has slept in a stuffy room. What extra effort adenoids mean can be ascertained by closing the nostrils for a forenoon.

For many reasons it is perhaps unfortunate that we can breathe at all when the nose is stopped up. If we could see with our ears as well as with our eyes, we should probably not take as good care of our eyes. In this respect the whole race has experienced the misfortune of the man of whom the coroner reported, "Killed by falling too short a distance." Because we can breathe through the mouth we have neglected for centuries the nasal passages. When a cold stops the nose we necessarily breathe through the mouth. Unfortunately children make the necessary effort required to breathe through the nose long before other people notice the lines along the nose and the slow mind. Mouth breathing will show with the child asleep, before the child awake loses power to accommodate his effort to the task. Therefore the importance of a physical test at school to detect the beginnings of adenoids and large tonsils before these symptoms become obvious to others.

No child should be exempted from this examination because of apocryphal theories that only the poor, the slum child, the refractory, or the unclean have defects in breathing. This very afternoon a friend has told me of her year abroad with a girl of nine, whose parents are very wealthy. The girl is anæmic. Her backwardness humiliates her parents, especially because she gave great promise until two years ago. High-priced physicians have prescribed for her. It happens that they are too eminent to give attention to such simple troubles as adenoids that [51]can be felt and seen. They are looking for complications of the liver or inflammation of muscles at the base of the brain. One celebrated French savant found the adenoids, assured the mother that the child would outgrow them, and advised merely that she be compelled to breathe through the nose. The mother and nursemaids nag the child all day. The poor unwise mother sits up nights to hold the child's jaws tight in the hope that air coming through the nose will absorb the adenoids. The mother is made nervous. Of course this makes the child more nervous and adds to the evil effects of adenoids. If the mother had the good fortune to be very poor, she could not sit up nights, and would long ago have decided either to let the child alone or else to have the trouble removed.

Adenoids are not a city specialty. Country earache is largely due to adenoids or to inflammation that quickly leads to adenoids. In 415 villages of New York state twelve per cent were found to be mouth breathers. For two summers I have known a lad named Fred. He lives at the seashore. Throughout his twelve years he has lived in a veritable El Dorado of health and nature beauty. Groves and dunes and flora vie with the blues of ocean and sky in resting the eye and in filling the soul with that harmony which is said to make for sound living. Yet to a child, Fred's schoolmates are experts on patent medicines and on the heredity that is alleged to be responsible for bad temper, running sores, tuberculosis, anæmia, and weak eyes. Freddie is particularly favored. His well-to-do parents have supplied him with ponies, games, and bicycles. Nothing prevents his breathing salt air fresh from the north pole but hermetically sealed windows. The father thinks it absurd to make a fuss over adenoids. Didn't he have them when a boy, and doesn't he weigh two hundred pounds and "make good money"? The mother never knew of operations for such trifles when [52]she taught school; she supposes her boy needs an operation, but "just can't bear to see the dear child hurt." As for Fred, he breathes through his mouth, talks through his nose, grows indifferent to boy's fun, fails to earn promotion at school, and fears that "I won't be strong in spite of all the patent medicine I've taken." Father, mother, and Fred feel profound pity for the city child living so far from nature.

Adenoids are not monopolized by children whose parents are ignorant of the importance of them and of physical examination. Last summer I was asked by a small boy to buy some chocolate. A glance at his cigar box with its two or three uninviting things for sale showed that the boy was really begging. He had thick lips, open mouth, "misty" eyes, and a nasal twang. I asked him if his teacher had not told him he had lumps back of his nose and could not breathe right. He said, "No." I explained then that he could make a great deal more money if he talked like other boys, stepped livelier, and breathed as other people breathe. He said he had "been by a doctor onct but didn't want to be op'rated." I turned to my companion and asked, "Have you never noted those same lines on your boy's face?" Although he had been lecturing on mouth breathers, he had never noticed his own boy's trouble. He hastened home and found the infallible signs. The mother declared it could not be true of her boy. About five months before, their family physician had said of the child's earache, "The same inflammation of the nasal passages that causes earache causes adenoids; you must be on the lookout." Although in the country, the boy's appetite was not good and his zest for play had flagged. They had looked for the trouble to back generations and in psychology books,—everywhere but at the boy's face, in his mouth, and in his nose. After the operation, which took less than two minutes, the appetite was [53]ravenous, the eyes cleared, and the spirit rebounded to its old buoyancy that craved worlds to conquer.

The new personal experience made a deep impression upon my friend's mind. He wanted everybody to know how easy it was to overlook a child's distress. One person after another had a story to tell him; even the janitor said: "You'd ought to have seen our John at sixteen. He spent a week by the hospital." The only people who do not seem to know more than the new convert are the mouth breathers whom he religiously stops on the street.

The indexes to adenoids and large tonsils for the teacher to read at school are:

1. Inability to breathe through the nose.

2. A chronically running nose, accompanied by frequent nose-bleeds and a cough to clear the throat.

3. Stuffy speech and delayed learning to talk. "Common" is pronounced "cobbéd"; "nose," "dose"; and "song," "sogg."

4. A narrow upper jaw and irregular crowding of the teeth.

5. Deafness.

6. Chorea or nervousness.

7. Inflamed eyes and conjunctivitis.

The adenoids and large tonsils discovered at school are an index:

1. To children needlessly handicapped in school work.

2. To teachers needlessly burdened.

3. To whole classes held back by afflicted children.

4. To breeding grounds for disease.

5. To homes where children's diseases and tuberculosis are most likely to break out and flourish.

6. To parents who need instruction in their duty to their children, to themselves, and to their neighbors, and who are ignorant of the way in which "catching" diseases originate and spread.

The riot that occurred when the adenoids of children in a school on the "East Side" in New York City were [54]removed without the preliminary of convincing the parents as to the advantages of the operation was merely a demand for the "right to knowledge," which is never overlooked with impunity. Reluctance to permit operation on a young child, and the natural shrinking of a parent at seeing a child under the surgeon's knife, require the teacher or school physician or nurse to answer fully the usual questions of the hesitant mother and father.

1. Is the operation necessary? Will the child not outgrow its adenoids? Usually the adenoid growths atrophy or dry up after the age of puberty. Adenoids are not uncommon in adults, however. The surgeon general of the army reports that during the year 1905, out of 3004 operations on officers and enlisted men in service, there were 225 operations on the nose, mouth, and pharynx, 103 of which were operations for adenoids and enlarged or hypertrophied tonsils. Allowing the child to "outgrow" adenoids may mean not only that he is being subjected to infection chronically but that his body is allowed to be permanently deformed and his health endangered. Beginning at the age of the second dentition, the bones of jaw, nose, throat, and chest are undergoing important changes—nasal occlusion. Adenoids left to atrophy—if large enough to cause mouth breathing—may mean atrophy of this developing process, permanent disfiguration of face, and permanent deformity of chest and lungs.

2. Will the growth recur? In a few cases it does recur; frequently either because it was not desirable to make a complete removal of the adenoid tissue or because the surgeon was careless. If the growths do recur, then they must be removed again.

3. Is the operation a dangerous one?

4. Is an anæsthetic necessary?

5. Will the operation cure the child of all its troubles? These questions are best answered by the process and [55]results of an "adenoid party," which was given especially for the benefit of this book, every step and symptom of which were carefully studied.

The seven children pictured here were discovered by their school physician to have moderately large adenoid growths,—one boy having enlarged tonsils also.

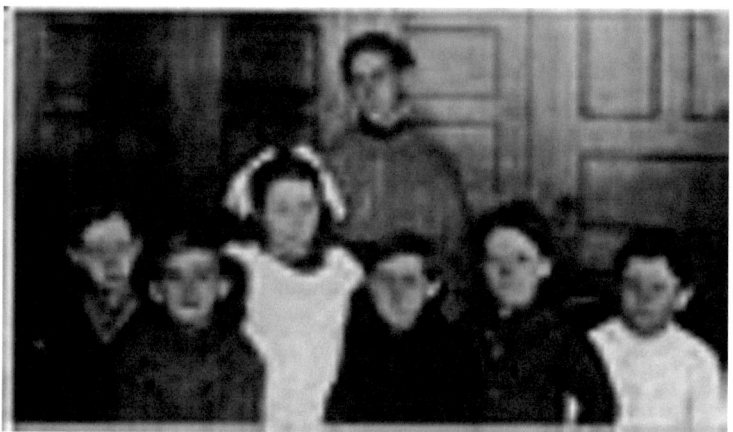

MOUTH BREATHERS IMMEDIATELY AFTER "ADENOID PARTY"

The picture on page 46 was taken by flash light at 2.30 P.M., January 15, 1908. At 3 P.M. the principal escorted these children into the operating room at Vanderbilt Clinic. The doctor examined the throat and nose of each child, entered the name and age of each, together with his diagnosis, on a clinic card, sending each child into the next room after examination. He then called the first boy and explained that it would hurt, but that it would be over in a minute. The principal stood by and told him to be brave and remember the five cents he could have for ice cream afterwards. The clinic nurse tied a large towel about him and put him in her lap; with one hand she held his clasped hands, while the other held his head back. The doctor then took the little instrument—the curette—and pushed it up back of the soft palate, and with one twist [56]brought out the offending spongy lump. The boy's head was immediately held over a basin of running water. He was so occupied with spitting out the blood that rushed down to choke him that he hadn't time to cry before the acute pain had ceased. The rush of cool air through his nostrils was such a pleasurable sensation that he smiled as the school nurse escorted him out into the hall to wait for his companions. At 3.30 P.M. all seven children were out in the hall, all seven mouths were closed, and all seven faces were clothed with the sleepy, peaceful expression that comes with rest from the prolonged labor of trying to get enough air. At 3.45 P.M. they had been all reëxamined by the doctor, and a few tag ends were picked out of the nasopharynx of one child. At 4 P.M. the "party" had returned to the Children's Aid Society's school and to the ice cream that follows each adenoid party.

It is worth while to tell mothers stories of the "marvelous improvement in school progress of those children whose brains have been poisoned and starved by the accursed adenoid growths, and how their bodies fairly bloom when the mysterious and awful incubus is removed," to use the words of one school principal. It is worth while to show them "before" and "after" pictures, and "before" and "after" children, and "before" and "after" school marks.

[57]

CHAPTER VIToC

CATCHING DISEASES, COLDS, DISEASED GLANDS

Deadly fevers, the plague, black death, cholera, malaria, small-pox, taught mankind invaluable lessons. Millions of human beings died before the mind of man devoted itself to preventing the diseases for which no sure cure had been found. Efforts to conquer these diseases were tardy because men were taught that some unseen power was punishing men and governments for their sins. The difference between the old and the new way is shown powerfully by a painting in the Liverpool Gallery entitled "The Plague." A mediæval village is strewn with the dead and dying. Bloated, spotted faces look into the eyes of ghouls as laces and jewelry are torn from bodies not yet cold. In the foreground a muscular giant, paragon of conscious virtue, clad like John the Baptist and Bible in hand, finds his way among his plague-stricken fellow-townsmen, urging them to turn from their sins. Modern efficiency learns of the first outbreak of the plague, isolates the patient, kills rats and their fleas which spread the disease, thoroughly cleanses or destroys, if necessary, all infected clothing, bedding, floors, and walls, and makes it possible for us to go on living for each other with a better chance of "bringing forth fruits worthy for repentance."

Where boards of health make it compulsory to report cases of sickness due to contagion, health records are a reliable index to "catching" diseases. But now that the chief infection is the kind that afflicts children, we can read the index before the outbreak that calls in a physician to diagnose the case. School examination shows which [58]children have defects that welcome and encourage disease germs. It points to homes that cultivate germs, and consequently menace other homes. To locate children who have enlarged tonsils may prevent a diphtheria epidemic. To detect in September those who are undernourished, who have bad teeth, and who breathe through the mouth will help forecast winter's outbreaks of scarlet fever and measles. One dollar spent at this season in examination for soil hospitable to disease germs may save fifty dollars otherwise necessary for inspection and cure of contagious diseases.

It is harder at first to interest a community in medical examination than in medical inspection, because we are all afraid of "catching" diseases, while few of us know how they originate and how they can be prevented by correcting the unfavorable conditions which physical examination of school children will bring to light.

Courses in germ sociology are therefore of prime necessity. How do germs act? On what do they live? Why do they move from place to place? What causes them to become extinct? With few exceptions, germs migrate for the same reason as man, — search for food, love of conquest, and love of adventure. When there is plenty of food they multiply rapidly. Full of life, overflowing with vitality, they move out for new worlds to conquer. Like human beings, they will do their best to get away from a country that provides a scanty food supply. Like men and women, they starve if they cannot eat. Like boys and girls, they avoid enemies; the weak give way to the strong, the slow to the swift, the devitalized to the vitalized.

Human sociology imprisons, puts to death, deprives of opportunity to do evil, or reforms those who murder, steal, or slander. Germ sociology teaches us to do the same with injurious germs. We imprison them, we take away their food supply, we kill them outright, or we starve them slowly. They have a peculiar diet, being especially [59]partial to decomposing vegetable and animal matter and to what human beings call dirt. By putting this diet out of their reach we make it impossible for them to propagate their kind. By placing poison within their reach or by forcing it upon them we can successfully eliminate them as enemies. As the president of Mexico restored order "by setting a thief to catch a thief," so modern science is setting germs to kill germs that harm crops and human stock. Of utmost consequence is it that the body's germ consumer — its pretorian guard — be always armed with vitality ready to vanquish every intruding hostile germ. If we are false to our guard, it will turn traitor and join invaders in attacking us. But here, as in dealing with evils that originate with human beings, an ounce of prevention is worth a ton of cure. The most effectual way to eliminate germ diseases is to remove the cause—the food supply of disease germs. The fact that many germs are plants, not animals, does not weaken the analogy, for weeds do not get a chance in well-tilled soil.

Perhaps the most notable recent example of government germ extermination is the triumph over the yellow-fever and malaria mosquito in Panama. When the French started to build a canal in Panama, the first thing they did was to build a hospital. The hospital was always full and the canal was given up. At the time the United States proposed to re-attempt the work, it was thought that it could not be done without great loss of life and without great labor difficulties. Instead of taking the sickness for granted and enlarging the French hospital, the chief medical inspector, Gorgas, took for granted that there need be no unusual sickness if proper preventive measures were taken. He knew what the French had not known, that the yellow-fever scourge depends for its terrors upon mosquitoes. Accordingly, with the aid of six thousand men and five million dollars he set about to starve [60]out the few infected and infectious kinds of mosquito,—the yellow-fever or house mosquito and the malaria or meadow mosquito. He introduced waterworks and hydrants, paved the streets, drained the swamps and pools in which they breed, and instituted a weekly house-to-house inspection to prevent even so much as a pail of stagnant water offering harbor to these enemies. The grass of the meadows where the malaria mosquito breeds was cut short and kept short within three hundred feet of dwellers,—as far as the mosquito can fly. All ditches were disinfected with paraffin, and the natives were forced to observe sanitary laws. President Roosevelt, in his special message to Congress on the Panama Canal in 1906, stated that in the weekly house-to-house visit of the inspectors at the time he was in Panama but two mosquitoes were found. These were not of the dangerous type. As a consequence of this sanitary engineering there is very little sickness in Panama, the hospital is seldom one third full, and the canal is progressing very much faster than was expected. Panama, like Havana, is now safer than many American cities, because cleaner and less hospitable to disease germs.

Any place where numbers of people are accustomed to assemble favors the propagation of germs,—whether it be the meetinghouse, the townhall, the theater, or the school. Every teacher can be the sanitary engineer of her own schoolroom, school, or community by coöperating with the school doctor, the town board of health, family physicians, and mothers. Every teacher can exterminate disease by applying the very same principles to her schoolroom as Chief Medical Inspector Gorgas applied to Panama. Knowledge, disinfection, absolute cleanliness, education, and inspection are the essential steps. First she must know that "children's diseases" are not necessary. She should discountenance the old superstition that every child [61]must run the gamut of children's diseases, that every child must sooner or later have whooping cough, measles, chicken pox, mumps, scarlet fever, just as they used to think yellow fever and cholera inevitable. The price of this terrible ignorance has been not only expense, loss of time, acquisition of permanent physical defects, and loss of vitality, but, for the majority of children, death before reaching five years of age. All these "catching" diseases are germ diseases, which disinfection can eliminate. The free use of strong yellow soap and disinfectants on the school floor, windows, benches, desks, blackboards, pencils, in the coat closets and toilets, plus the natural disinfectants, hot sun and oxygen, will prevent the schoolroom from being a source of danger. One or more of these germ-killing remedies must be constantly applied; cleansing deserves a larger part in every school budget.

Often country towns are as ignorant of the existence of germs and of the means of preventing the spread of disease as the woman in a small country town who used daily to astound the neighbors by the "shower of snow" she produced by shaking the bedding of her sick child out of the window. Their astonishment was soon changed to panic when that shower of snow resulted in a deadly epidemic of scarlet fever. Medical inspection of New York City's schools was begun after an epidemic of scarlet fever was traced to a popular boy who passed around among his schoolmates long rolls of skin from his fingers.

Much of the care exercised at school to prevent children's diseases is counteracted because children are exposed at home and in public places to contagion, where ignorance more often than carelessness is the cause of uncleanliness. By hygiene lessons, illustrating practically the proper methods of cleaning a room, much may be done to enlist school children in the battle against germs. Through the enthusiasm of the children as well as through [62]visits to the homes parents may be instructed as to the danger of letting well children sleep with sick children; the wisdom of vaccination to prevent smallpox, of antitoxin to prevent serious diphtheria, of tuberculin tests to settle the question whether tuberculosis is present; why anything that gathers dust is dangerous unless cleansed and aired properly; and why bedding, furniture, floor coverings, and curtains that can be cleansed and aired are more beautiful and more safe than carpets, feather beds, upholstery, and curtains that are spoiled by water and sunshine; how to care for the tuberculous member of the family, etc. Anti-social acts may be prevented, such as carrying an infected child to the doctor in a public conveyance, thereby infecting numberless other people; sending infected linen to a common laundry; mailing a letter written by an infected person without first disinfecting it; sending a child with diphtheria to the store; returning to the dairy unscalded milk bottles from a sick room.

The daily inspection of school children for contagious diseases by the school physician has, where tried, been found to reduce considerably the amount of sickness in a town. Such inspection should be universally adopted. Moreover, the teacher should be conversant with the early symptoms of these diseases so that on the slightest suspicion the child may be sent home without waiting for the physician's call. Like the little girl who never stuttered except when she talked, school children and school-teachers are rarely frightened until too late to prevent trouble. The "easy" diseases such as measles, whooping cough, etc., cost our communities more than the more terrible diseases like typhoid and smallpox. During one typical week ending May 18, 630 new cases of measles were reported to one department of health. Obviously the nineteen deaths reported give no conception of the suffering, the cost, the anxiety caused by this preventable disease. The same [63]may be said of diphtheria and croup, of which only thirty-two deaths are reported, but 306 cases of sickness. Yet no one to-day will send a child to sleep with a playmate so as to catch diphtheria and "be done with it."

The most strategic point of attack is almost universally unrecognized. That is the child's mouth. Here the germs find lodgment, here they find a culture medium—at the gateway of the human system.

The mouth is never out of service and is almost never in a state of true cleanliness. Solid particles from the breath, saliva, food between the teeth, and other débris form a deposit on the teeth and decompose in a constant temperature of ninety-eight degrees Fahrenheit. In the normal mouth from eight to twenty years of age the teeth present from twenty to thirty square inches of dentate surface, constantly exposed to ever-changing, often inimical, conditions. This bacterially infected surface makes a fairly large garden plot. Every cavity adds to the germ-nourishing soil. Dental caries—tooth decay—is a disease hitherto almost universal from birth to death. Thus the air taken in through the mouth becomes a purveyor of its poisonous emanations and affects the lung tissues and the blood. Food and water carry hostile germs down into the stomach. Thence they may be carried into any organ or tissue, just as nourishment or poison is carried.

Moreover, the child with an unclean mouth not only infects and reinfects himself but scatters germs in the air whenever he sneezes or coughs. In a cold apartment where there is no appreciable current of air a person can scatter germs for a distance of more than twenty-two feet. Germs are also scattered through the air by means of salivary or mucous droplets. It is this fact that makes colds so dangerous.

[64]

Table VIII

City of Manchester Education Committee

INFECTIOUS OR CONTAGIOUS DISEASES IN SCHOOLS INFORMATION FOR TEACHERS

Four columns are omitted: (1) Interval between Exposure to Infection and the First Signs of the Disease; (2) Day from Onset of Illness on which Rash appears; (3) Period of Exclusion from School after Exposure to Infection; (4) Period of Exclusion from School of Person suffering from the Disease

DISEASE	PRINCIPAL SIGNS AND SYMPTOMS	Method of Infection	REMARKS

Measles	*Begins like cold in the head*, with *feverishness, running nose, inflamed and watery eyes, and sneezing;* small crescentic groups of *mulberry-tinted spots* appear about the third day; *rash first seen on forehead and face.* The rash varies with heat; may almost disappear if the air is cold, and come out again with warmth.	Breath and discharges from nose and mouth.	After effects often severe. Period of greatest risk of infection first three or four days, before the rash appears. May have repeated attacks. Great variation in type of disease.
German Measles	Illness usually slight. Onset sudden. *Rash often first thing noticed;* no cold in head. Usually have *feverishness* and *sore throat*, and the *eyes may be inflamed. Rash* something between Measles and Scarlet Fever, variable.	Breath and discharges from nose and mouth	After effects slight.
Chicken Pox	Sometimes begins with feverishness, but is *usually very mild* and without sign of fever. *Rash* appears on second	Breath and crust of spots.	When children return, examine head for overlooked spots. All spots should have disap-

	day as *small pimples*, which in about a day become filled with *clear fluid*. This fluid then becomes *matter*, and then the *spot dries up* and *the crust falls off.* May have *successive crops of of rash* until tenth day.		peared before child returns. A mild disease and seldom any after effects.
Whooping Cough	*Begins like cold in the head*, with *bronchitis* and *sore throat*, and a *cough* which is *worse at night.* Symptoms may at first be very mild. Characteristic *"whooping" cough* develops in about a fortnight, and the spasm of coughing often ends with *vomiting.*	Breath and discharges from nose and mouth.	After effects often very severe and the disease causes great debility. Relapses are apt to occur. Second attack rare. Specially infectious for first week or two. If a child is sick after a bout of coughing, it is most probably suffering from whooping cough. Great variation in type of disease.
Mumps	Onset may be sudden, beginning with	Breath and discharges	Seldom leaves after effects.

	sickness and fever, and *pain about the angle of the jaw*. The *glands become swollen and tender*, and the *jaws stiff*, and the *saliva sticky*.	from nose and mouth.	Very infectious.
Scarlet Fever or Scarlatina[65]	The *onset is usually sudden*, with *headache, languor, feverishness, sore throat*, and often the child is *sick*. Usually within twenty-four hours the *rash* appears, and is *finely spotted, evenly diffused*, and *bright red*. The *rash* is seen first on the *neck and upper part of chest*, and lasts three to ten days, when it fades and the *skin peels in scales, flakes*, or even *large pieces*. The *tongue* becomes whitish, with bright red spots. The eyes are not watery or congested.	Breath, discharges from nose and mouth, particles of skin, and discharges from suppuratory glands or ears. Milk specially apt to convey infection.	Dangerous both during attack and from after effects. Great variation in type of disease. Slight attacks as infectious as severe ones. Many mild cases not diagnosed and many concealed. The peeling may last six to eight weeks. A second attack is rare. When scarlet fever is occurring in a school, all cases of sore throat should be sent home.
Diphtheria	Onset insidious, may be rapid or gradual. Typically *sore throat*, great	Breath and discharges from nose, mouth, and	Very dangerous both during attack and from after effects.

	weakness, and swelling of glands in the neck, about the angle of the jaw. The back of the throat, tonsils, or palate may show *patches* like pieces of yellowish-white kid. The most pronounced symptom is great debility and lassitude, and there may be little else noticeable. There may be hardly any symptoms at all.	ears.	When diphtheria is occurring in a school all children suffering from sore throat should be excluded. There is great variation of type, and mild cases are often not recognized but are as infectious as severe cases. There is no immunity from further attacks. Fact of existence of disease sometimes concealed.
Influenza	*Begins with feverishness, pain in head, back*, and *limbs*, and usually *cold in the head*.	Breath and discharges from nose and mouth.	Excessively infectious. After effects often very serious and accompanied with great prostration and nervous debility.
Smallpox	The illness is usually well marked and the onset rather sudden, with *feverishness, severe backache, and sickness*. About third day a *red rash* of *shotlike*	Breath, all discharges, and particles of skin or scabs.	Peculiarly infectious. When smallpox occurs in connection with a school or with any of the children's homes, an endeavor

pimples, felt below the skin, and seen first about the *face* and *wrists. Spots develop* in *two days*, then form *little blisters*, and in other two days become *yellowish* and filled with matter. *Scabs* then form, and these fall off about the fourteenth day.

should be made to have all persons over seven years of age re-vaccinated.

Cases of modified smallpox — in vaccinated persons — may be, and often are, so slight as to escape detection. Fact of existence of disease may be concealed. Mild or modified infectious as severe type.

In the following diseases only the affected child is excluded

Erysipelas. Child should not return till all swelling and peeling of skin has disappeared.

Ophthalmia. Child should not return till all traces have disappeared.

Scabies or Itch. Child should be excluded until cured.

Ringworm on Skin. Child should be excluded till cured. This takes only a few days if properly treated.

Ringworm on Scalp. Child should be excluded till cured. Very difficult to cure and often takes a very long time.

Phthisis (**Consumption**). If in advanced stage and coughing much *or spitting*, child should be excluded. (Infection from breath and dried spit floating in the air as dust.)

Impetigo (**Contagious Sore**). Child should be excluded until cured. A week or ten days should suffice.

A. BROWN RITCHIE, *Medical Officer to Education Committee.*

[66]Most people still think that colds are due to cold air or draughts rather than to a cold germ, which finds a body unequipped with resisting power, with its germ police off guard, exhausted from overwork, or disaffected and ready to turn traitor if the enemy seems stronger than our vitality. Sometimes it seems as if we contracted it from a sneezing fellow-passenger, sometimes from a draught from an open car window. An uninformed opponent of the theory that colds are a germ disease wrote the following letter last winter to a New York newspaper:

In addition to the Society for the Suppression of Noises there should be in this town a Society for the Suppression of "Fresh-Air" Fiends. The newspapers report an epidemic of pneumonia, grippe, and colds. It is almost entirely due to the fact that the average New Yorker is compelled to live, move, and have his being from daylight to midnight in a succession of draughts of cold air caused by the insanity of overfed male and female hogs, who, with blood almost bursting through their skins, demand "fresh air" in order to keep from suffocating. Everywhere a man goes, day or night, he is in a draught caused by the crazy ideas about fresh air.

Our wise ancestors, who as a rule lived much longer than we do, and had much better health, said:

> "If the wind should blow through a hole,
> God have mercy on your soul."

After the correspondent has learned that our ancestors had more colds than we, had poorer health, and died twenty years younger, perhaps he will listen to proof that his unclean warm air weakens the body and makes it an easy prey to cold germs.

Many physicians preach and practice this fallacy as to fresh air and colds, but few physicians now deny that influenza is a germ disease or that a nose so irritated and so neglected as to secrete large quantities of mucus is a better place for breeding disease germs than a nose whose membranes are clean and not thus irritated.

[67]Until medical specialists are agreed, and until they have definitely located the cold germ, we laymen must choose for ourselves a working theory. The weight of opinion at the present time declares that colds are due to germs. Strong membranes with good circulation and drainage provide poor food for germs. Congested membranes furnish proper conditions for propagation. The germ theory explains the spread of germs from the nose to the passages of the head, and from head to arteries and lungs.

A cold can always be charged to some one else. How many can be laid to our account? There is one right that is universally not recognized, and that is the right of protection from the germs showered in the air we breathe, over the food we eat, by the sneezes of our unfortunate neighbor at school, in the street car, at the restaurant. The chief danger of a cold is to our neighbor, not to ourselves. A cold which a strong person may throw off in a day or two may mean death to his tuberculous neighbor. Though for our own health "lying up for a mere cold" is an unnecessary bore, the failure to do so may deprive our neighbor of a right greater than the right to protection against scarlet fever or smallpox. Though formerly this statement would [68]not have been true, rights change with conditions, and the fact that to-day the three most deadly diseases are pneumonia, tuberculosis, and diphtheria,—all diseases of the respiratory organs,—justifies the assertion that we have a right to protection against colds. The prevalence of colds, sore throats, irritated vocal cords, bad voices, catarrh, bronchitis, laryngitis, and asthma in America to-day demands summary measures. One can learn to sneeze into a handkerchief, not into a companion's face or into a room. School children can be taught to avoid handkerchiefs on which mucus has dried. In the far distant future we may be willing to use cheesecloth, and boil it or throw it away, or, like the Japanese, use soft paper handkerchiefs and burn them after using.

Table IX

Death Rate per 10,000 Population, Pneumonia and Bronchitis
Five-Year Period, 1896-1900

England and Wales	22.70
Scotland	27.40
Stockholm	26.70
London	31.20
Berlin	16.10
Vienna	39.70
Christiania	21.30
Boston	30.60
Chicago	24.20
Philadelphia	25.10
New York City	36.60

One child with a cold can infect a whole class or family, thus depriving the class and family of the top of their vitality and efficiency without their consent. Because a person is thought a weakling who lies up for a "mere cold," one is inclined to wish that colds were as prostrating as typhoid, in which case there would be some hope of their extermination.

The exclusion of children with colds from school deserves trial as a check to children's diseases. Many of these "catching" diseases start with a cold in the head, as, for instance, measles, influenza, and whooping cough. The first symptom of mumps, diphtheria, and scarlet fever is a sore throat or swollen glands, which, because they commonly accompany a cold, are not at first distinguished from it.

The first step for the teacher or mother in reading the index for colds is to look into the coat closet for evidence of warm clothing and overshoes, then to note whether the children put them on when they go out for lunch or recess. Whether "cold" settles in the nasal passages, ear, or stomach depends upon which is the weak spot. Draughts, [69]thin soles, wet soles, exposure when perspiring, may be the immediate cause of the nutritional or respiratory disturbances that give cold germs a foothold. Adenoids, diseased teeth, inflamed ears, may furnish the food supply. "There is no use treating children and sending them on fresh-air trips as long as they have nutritional and digestive disturbances due to bad teeth, or colds due to adenoids," said a physician when examining a party of children for a summer outing. The great preventive measure to be taken for catching diseases, colds, diseased glands, — in fact all germ diseases, — is the repeated cleansing of those portions of the human body in which germs may find lodgment, — the mouth, the nose, the eyes, and the ears.

In caring for young infants great pains is taken to cleanse all the orifices daily, but as soon as the child washes himself this practice is usually abandoned. Washing these gateways is far more important than washing the surface of the body through which germs could not possibly gain entrance into the system except through wounds. Oftentimes the douching of the nostrils with salt water will stop a cold at once. The mouth is the most important place of all, and the teacher should take care of her pupils' mouths first and foremost. As bad teeth, enlarged tonsils, and adenoids harbor germs and putrescent matter that vitiate every incoming and outgoing breath, these defects should be immediately corrected. Are we coming to a time when a thorough house-cleaning in the mouth of every child will take place before he enters the schoolroom, preferably in the presence of the teacher?

Two other "catching" diseases cause city schools a great deal of trouble,—trachoma and pediculosis (head lice). There are probably no two diseases more quickly transmitted from one person to another. Almost before their presence is known, all children of a school or all [70]persons of a group have contracted them. When at college twenty men of my fraternity discovered almost at the same time that they had an infectious eye trouble; yet we thought we were using different towels and otherwise taking sanitary precautions. Last summer a Vassar graduate took a party of tenement children for a country picnic. She returned with head lice that required constant attention for weeks. What then may we expect of children who live in homes where there is neither water, time, nor privacy for bathing, where one towel must serve a family of six, where mothers work for wages away from home and see their children only before seven and after six?

Unfortunately for thousands of children, many parents still believe these troubles will be outgrown. Last summer a fresh-air agency in New York City arranged for several hundred school girls to go to a certain camp for ten days each. The only condition was that the heads should be free from lice and nits (eggs). From the list furnished by school-teachers—girls supposed to have been cured by school nurses—not one in five was accepted. A baby two weeks old, brought to Caroline Rest, had already begun to suffer from this easily preventable scourge. Of 1219 children examined in Edinburgh, Scotland, 909, or 69 per cent, had some skin disease, and 60 per cent had sores due to head lice. Even when neglect has caused the loss of hair and ugly sores on the head, mothers deceive themselves into believing that some other cause is responsible.

Trachoma, if neglected, not only impairs the health of the eye, but may cause blindness. Tears carry the germs from the eye to the face, where they are taken up on handkerchiefs, towels, and fingers and infect other eyes. Of late, thanks to school nurses and physicians and hygiene instruction, American cities have found relatively little trachoma except among recent immigrants. So dangerous is the germ and so insidious its methods of propagation, [71]that a physician should be summoned at once at the first sign of inflammation. Conjunctivitis is due to a germ, and will spread unless checked. Since the board of health of New York City has instituted the systematic examination of the eyes of the children in the public schools, it has found fully one third affected with some form of conjunctivitis. Many of these cases are out-and-out trachoma, others acute conjunctivitis, and a larger proportion are "mild trachoma." This last form of the disease is found to a great extent among children who have adenoids. The adenoids should be regarded as a predisposing factor rather than a direct cause. Therefore sore eyes are given as one of the indexes of adenoids. When we consider that adenoids are made up of lymphoid material, and that trachoma follicles are made up of the same sort of tissue, it is not surprising that the two conditions are found in the same child. The catarrhal inflammation produced by adenoids in the nasal mucous membrane travels up the lachrymal duct and thus infects the conjunctiva by contiguity.

In preventing pediculosis and infection of the eye vigilance and cleanliness are indispensable. After the diseases are advanced, after the germ colonies have taken title, some antiseptic or germ killer more violent than water is needed,—kerosene for the hair or strong green oil soap; for the eye, only what a physician prescribes.

[72]

EYE STRAIN

Wherever school children's eyes have been examined, from six to nine out of thirty are found to be nearsighted, farsighted, or otherwise in need of attention. A child is dismissed from school for obstinately declaring that the letter between *c* and *t* in "cat" is an *o*; "a pupil in her fourth school year was recently brought to me by her teacher with the statement that she did unreasonably poor work in reading for an intelligent and willing child;" a boy is punished for being backward. These three cases are typical. Examinations showed that the first child was astigmatic and not obstinate; the boy had run a pin into one eye ten years before and destroyed its sight; while the second girl was found to be afflicted with diplopia, and in a friendly chat told the following story: "I very often see two words where there is only one. When I was a very little girl I used to write every word twice. Then I was scolded for being careless. *So I learned that I must not say two words even when I saw them.*" As Miss Alida S. Williams, principal of Public School 33 in New York City, has in many articles and addresses freely illustrated from school experience, the art of seeing is acquired, not congenital, and every human being who possesses it has learned it.

The large proportion of children suffering more or less seriously from eye trouble has led many persons to suggest physical deterioration as the cause. Eye specialists, however, assure us that eye troubles are probably as old as man. Our tardiness in learning the facts regarding these [73]troubles is due in part to the lack, until recently, of instruments for examining the eye and for manufacturing glasses to correct eye defects; in part, also, to the tendency of the medical profession, which I shall repeatedly mention, to explain disorders by causes remote and hard to find rather than by those near at hand.

About 1870 Dr. S. Weir Mitchell's attention was called "to the marked relief of headache, insomnia, and other reflex symptoms following the correction of optical defects by glasses." In 1874 and 1876 he wrote two articles that "impressed upon the general profession the grave significance of eye strain." Since that time, "in Philadelphia at least, no study of the rebellious cause of headache or of the obscure nervous diseases has ever been considered complete until a careful examination of the eyes has included them as a possible cause of the disturbance."

The new fact, therefore, is not weak eyes or strained eyes, but rather (1) an increase in the regular misuse of eyes by school children, seamstresses, stenographers, lawyers, etc.; and (2) the incipient propaganda growing out of school tests that show the relation of eye strain to headache, nervous diseases, stomach disorder, truancy, backwardness.

Every school, private and parochial as well as public, should supply itself with the Snellen card for testing eyes. Employers would do well to have these cards in evidence also, for they may greatly increase profits by decreasing inefficiency and risks. If there is no expert optician near, apply for cards to your health board or school board; failing there, write to your state health and school boards. In many states rural teachers are already supplied with these cards by state boards. In October, 1907, the New York state board of health sent out cards, with instructions for their use, to 446 incorporated towns. The state commissioner of education also sent a letter giving school reasons for using the cards. Results from 415 schools having [74]shown that nearly half the children had optical defects, it is proposed to secure state legislation that will make eye tests obligatory in all schools. Such a test in Massachusetts recently discovered twenty-two per cent of the school children with defective vision, and from forty to fifty thousand in need of immediate care by specialists.

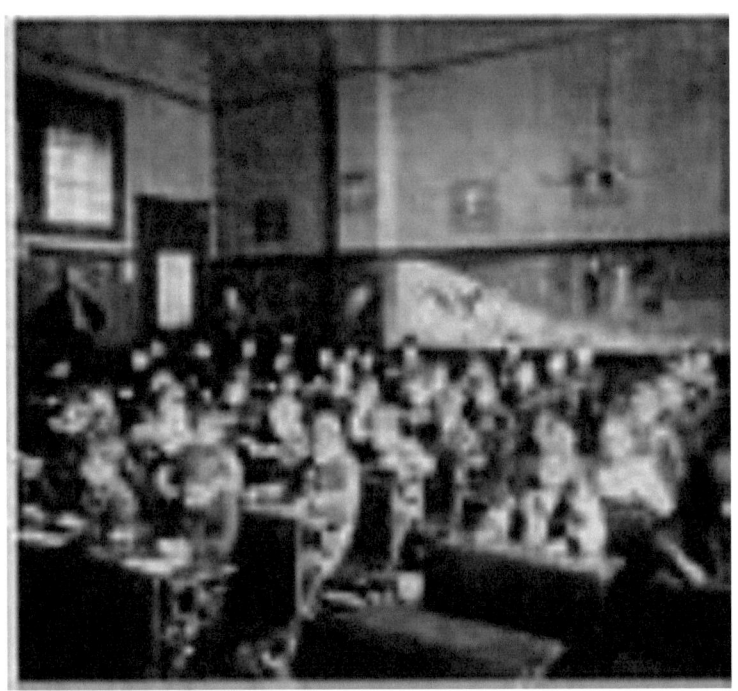

POSITIONS OFTEN SUGGEST EYE STRAIN

Of course eye specialists, — oculists, — if skillful, know more about eyes and eye troubles than general medical practitioners or teachers. Preliminary eye tests, however, may be made by any accurate person who can read. The Massachusetts state board of health reports that tests made by teachers were "not less efficient" than tests made by specialists. In June, 1907, a group of eminent oculists recommended to the school board of New York [75]City that teachers make this first test after being instructed by oculists. Persons interested in the schools nearest them can quickly interest teachers and pupils by starting tests with this card. In cities oculists can be found who will be glad to explain to teachers, individually or in groups, how the cards should be used and what dangers to avoid.

Nature intended the human eye to read the last line of this card at a distance of ten feet. This conclusion is not a guess, but is based upon the examination of thousands of eyes. In making the test, the number of feet the eye ought to see is written as the denominator of the fraction; the distance the eye can see clearly is the numerator. If the child's card reads, "Right eye 10/10, left eye 10/20," it means that the right eye sees without conscious strain the distance it is intended to see, while the left eye must be within ten feet to see what it ought to see twenty feet away.

The practical steps for a teacher to take in making eye tests are:

1. Scrutinize the faces for a strained or worried expression while reading or writing, for squint eyes, for unnatural positions, and for improper distances (more or less than nine inches) from eye to book.

2. Select for first tests the children who obviously need attention and will be obviously benefited. Use the eye test to help trace the cause of headaches, nervousness, inattention.

3. Let the children mark off the distances with a foot rule and chalk, going as high as twenty. Be sure to get the best light in the room.

4. Start all children on the ten-foot line. If a child cannot read at ten feet the letter which should be seen at that distance, move the child forward, have it step forward and backward, and note the result carefully. It is better to have ten separate letters of exactly the right size and the same size than a row of letters on one card, as in the Snellen test, otherwise memory will aid the eye, or, as happened recently, a whole class may agree to feign remarkable [76]nearsightedness or farsightedness by confusing letters learned in advance from the card. If the Snellen card is used, and if it is more convenient to have both child and card stationary, satisfactory results will be obtained by having the child read from large letters down as far as he can see.

5. Have the child read from right to left, from left to right, or skip about so that memory cannot aid the eye.

6. Test each eye separately. I was twenty-five years old before I learned that my left eye did practically all of the close sight work. A grown woman discovered just a few days ago that she was almost blind in the left eye; when she rubbed the right one while reading she was shocked to find that she could see nothing with the left eye.

7. If the card is stationary and the child moved, and if only one size of the letter is used, put in the denominator the number of feet at which the normal eye should see clearly, and in the numerator the distance at which each eye and both together can easily see. If the regular Snellen card is used containing letters of different size, place in the denominator the number of the lowest line each eye and both eyes together can read easily, and in the numerator the number of feet from card to eye.

8. Explain the result to the child, to his fellows, to his parents. If the left eye reads 10/20 and the right eye 10/30, it means that neither eye is normal, and that reading small type is a constant strain, even though unnoticed. The right eye must be within ten feet to read what it should read at twenty feet. The left eye must be within ten feet to read what it should read at thirty feet. If the two eyes read at ten, it means that in working together they successfully strain for a result that is not worth what it is costing. When eyes thus unconsciously see what they are not intended to see, it is only a matter of time when stomach and nervous system will announce that the strain can no longer be borne. Indigestion, dislike of study, restlessness follow. If, however, the eyes are so near the normal that their story reads 12/10 or 8/10, the strain will be negligible *for the present*. If, on the other hand, the only difficulty is a confusion of x and z with c and g, it means that there is a strain due to astigmatism, and that the child should be sent to an oculist.

[77]9. Teach children and parents (and practice what you preach) the urgent importance of periodic reëxamination, just as you would teach them to visit a dentist twice a year. This is needed by those who wear eyeglasses, and more particularly by those who have recently put them on. Moreover, as shown below, it is needed by children able to pass satisfactorily the Snellen test.

10. Acquire the habit of reading the eye for evidence of temperate or intemperate living, sleeping, eating, dancing, drinking, and smoking. Inflamed eyes are *results*,—signals of danger. "The organ may be faultless in construction and in its work poor, because of nerve exhaustion, or, in a less and more easily recoverable degree, nerve fatigue." If unusual eye conditions are not readily explained by mode of living or by eye tests, an oculist should be consulted.

The limits of the card test must be constantly kept in mind: (1) it does not register eye sickness due to dust, smoke, or disease germs; (2) it does not show unconscious eye strain due to successful accommodation. But it will discover a great part of the children who most need care. Sooner or later, too, inflammation of the eyelids, due to external causes, will affect the nerves of the eye and their power to conceal by accommodation the eye's defects. Just as we unconsciously open the mouth when a cold stops up the nose, the eye adapts itself to our needs without our realizing it. We expect it to see. It sees. If our eyes are not made alike, they do their best to work together. Like a good team of horses, the slow one hurries, the fast one holds back a little. But if one eye is 10/15 and the other 10/10, they will both be unnatural and strained if both read the same type. The effects of this strain frequently upset the stomach before the eyes rebel. I learned that I needed eyeglasses after a case of protracted indigestion, first diagnosed as "nervous" and later traced to eyes. Thousands of upper-grade children and college students are dieting for stomach trouble that will last until the eyes are relieved of the undue and unrecognized strain. [78]To prove the influence of eye strain on indigestion, persuade some obstinate parent to wear improperly focused glasses for a day; she will then be willing to have her child's eyes attended to.

It is unfortunate that the eyes will overwork without protesting. For years many persons suffer without learning that their eyes are unlike, or, as often happens, that one eye does all the close range work. Even when being tested, eyes will seem to see easily what requires a great effort of "accommodation." To prevent this self-deception skilled oculists do not trust the eye card, but put a drug in the eye that benumbs the muscles of accommodation. They cannot contract or expand if they want to. The oculist then studies the length of the eye and the muscle of accommodation. With this absolute knowledge of how each eye is made he knows what is wrong, exactly at what angle light enters the eye, whether objects are focused too soon or too late, exactly what kind of eyeglasses or what operation upon the eye is needed to enable it to do its work without undue straining or accommodation. So unconsciously do the eyes accommodate themselves to the work expected of them that not infrequently a child with seemingly perfect sight may be more in need of glasses than the child with imperfect sight. Practically, however, it is out of the question at the present time to have the majority of children given a more thorough test than that provided by the Snellen card. Where eye strains escape this test teachers will find evidence in complaints of headache, nervousness, sick stomach, chorea, or even epilepsy. The constant strain may also cause red or inflamed lids. Parents and teachers must be on the constant lookout for these symptoms of good sight persisting in spite of imperfect eyes.

An epidemic of eyeglasses is usually the consequence of eye tests. So naturally do we associate eyeglasses with [79]eye defects that some people assert that the eye tests at school originate with opticians more intent upon selling spectacles than upon helping children. In fact, even among educators who proclaim the need for eye tests there has been far more talk of eyeglasses than of removable conditions that cause eye strain. The women principals of New York City have sounded an alarm, and urge more attention to light and to reading position, more rest, more play, more hand work, less home study and less eye work at school, rather than more eyeglasses to conceal temporarily the effect of abusing children's eyes. Putting glasses on children without changing causal conditions is like giving alcohol to consumptives. The feeling of relief is deceptive. The trouble grows worse.

For some time to come eye tests will find eye troubles by the wholesale in every industrial and social class, in country as well as city schools. In 415 New York villages 48.7 per cent of school children had defects of vision,—this without testing children under seven,—while 11.3 per cent had sore eyes.

There are three possible ways of remedying defects: (1) changing the eye by operation; (2) changing the light as it enters the eye by eyeglasses; (3) decreasing the demands made upon the eye. To change eyes or light requires a technical skill which few physicians as yet possess. It will be remembered that it is but thirty years since the medical profession in America first began to understand the relation of eye defects to other defects. Until a generation of physicians has been trained by medical colleges to learn the facts about the eye and to apply scientific remedies, it is especially necessary that teachers and parents reduce the demands made upon children's eyes; oral can be substituted for written work, manual for optical work, relaxed and natural movement for discipline, outdoor exercise for less home study. Other requirements are [80]suitable light and proper position, and abolition of shiny paper, shiny blackboard, and fine print. Even after it is easy to obtain the correction of eye defects it will still be necessary to adapt the demands upon children's eyes to the strength and shape of those eyes. Because we are born farsighted, nearsighted, and astigmatic, we must be watchful to eradicate conditions that aggravate these troubles. Finally, there is no excuse whatever for permitting the parent of any school child in the United States to remain ignorant of the fact that it is just as absurd to go to the druggist or jeweler for eyeglasses as to the hardware store for false teeth.

The education of physician, oculist, and optician can be expedited by eye tests in school and by the follow-up work of schools in removing the prejudice of parents against glasses when needed. Because knowledge of chemistry preceded knowledge of the human body, the teaching of medicine still shows the effect of predilection for the remote, the problematical, the impossible. This predilection has influenced many specialists as well as many general practitioners, both overlooking too frequently obvious causes that even intelligent laymen can be taught to detect. Very naturally the man who makes money out of attention to simple troubles has stepped into the field not as yet occupied by the general practitioner and the specialist. Thus we have the optician, the painless tooth extractor, and quack cures for consumption. Opticians are placing before hundreds of thousands simple truths about the eye not otherwise taught as yet. Because they make their money by selling eyeglasses and because their special knowledge pertains to glasses rather than to eyes they frequently fail to recognize their limitations.

Physicians feel very strongly that it is as unethical for an optician to fit eyeglasses without a physician's prescription as for a pharmacist to give drugs without a physician's [81]prescription. The justification for this feeling should be based not upon the commercial motive of the optician but upon his ignorance. A physician uninformed as to eye troubles is just as unsafe as an optician determined to sell glasses. It must be made unethical and unprofessional for physician and optician alike to prescribe in the dark. Laymen and physicians must be taught that it is just as unethical and unprofessional for oculists and physicians to fail to bring their knowledge within the practical reach of the masses as for the optician to advertise his wares. School tests will not have been used to their utmost possibilities until optician and physician alike take the ethical position that the first consideration is the patient's welfare, not their own profits. It must soon be recognized as unethical and unprofessional for an optician who is also a skilled physician to refer patients to a medical practitioner ignorant as to optical science.

Whether opticians and physicians are unprofessional or unethical may be told by reëxamination if the *examiner* is himself competent and ethical. There is no better judge of their efficiency than the patient himself, who can tell whether the results promised have been effected. Whether the work of a country oculist is efficient and ethical can be learned: (1) by teaching country school children to recognize eye strain; (2) by comparing his results with those of other physicians. As soon as one or two states have tested eyes, we shall have an average by which to compare each class, school, and city with others of their size under similar conditions. If a particular physician finds half as many more or only half the average number, the presumption will be that his results are inaccurate and warrant an investigation. The interested teacher or parent can render an inestimable service to her local school and to the children of her state by taking steps to secure state laws compelling eye tests in all schools.

[82]Finally, it must be remembered by teachers, employers, parents, and all eye users that eyes are constantly changing; that eyes may need glasses six months after they are examined and found sound; that glasses change or develop the eye, so that they may be unnecessary and harmful six months after they are prescribed, or the eye may require a stronger glass; that eyeglasses become bent and scratched, so that they worry and strain the eye; that a periodic examination is essential to the health of the eye.

In caring for the health of the eye, we should also remember that our eyes are our chief interpreters of the world that gives us problems, profits, and pleasures. Out of gratitude, if not out of enlight-

ened self-interest, we owe our eyes protection, attention, and training, so that without straining we shall always be able to see truth
and beauty.

[83]

CHAPTER VIIIToC

EAR TROUBLE, MALNUTRITION, DEFORM-ITIES

The presence of adenoids is a frequent cause of both slight and aggravated deafness. Of 156 deaf mutes examined 59 per cent had adenoids, while only 6 per cent of the general run of the children in the neighborhood had this trouble. In mouth breathing, the current of air entering the mouth draws out some of the air from the Eustachian tube which ventilates the middle ear and unequalizes the atmospheric pressure on the eardrum, causing it to sink in and to blunt the hearing. An examination of the eardrums of school children in New York who are mouth breathers showed a high percentage of deafness, incipient or pronounced, accompanying adenoids. For example, of 9 mouth breathers selected from one class (average age 7-8 years), 6 were well-marked cases of deafness. Of 8 mouth breathers (average age 8-9 years), and of 5 mouth breathers (average age 5-6 years), all had noticeable defects of hearing. Many adults that suffer from deafness maintain that they never had any trouble in childhood. Yet the evidences of nose and throat trouble in childhood persist and disprove such statements. *The foundations of deafness in later life are, in most instances, laid in childhood.* Since the majority of cases of ear trouble occurring in school children accompany diseased conditions of the nose and throat, the proper care of nose and throat will, in large measure, balance the shortcomings of the aural examinations. Since the examination of the drum itself is not practicable, especial care should be given to the examination of the nose and throat.

[84]The figures published by New York City's department of health show that of 274,641 children examined from March, 1905, to January, 1908, 3540, or 1.2 per cent, gave evidence of defective hearing. Ear specialists suggest that this small percentage results from employing the whisper test at twenty feet. The whisper test at sixty

feet has been set by experts as a test of normal hearing. But preciseness with this test is well-nigh impossible when we consider that the acoustics, the quality of the examiner's voice, the weather, the vowel or consonant sounds, all are variable quantities. The watch test is frequently used, but since a young teacher in her enthusiasm used an alarm clock to make the test, specialists have decided that the volume of sound differs in watches to such a degree as to make the watch test unreliable. The examination of the eye has been reduced to mathematical precision, due altogether to the anatomy of that organ. As yet there is no instrument for the ear comparable to the ophthalmoscope. The acoumeter is largely used by aurists and can be obtained from the optician. This instrument has an advantage over the whisper or watch tests in that its tick is uniform.

Each ear should be tested separately. Let the child place his finger against the flap of one ear while the other is being tested. Then compare the farthest distance from the ear at which the tick can be heard with the normal, standard distance. During the test all sound should be eliminated as far as possible and the eyes should be closed. At a demonstration of ear testing at Teachers College, one student stated that she could not hear the tick of the watch at a distance greater than twenty inches. Then the tester walked noisily toward her, leaving the watch on the desk, five feet away from the patient. She heard it now. When the class burst out laughing she opened her eyes, and, seeing the watch so far away, exclaimed, "Why, [85]I thought I imagined it." Be careful in testing a child to distinguish between what he "thinks he imagines" and what he really hears. Because of the difficulties of this test a doubt should be sufficient to warn the teacher to send the child to be tested by an expert. Detection of slight deafness may lead to the discovery of serious defects of nose or throat. Inflammation from cold or catarrh may cause deafness, which if neglected may permanently injure the ear. Often deafness is due to an accumulation of wax. A running ear should receive immediate attention, as it is an indication of inflammation which may imperil the integrity of the eardrum, and, if neglected, may eat its way through the thin partition between the ear and the brain and cause death.

It should never be assumed that deafness is incurable. Stupidity, inattention, and slowness to grasp a situation accompany difficulty of hearing and should cause the teacher to examine the ears. No ear trouble is negligible. Children and parents should be taught that the normal ear is intended to hear for us, not to divert our attention to itself. When the ear aches or "runs" or rumbles there is something wrong, and it should be examined together with the throat and nose.

Nervousness

In New York City one child in ninety-one already examined has had the form of nervous disease known as St. Vitus's Dance, or chorea. So prone are we to overlook moderate evils and moderate needs that the child with aggravated St. Vitus's Dance is apt to be cured sooner than the child who is just "nervous." Teachers cannot know whether twitching eyes, emotional storms, constant motion of the fingers or feet are due to chorea, to malnutrition, to eye strain, or to habits acquired in babyhood or early childhood and continued for the advantage that [86]accrues when discipline impends. Many a child treasures as his chief asset in time of trouble the ability to lose his temper, to have a "fit," to exhibit nervousness that frightens parent, teacher, or playmate, incites their pity, and wards off punishment. The school examination will settle once for all whether the trouble can be cured. The family physician will explain what steps to take.

Tests of Malnutrition

We Americans were first interested in the physical examination of school children by exaggerated estimates of the number of children who are underfed. As fast as figures were obtained for eye defects, breathing defects, bad teeth, some one was ready to declare that these were results of underfeeding. Hence the conclusion: give children at least one meal a day at school. Scientific men began to set us straight and to give undernourishment a technical meaning,—soft bones, flabby tissue, under size, anæmia. While too little food might cause this condition, it was also explained that too much food of the wrong sort, or even food of the right sort eaten irregularly or hurriedly or poisoned by bad teeth, might also cause undernourishment, including the extreme type known as malnutrition. In extreme instances the symptoms enable an observant teacher who has learned to distinguish between the pretty hair ribbon and clean collar and the sunken, pale, or hectic cheek and lusterless eyes to detect the cause. But as with eyes and nose, an unhealthy condition [87]of nourishment may exist long before outward symptoms are noticeable. Therefore the value of the periodic searching examination by the school physician.

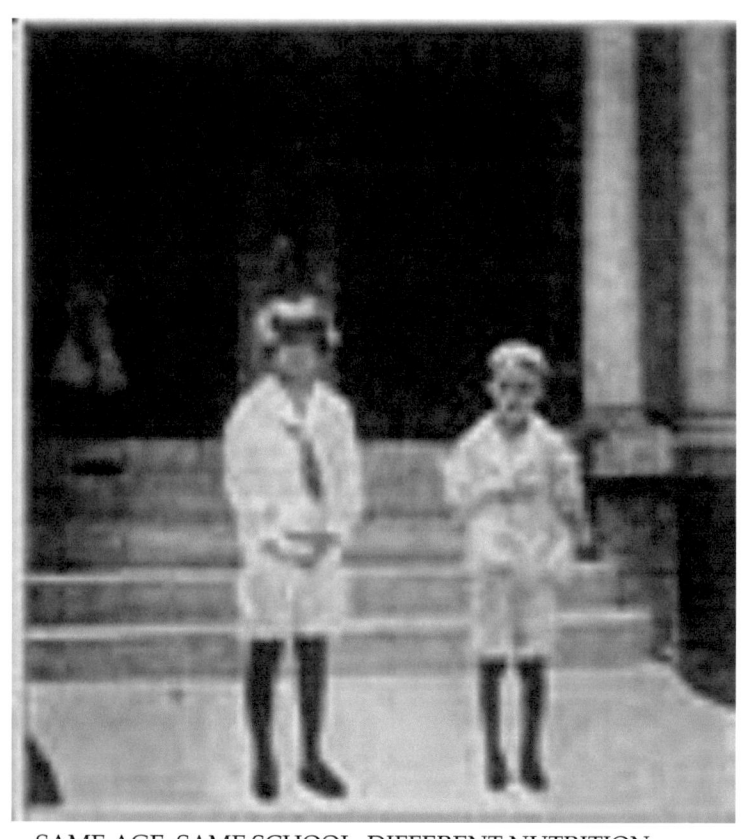

SAME AGE, SAME SCHOOL, DIFFERENT NUTRITION

Bone Tuberculosis; Orthopedic Tests

Only recently have we laymen learned that knee trouble, club-foot, ankle sores, spine and hip troubles, scrofula, running sores at joints, etc., are not hereditary and inevitable, but are rather the direct result of carelessness on the part of adult consumptives. These conditions in school are indices of homes and houses where tuberculosis is or has been active, and of health boards that are or have been inactive in checking the white plague. Early examination may disclose the small lump on the child's spine,—which one mother diagnosed as inherited "round shoulders,"—and save a child from being a humpback for life. Moreover, the examination of the crippled child's brothers and sisters will often show the beginnings of pulmonary tuberculosis.

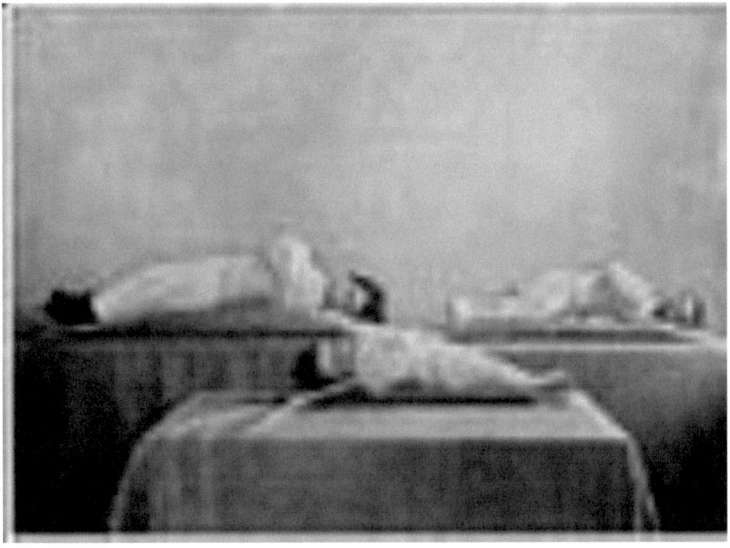

A GRIEVOUS PENALTY FOR NEGLECT BY ADULT CONSUMPTIVES

[88]

Enlarged Glands — Tuberculosis

In almost every class are one or more children who are proud of small or big lumps under one or more jaws. Only physicians can find very small lumps. Many family doctors will say, "Oh, he will outgrow those," or "Those lumps will be absorbed." Like most other evils that we "outgrow" or that pass away, these lumps shriek not to be neglected. They mean interference with nourishment and prevent proper action of the lymphatic system, as adenoids prevent free breathing. Even when not actually infected with tubercle bacilli, they are fertile soil for the production of these germs. If detected early, they point to home conditions and personal habits that can be easily corrected. In New York one child in four has these enlarged glands. If the same proportion prevails in other parts of the United States, there are 5,400,000 children whose strength is being needlessly drained, many of whom, if neglected, will need repeated operations.

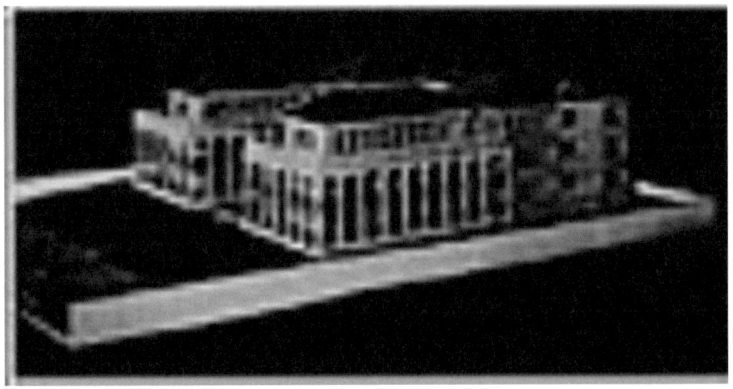

MODEL OF AMERICA'S FIRST HOSPITAL FOR SEASHORE FRESH-AIR
TREATMENT OF NONPULMONARY TUBERCULOSIS IN CHILDREN
To be erected at Rockaway Beach, New York City

DENTAL SANITATION

"Have their teeth attended to first, and many of the eye defects will disappear." This was an unexpected contribution to the debate upon free eyeglasses for the school children of New York City. So little do most of us realize the importance of sound, clean teeth, and the interrelation of stomach and sense nerves, that even the school principals thought the eye specialist was exaggerating when he declared that bad teeth cause indigestion and indigestion causes eye strain.

"Bad" teeth mean to most people dirty teeth and offensive odors, loose, crooked, or isolated teeth, or black stumps. Even among dentists a great many, probably the majority, do not appreciate that "bad" teeth mean indigestion, lowered vitality, plague spots for contaminating sound teeth and for breeding disease germs. Until recently the only rule about the teeth of new recruits in the United States army was: "There must be two opposing molars on each side of the mouth. It doesn't matter how rotten these molars may be." The surgeon general was persuaded to change to "four opposing molars on each side"; still nothing as to the condition of the two additional molars! In the German army there is a regular morning inspection of teeth and toothbrushes. Several German insurance companies give free dental treatment to policy holders, not to bestow charity but to increase profits.

Neglecting "baby teeth" and adenoids may mean crooked second teeth that will cause: (1) hundreds of dollars for straightening; (2) permanent business handicap because crooked teeth are disagreeable to others, because mastication [90]is less perfect, and because a disfigured mouth means dis-arranged nerves; or perhaps (3) large dental bills because it is difficult to clean between cramped, crooked teeth.

Unfortunately the great majority of parents rarely think of their children's teeth until too late to preserve them intact. Even among families where the rule of brushing the teeth twice daily prevails, regular dental examination is often not required. Doctors and dentists themselves have not been trained to realize that the teeth are a most dangerous source of infection when unclean. Does your dentist insist upon removing tartar and food particles beyond your reach, upon polishing and cleansing, or does he regard these as vanity touches, to be omitted if you are in a hurry?

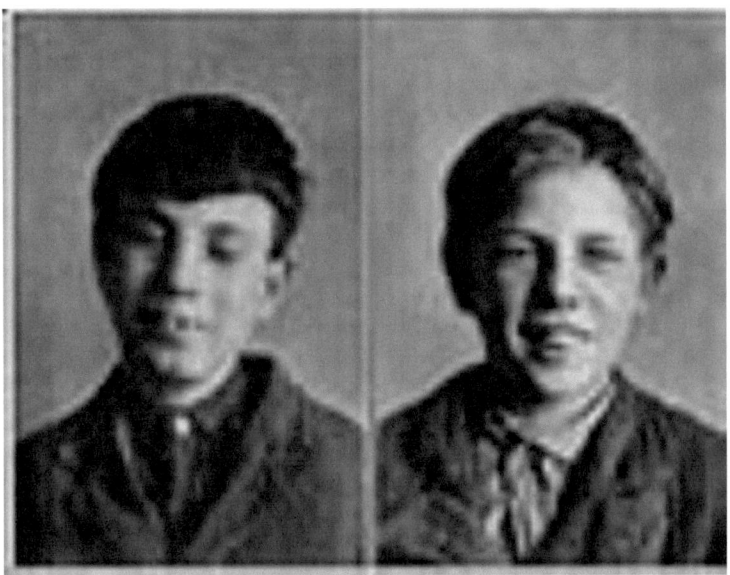

INDUSTRIAL HANDICAPS DISCOVERED AT SCHOOL

Physicians send tuberculosis patients to hospitals or camps without correcting the mouth conditions that make it impossible for the patient to eat or swallow without infecting [91]himself. Tonics are given to women whose teeth are breeding and harboring disease germs that tear down vitality. Nurses watch their suffering patients and do the heavier tasks heroically, but are not trained to teach the simple truths about dental hygiene. The far-reaching results of neglect of teeth will not be understood until greater emphasis is placed on the bacteriology, the economics, the sociology, and the æsthetics of clean, sound teeth. Whether or not there is at present a tendency to exaggerate the importance of sound teeth, there is no difference of opinion as to the fact that the teeth harbor virulent germs, that the high temperature of the mouth favors germ propagation, that the twenty to thirty square inches of surface constantly open to bacterial infection offer an extensive breeding ground, and that the formation of the teeth invites the lodgment of germs and of particles of food injurious both to teeth and to other organs.

By scraping the teeth with the finger nail and noticing the odor you can convince yourself of the presence of decomposing organic matter not healthful to be carried into the stomach. By applying a little iodine and then washing it off with water, your teeth may show stains. These stains are called gelatinous plaques, which are transparent and invisible to the naked eye except when colored by iodine. These plaques protect the germs, which ferment and create the acid which destroys tooth structure. Their formation can be prevented by vigorous brushing and by eating hard food.

The individual with decayed teeth, even with unclean teeth, is open to infection of the lungs, tonsils, stomach, glands, ears, nose, and adenoid tissues. Every time food is taken, and at every act of swallowing, germs flow over the tonsils into the stomach. Mouth breathers with teeth in this condition cannot get one breath of uncontaminated air, for every breath becomes infected with poisonous emanations from the teeth. Bad teeth are frequently the sole [92]cause of bad breath and dyspepsia, and can convey to the system tuberculosis of the lungs, glands, stomach, or nose, and many other transmissible diseases. They may also cause enlarged tonsils and ear trouble.

Apart from decomposing food and stagnant septic matter from saliva injured by indigestion, and by sputum which collects in the healthy mouth, there are in many infected mouths pus, exudations from the irritated and inflamed gum margins, gaseous emanations from decaying teeth, putrescent pulp tissue, tartar, and chemical poisons. Every spray from such a mouth in coughing, sneezing, or even talking or reading, is laden with microbes which vitiate the air to be breathed by others. Indigestion from imperfect mastication and imperfect salivation (themselves often due solely to bad teeth) is far less serious than indigestion from germ infection. Germs taken into the stomach can so change the composition of saliva (a natural disinfectant when healthy) as to render it no longer able to kill germs. Indigestion may result in excess of uric acid and toxic material, so that the individual becomes subject to gout and rheumatism, which in turn frequently destroy the bony support of the teeth and bring about Riggs's Disease. The last named is a prevalent and disfiguring disease, whose symptom is receding gums. The irritating toxins deposited on the teeth cause inflammation of the tissues at the gum margins. The gums withdraw more and more from sections of the teeth; the poisons get underneath and work back toward the roots; the infection increases and hastens the loosening of the teeth. I know of a man who had all of his teeth extracted at twenty-one years of age, because he was told that this was the only treatment for this disease, which was formerly thought to be incurable. Yet thorough cleansing and removal of this matter from under the edges of the gums, disinfection, a few visits to the dentist, will stop the recession but cannot regain lost ground.

[93]Among those who regularly use the toothbrush, instinct, comfort, or display is the ruling motive, while a small percentage have evolved to the anti-nuisance stage, where the æsthetic standard of their group forbids any member to neglect his teeth. The anti-slum and pro-slum motives for mouth cleanliness and dental sanitation have been awakened in but one or two places. A significant pro-slum activity is the dental clinic organized by forty volunteer dentists, acting for an industrial school maintained by the New York Children's Aid Society.

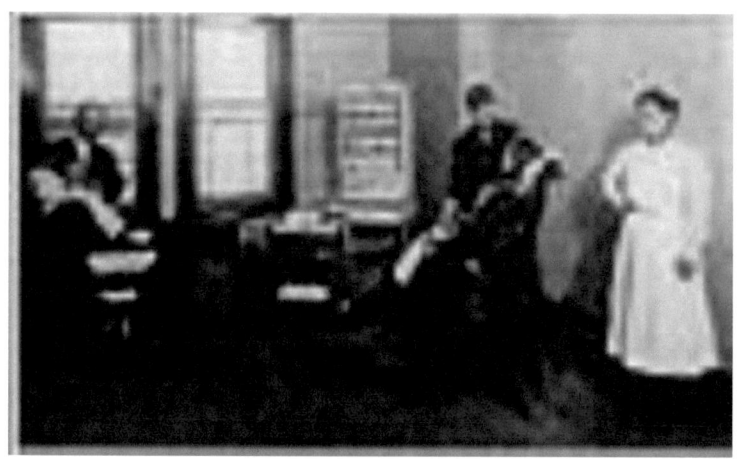

NEW YORK CHILDREN'S AID SOCIETY'S DENTAL CLINIC FOR SCHOOL CHILDREN

Here 550 children have been examined, 447 teeth extracted, 284 teeth filled, 200 teeth treated for diseased pulp (and only 24 sets cleaned), 40 dentists taking turns in giving time to this work. The equipment cost but $239; cards and stationery, $72; incidentals, $33. The principal attends the clinic, because in her presence no child is willing to confess fear or unwillingness. To supplement this work, the dentists have prepared for free distribution a leaflet which tells in short, clear sentences how to care for the teeth.

[94]

A DENTAL CATECHISM

What are the teeth for?
To masticate food; that is, grind it into fine particles, mix it with saliva, and so begin its digestion; also to aid in speaking and singing.

How long should they last?
To the very end of life.

How do we lose them?
By decay, by loosening, and by accident.

What causes teeth to decay?
Particles of food decaying in contact with them.

Where does food lodge?
All along the edges of the gums, in the spaces between the teeth, and in the crevices of their grinding surfaces.

Can we prevent this loss?
Yes, to a large extent.

How can we do it?
By using the teeth properly and by keeping them clean and the gums healthy.

What does using them properly mean?
1. Using sufficient hard or fibrous food to give the teeth and gums full exercise.
2. Taking time enough to masticate food thoroughly before swallowing.

How often should teeth be cleansed?
As often as they are used.

When should they be cleansed?
Immediately after the morning and noonday meals and before going to bed.

By what means should they be cleansed?
By a moderately stiff brush, water, and floss silk.

How should these be used?
The brush should be first used in a general way, high up on the gums lengthwise of the jaws, to remove large particles and stimulate the gums, then the brush and the teeth should be carefully rinsed with water. The brush should next be used with a rolling or circular motion, so that the bristles will follow the lines of all the grooves and spaces in which the particles of food have lodged, and so brush them out. Then again the mouth should be rinsed with water.

Should the gums be brushed?
Yes, moderate friction helps to keep them healthy.

How can the spaces between the teeth be reached?
By dental floss silk passed between the teeth, drawn carefully back and forth till it reaches the gum, pressed firmly against the side of each tooth in turn and drawn out towards the grinding end of the tooth, and this repeated several times in each space.

Should tooth powder or paste be used?
Usually once a day.

Such a leaflet should be given out at dispensaries, hospitals, dental offices, schools, and from many Sunday schools and missions.[5]

[95]The time for the schools to begin is when the child is first registered. Examination and reëxamination must be accompanied by explanation of the serious disadvantages of neglected teeth, and the physical, social, and economic advantages of clean, sound teeth. Instruction at school must be followed by education of parents. The school or health authorities should examine the teeth of all children before issuing work certificates. Finally, the dental, medical, and

nursing professions and the press must be enlisted in the school's campaign for dental hygiene. The Dental Hygiene Council of Massachusetts should be copied in all states.

A preliminary examination of teeth can be made by parent or teacher. Crooked, loose, dirty, or black teeth or receding gums can be detected by a layman's naked eye. In fact, children can be interested in finding the most obvious defects in their own or their brothers' teeth. There could be no better first lesson than to ask each pupil to look in a hand mirror and to count each tooth obviously needing a cleaning or a filling. The most urgent need can thus be ascertained without expert aid. But because parent, teacher, or child cannot discover defects does not prove that dental care is not imperative; hence the importance of examination by a dentist or by a physician competent to discover dental needs. If a private, public, or parochial school has no paid visiting dentist, a zealous school officer can, at least in large towns, persuade one or more dentists or physicians to make a few first tests to confirm the teacher's findings, and to persuade the community that regular examination and reëxamination are necessary and a saving of pain, beauty, and money.

Reëxamination is necessary because decay *may* start the day after a dentist has pronounced a tooth sound. For most of us twice a year is often enough. A reëxamination should be made upon the slightest suspicion of decay, breaking, or loosening.

[96]Educational use should be made by the teacher of the results of school examination. Children cannot be made self-conscious and cleanly by telling them that their teeth will ache three or five years from now. They can be made to brush or wash their teeth every morning and every night if they once realize that cavities can be caused only by *mouth garbage*. All decay of human teeth starts from the outside through the enamel that covers the soft bone of the tooth. This enamel can be destroyed by accidentally cracking or breaking it, or by acids eating into it. These acids come from (1) particles of food allowed to remain in the teeth; (2) tartar, etc., that adheres to the teeth and can be removed only by a dentist; (3) saliva brought up from an ill-conditioned stomach. Even where the enamel is destroyed, absolute cleanliness will prevent serious decay of the tooth. A perfectly clean tooth will not decay. Generally speak-

ing, unless particles of food or removable acids remain on or between the teeth long enough to decompose, teeth cannot decay. Decay always means, therefore, uncleanliness. To unclean teeth is due in large part the offensive odor of many schoolrooms.

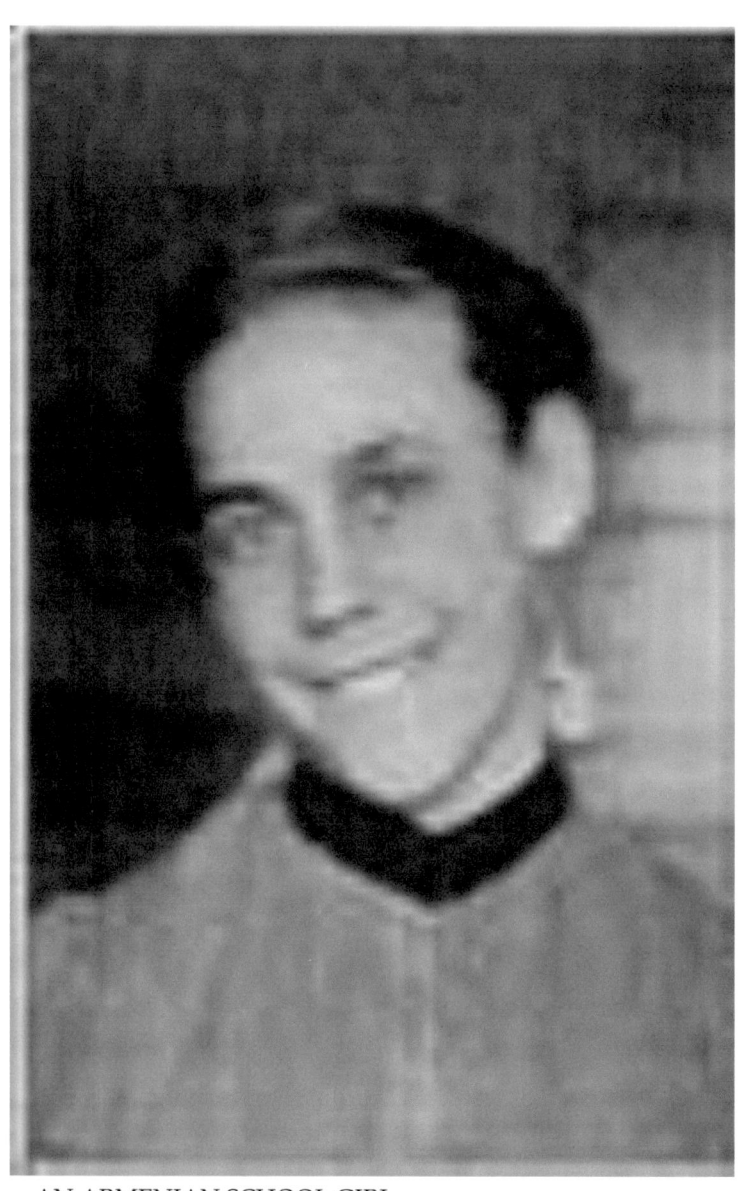

AN ARMENIAN SCHOOL GIRL

Uncleanliness becomes noticeable to our neighbors sooner or later. There is no offense we are so reluctant to commit as that of having uncleanliness of our bodies disagreeable to those about us. Very young children will make every effort in their power to live up to the school's standard of cleanliness. The other side to this reason for having clean teeth is vanity. Because all cleanliness is beautiful to us, clean teeth are one attribute of beauty that all of us can possess.

Habits of cleanliness are easily fixed. In the most crowded, most overworked section of large cities visitors from "uptown" are surprised by the children's bright hair ribbons, clean aprons, clean faces, and smoothly combed hair. It will be easy to add clean teeth to the list of things necessary to personal and family standing. Armenian children [97]are taught to clean their teeth after eating, even if only an apple between meals. They covet "beautiful teeth." American standards will soon prevent these Armenians from cleaning their teeth in public, but desire for beautiful teeth will stay, and will remind them to care for their teeth in private. As coarse food gives way to sugars and soft foods, stiff toothbrushes must supplement tongue and toothpicks.

Strong as are the instinct and display motives in cleaning teeth, both parents and children need to be reached through the commerce motive. Instinct makes children afraid of the dentist, or content when the tooth stops aching. Display may be satisfied with cleaning the front teeth, as many boys comb only the front hair or as girls hide dirty scalps under pompadours and pretty ribbons. Desire to save money may give stronger reasons for not going to the dentist than instinct and comfort can urge for going. But parents can be made to see, as can children after they begin to picture themselves as wage earners, that a dentist in time saves nine, and that no regular family investment will earn more money than the price of prompt and regular dental care. A problem in arithmetic would be convincing, if, by questions such as those on page 98, we could compare the family cost of neglecting teeth with the cost of toothbrushes, bicarbonate of soda, pulverized chalk or tooth powder, early and repeated examination by a dentist, and treatment when needed.

[98]

How many members in your family?

How many teeth have they?

How many teeth have they lost?

How many false teeth have they?

How many teeth have been filled?

What is the total cost to date?

How many days have been lost from work because of toothache?

How many teeth are now decayed?

What will it cost to have them attended to?

What does a toothbrush cost?

How many do you need in one year?

How much does tooth powder cost?

How much is needed for one year?

How much would two examinations a year by a dentist cost?

The result will show that the money spent for one good "house cleaning" of one child at fourteen or eighteen exceeds the cost of keeping clean and in repair the teeth of the entire family. How effective and economical is thorough cleaning is confessed by an eminent dentist, who taught an assistant to clean his patients' teeth. "Do you know," he said, "I had to stop it, so perceptibly did my work decrease." The total time required to examine school children for teeth needing attention is much less than the time now lost by absence from school or wasted at school on account of toothache.

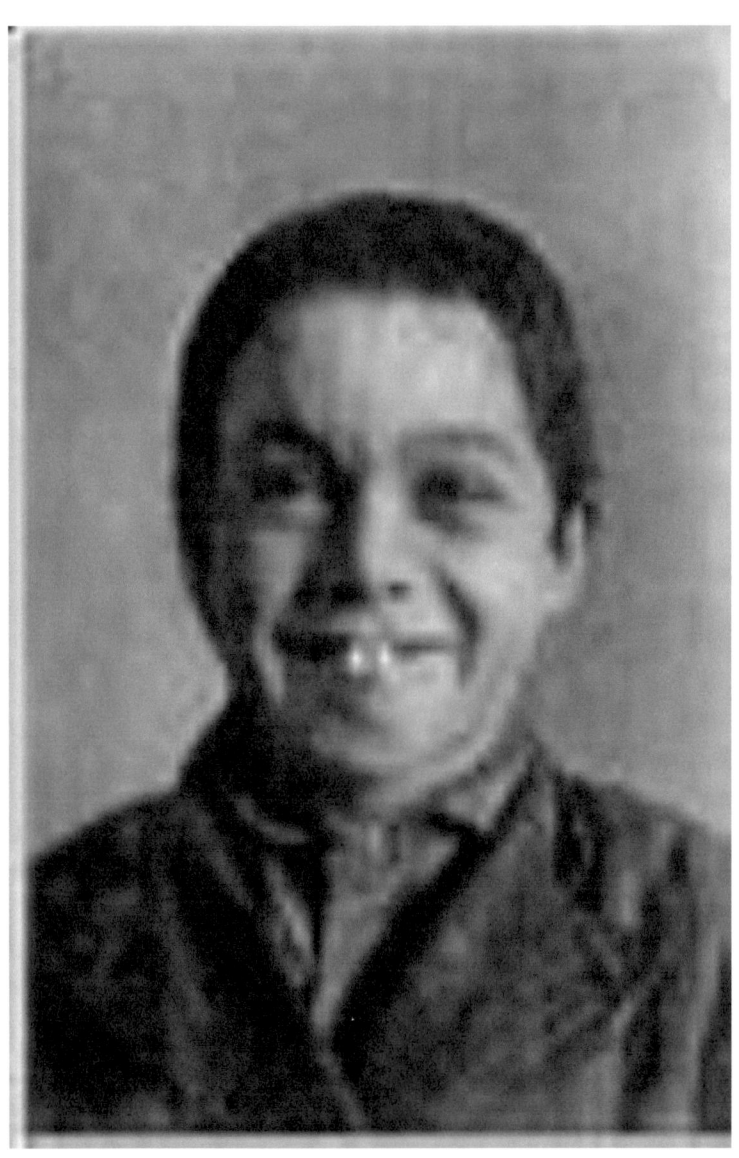

WON BY THE ECONOMIC ARGUMENT

To remind school children regularly of dental hygiene is not more important than for the school to remind parents repeatedly of the many reasons for attending to their children's teeth. It is not enough, however, to send one message to parents. Illustrated lectures, mothers' meetings, demonstrations at hospitals and fresh-air homes are all very serviceable, but listening is a poor substitute for understanding. Schools should see that parents understand the æsthetics, the economics, the humanity of dental hygiene. [99]The best test of whether the parent has understood is the child's tooth.

Dental examination of children applying for work certificates gives the health and school authorities a means of enforcing their precepts. When no child is allowed to go to work whose teeth cause malnutrition or disgust, the news will spread, and both child and parent will see clearly the grave need for dental care.

Finally, local papers can be interested. They will print almost anything the teacher sends about the need for dental care. They like particularly facts about the number of cavities found, the number of children needing care, efforts made to procure care, and new facts about diseases that can be caused by bad teeth or about diseases that can injure teeth. Teachers can persuade dentists and physicians to write stories. No newspaper will refuse to print such statements as this: "A tuberculous patient in six weeks lost ground steadily. I persuaded him to go to a dentist to clean the vestibule to his digestive system, and to have a set of false teeth. He enjoys his meals, and has gained twelve pounds in six weeks." Popular magazines and newspapers mention teeth seldom, because those who best know the interesting vital things are making money, not writing articles or otherwise concerning themselves with dental education. It is said that of forty thousand American dentists not over eleven thousand are readers of dental journals, and probably not three hundred contribute to professional [100]literature. One dentist who is working for the children's clinic described above, when asked by the board of education to lecture to the people on the care of the teeth and to recommend simple, readable books, told me that he knew no good books to suggest.

Five obstacles exist to practicing what is here preached:

1. The expensiveness of proper dentistry.

2. The untrustworthiness of cheap dental service and "painless" dental parlors; the domination of the supply houses wishing to sell instruments and other supplies.

3. The ethical objection to any kind of advertising or to work by wholesale.

4. The lack of dispensaries.

5. The profit-making basis of dental education.

Additional reasons these for cleanliness that will make the dentist serviceable for his knowledge rather than for his time and gold.

Good dentists really "come too high" for both the poor and the comfortably situated. Families in New York City that have four or five thousand dollars a year hesitate to go to a dentist whom they thoroughly trust, because his time is worth more than they feel they can afford to pay.

The "free-extraction" dental parlors undoubtedly are doing a vast amount of harm. In every city are dental quacks that injure wage-earning adults as much as soothing-sirup quacks injure babies. Instead of teaching people to preserve their teeth, they extract, and then, by dint of overpersuading by a pretty cashier hired for the purpose, make a contract for a gold crown or a false set at an exorbitant price. A reputable dentist has said that a dental parlor can do more damage to the welfare of the race in a few months than a well-intentioned man in the profession can repair in a lifetime. Its question is not, What can I do for this patient? but What is there in this mouth for me? Many "parlors" never expect to see the same [101]person twice, because they do not make him comfortable or gain his confidence; they put a filling in on top of decayed matter or even diseased pulp; put in plates and bridges that do not fit; charge more than the examination at first leads one to expect; refuse to correct mistakes; deny having ever seen the patient before. Yet true and severe as this arraignment is, many of these parlors, with their liveried "runners in," are doing an educational service not otherwise provided; it is conceivable that in many cities they are doing less harm by their malpractice than well-intentioned men in the profession by neglect of public needs or by failure to organize facilities for meeting those needs.

I realize that advertising is "unethical" among dentists as among physicians. Humbug and imposition are supposed to go inevitably with self-advertising by the methods used in selling shoes or automobiles. Therefore such advertising is prohibited. But what seems to be forgotten in this definition of ethics is that the need and the opportunity for dental care must be advertised in some way, if we are ever to control diseases and evils due to bad teeth. The rich that one dentist can help are able to pay for his good taste, his neat attendants, his automobile, his club dues, his vacations at fashionable resorts, his hours without work, his standard of living. All of these things advertise him, just as hospital appointments and social position may and do advertise successful physicians. The patients of moderate means that one dentist can treat cannot afford to pay for rent, time disengaged, and indirect advertising. Either they must have free treatment, must go without treatment, or must go to a dental parlor where dental needs are organized so that a very large number will contribute to rent and display. It is out of the question to have both dentists and patients so distributed and prices so adjusted that dentists can make a good living by charging what the patient can afford, and at the same time admit of every [102]patient being properly treated when necessary. Judging from every other branch of work, the solution of the problem lies partly in free care for those who can pay nothing or very little, and partly in coöperative treatment through the heretofore objectionable dental parlors. If instead of inveighing against advertisers, honorable and capable dentists worked through dental and medical societies to secure adequate public supervision of dental practice, more progress would be made against dental malpractice.

Dental clinics will quickly follow the publication of facts that schools should gather. In some places these should be separate; but at first the best thing is to make every hospital, every children's home, every settlement a clinic, and every school an examining center. A skilled dentist informs me: "The demand that will follow examination of school children's teeth will make it profitable for young dentists to adopt a coöperative scheme, where several young men hire a parlor in a cheap district, and, under the supervision of some experienced dentist, give good advice at reasonable rates. This is the best antidote to the dental parlor which exploits the public so shamelessly." Bellevue Hospital in New York is the first general hospital to establish regular dental examination; others will undoubtedly soon follow.

Dental education for profit rather than for instruction and for health has been the rule. Even where universities have put in dental courses, they have demanded a net profit from tuition. Instead of protecting society against men incapable of caring for teeth, the schools have marketed certificates to as large numbers as slowly enlightened self-interest would permit. Much progress has been made toward uniform standards of admission and graduation, but dental colleges sadly need the light and the inspiration of school facts about teeth.

Of fourteen dental journals in America, only one has the advancement of dental science as its first reason for [103]existence. Thirteen are trade journals. Not one of these would print articles proving that the supplies advertised by their backers were inimical to dental hygiene. Many dental colleges still retain on their faculties agents or editors in the pay of supply houses, Harvard's new dental school being a notable exception. This trade motive tolerates and encourages the disreputable practices of existing dental parlors. Largely because of this prostitution of the dental profession, patients generally neglect the repairing and cleansing of the teeth and the sterilizing of the mouth from which germs are carried to all parts of the body. Dental journalism for the sale of supplies cannot outlive the dentist's reading of the school's index.

Many dentists will say that they must learn dentistry before they learn the economics and sociology of clean teeth. Being a young profession, it is natural that dentistry should first devote itself to learning its own mechanics,—the tricks of the trade—how to fill teeth. But the fact that it took the medical profession centuries to begin to feel responsibility for community health is no reason why the social sense of the dentist should be dormant for centuries or decades. We need training and exercise to determine what kind of filling will be most comfortable and most serviceable; whether the pulp of the teeth needs treating or removing before the filling is inserted; whether it is worth while to fill a deciduous or baby tooth. Sociology will never take the place of dental technic. The few dentists who have studied the social significance and social responsibility of their profession declare, however, that careless workmanship and indifferent education of patients continue chiefly because dentists themselves do not see the community's interest in dental hygiene. The school can socialize or humanize the dental profession if teachers themselves possess the social sense and make known the facts about the need for dental care among school children.

FOOTNOTES:

[5]*The Teeth and Their Care*, by Thaddeus P. Hyatt, D.D.S., is a short, concise treatment of the principles of dental sanitation.

[104]

ABNORMALLY BRIGHT CHILDREN

What is commonly considered abnormal brightness in a school child is often a tendency to live an abnormal physical life. Being a child bookworm means that time is spent indoors that should be spent playing games with one's fellows. Excellence in the activities of children, not ability to imitate the activities of adults, should be the test of child brightness. To be able to hit a bull's-eye, to throw a ball accurately, to calculate the swing of a curve or the bound of a "grounder," these are tests of brightness quite as indicative of mental power as the ability to win highest marks in school, while less injurious to physical power. The child who is abnormally bright requires special treatment just as much as the child who is abnormally dull. The former as well as the latter must have his abnormal condition corrected if he is to grow into a normally bright man.

The college man who sacrifices health to "marks" is thus described by the director of physical training at Harvard University:

A drooping head, a pale face, dull, sunken eyes, flat chest and rounded shoulders, with emaciated limbs, soft flabby muscles, and general lack of good physical, mental, and moral tone.

For the protection of these physical defective grinds it is suggested to put a physical qualification upon the candidates of Phi Beta Kappa and their awards of scholarship. If scholarship men cannot be induced to take time to improve their physique for fear of lowering their college standing, then give them credit for standing in physical work.

[105]The abnormally bright, at whatever age, is as much a subject for examination and treatment as the child with adenoids and pulmonary tuberculosis. Such attention will increase the percentage of abnormally bright schoolmates who figure in active business in later

life. Moreover, it will decrease the number of high school superintendents who declare that their honor pupils are physical wrecks.

There are children who develop very rapidly, both physically and mentally, and whose mental superiority is not at the expense of their bodies. Protection of such children requires that their minds be permitted to progress as rapidly as bodily health justifies. It is as cruel to keep back a physically and mentally superior child, as to push the physically or mentally defective beyond his powers. Worry and fatigue can be produced by lack of interest as well as by overwork. "Normal" should not be confused with "average." To keep a bright child back with the average child—marking time till the dull ones catch up—is to make him abnormal. The tests that we have employed for grading pupils are either the tests of age in years or of mental capacity. The first takes no account of slowness or rapidity of physiological development,—of physiological age. The second encourages mental activity at the expense of physique. The entrance of a child into school, the promotion from one class to another, the entrance into college, are thus determined either by the purely artificial test of age or by the individual teacher's discretion. There is nothing to prevent the ambitious teacher or the ambitious parent from pushing a child into kindergarten at four, high school at twelve, college at fifteen. If this cannot be done at the public school, a private school is resorted to. A community of college professors once started a school for faculty children. A tremendous pressure was put upon these scions of intellectual aristocracy to enter the high school at twelve. No thought was given to the ventilation of the school. The [106]windows were so arranged that they could not be opened without the air blowing on some child's back. "You could cut the air with a knife" was a description given by one sensible professor who had taken his sturdy girl of seven away from the school, because he feared that in this environment she would become like the other little puny, pale, undersized children of that school.

The University of Pennsylvania has instituted a psychological clinic. Parents and teachers are invited to bring any deviation from the usual or the expected to the attention of this clinic. Every month a bulletin is published called the *Psychological Clinic*, which will be found of great service in dealing with the abnormally bright as well as with the abnormally dull. Naturally the well-to-do and the rich are the first to take advantage of these special facilities for ascertaining just what work should be done by a precocious child or by the mentally and morally retarded.

Abnormal brightness means power to be happy and to be serviceable that is above the average. Every school can be a miniature psychological clinic. While every teacher cannot be an expert, national and state superintendents can constantly remind teachers that the abnormally bright are also abnormally apt to neglect physical welfare and to endanger future mental power.

[107]

NERVOUSNESS OF TEACHER AND PUPIL

Nervousness of teacher and pupil deserves special mention. So universal is this physical defect that we take it for granted, especially for teachers. Teachers themselves feel that they need not even apologize for nervousness, in fact they too frequently use it as an excuse for impatience, ugly temper, discourtesy, and unfairness. Children, slates, papers, parents, blackboards "get on their nerves." Nervousness of teacher causes nervousness of pupils and adds to the evil results of mouth breathing, bad teeth, eye strain, and malnutrition. These conditions, added to bad ventilation, bad light, and an overcrowded schoolroom, render the atmosphere thoroughly charged with electricity—nerves—toward the end of the day. Lack of oxygen to breathe as well as inability to breathe it; lack of well-printed books and good light, as well as lack of the power to use them; toothache, earache, headache, deplete the vitality of both teacher and pupil.

Most of the disturbances at school are but outward signs of unwholesome physical conditions. If the teacher attempts to treat these causes by crushing the child, she makes confession of her own nervousness and inadequacy and visits her own suffering upon her pupils. A transfixing glance prolonged into an overbearing stare, a loud, sharp voice, a rough manner, are successful only so far as they work on the nervousness of her pupil. She finds that it is temporarily effective, and so by her example and practice sets the child an example in losing control of himself. The position often assumed by school children when before authority, [108]of hands held stiffly at the side, head drooped, and roving eye, does not mean control: it means a crushed spirit, hypocrisy, or brooding anarchy. The mother or teacher who obtains obedience by clapping her hands, pointing her finger, distorting her face, is copying in her own home the attitudes of caste in India, of serfdom in Russia, the discipline of the prison the world over, a modern reminder of the power of life and death or of physical torture.

A young college girl unfamiliar with the ways of the public school was substituting in the highest grammar grade. The time for civics arrived. Here, she thought, is a subject in which I can interest them. The boys showed a vast amount of press information, as well as decided opinions on the politics of the day. The candidates which they elected for the position of ideal American patriot were Rockefeller, Lincoln, and Sharkey the prize fighter. During the ensuing debate, which gave back to Lincoln his proper rank, the boys in the back of the room had moved forward and were sharing seats with the boys in the front. Every boy was engrossed in the discussion. The room was in perfect order,—not, however, according to the ideas of the principal, who entered at that moment to see how the new substitute was managing the class, famed for its bad boys. With the stern look of a Simon Legree she demanded, "How dare you leave your seats!" When one child started to explain she shouted: "How dare you speak without permission! Don't you know your teacher never permits it? Every boy take his own seat at his own desk." This principal was far more to be pitied than the boys, for they had before them the prospect of "work papers" and a grind less monotonous and more productive than the principal's discipline. She was a victim of a nerve-racking system, more sinned against than sinning.

There is nothing in school life *per se* to cause nervousness. Given a well-aired, sunny room, where every child [109]has enough fresh air to breathe, where he can see without strain, where he has a desk fitted to his body and work fitted to his maximum abilities, a teacher who is physically strong and mentally inspiring, and plenty of play space and play time, there will be no nervousness. One who visits vacation schools is struck with the difference in the atmosphere from that of the winter day schools. Here are the same rooms, the same children, and in many cases the same teachers, but different work. Each child is busy with a bright, interested, happy expression and easy attitude. Some are at nature study, some are weaving baskets, making dresses, trimming hats, knitting bright worsted sacks and mittens for the winter. Boys are at carpentering, raffia, or wrought-iron work. In none of the rooms is the absolute unity or the methodical order of the winter schoolroom, but rather the hum of the workroom and the order that comes from a roomful of children interested in the progress of their work. This condition only illustrates what a winter schoolroom might be were physical defects corrected or segregated, windows open, light good, and work adapted to the child.

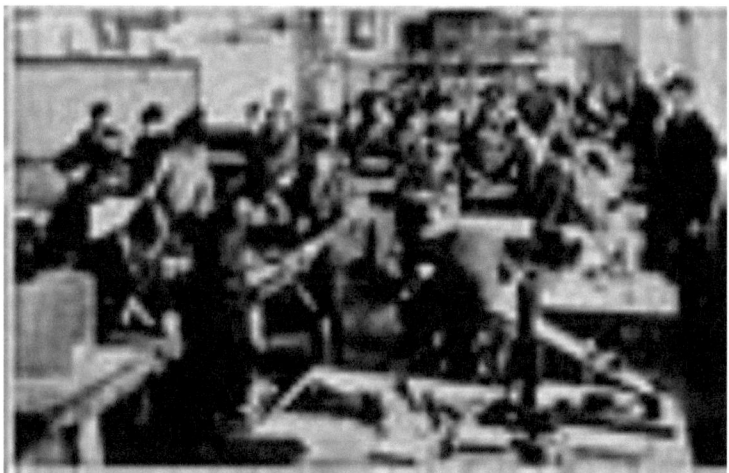

VACATION SCHOOL INTEREST: AN ANTIDOTE TO NERVOUSNESS

[110]Nervousness is not a monopoly of city teachers and city pupils. In country schools that I have happened to know, nervous children were the chief problem. Nervousness led in scholarship, in disorder, in absences, in truancy, and in backwardness. After reading MacDonald's *Annals of a Quiet Neighborhood*, I became interested in one or two particularly nervous children, just to see if I could overcome my strong dislike for them. To one boy I gave permission to leave the room or to go to the library whenever he began to lose his self-control. My predecessors had not been able to control him by the rod. A few weeks after Willie's emancipation from rules, the county superintendent was astonished to see that the county terror led my school in history, reading, and geography.

Had I known what every teacher should be taught in preparation,—the relation of eye strain, bad teeth, adenoids, "overattention," and malnutrition to nervousness and bad behavior,—I could have restored many "incorrigibles" to nerve control. Had I been led at college to study child psychology and child physiology, I should not have expected a control that was possible only in a normal adult.[6] In its primary aspect the question of nervousness in the schoolroom is purely physiological, and the majority of principals and teachers are not trained by professional schools how to deal with it. Normal schools should teach the physical laws which govern the child's development; should show that the pupil's mental, moral, and physical nature are one and inseparable; that children cannot at one time be docile, sickly, and intelligent,—perfect mentally and imperfect physically. Until teachers are so taught, the condition cannot be changed that makes of our schools manufactories of nervous teachers and pupils.

[111]Country nervousness, like city nervousness, is of three kinds: (1) that caused by defective nervous systems; (2) that resulting from physical defects other than defects of the nervous system, but reacting upon it; (3) that due to habit or to lack of self-control. Children who suffer from a defective nervous system should, in city schools, be segregated where they can have special care under constant medical supervision. Such children in schools too small for special classes should be given special treatment. Their parents should know that they have chorea, which is the same trouble as St. Vitus's Dance, although often existing in a degree too mild to attract attention. Special treatment does not mean that such children should be permitted to interfere with the school progress of other children. In many rural schools, where special privileges cannot be given children suffering with chorea without injury to other children, it would be a kindness to the unfortunates, to their parents, and to all other children, were the parents requested to keep such children at home.

Nervousness that results from removable physical defects—eye strain, adenoids, indigestion, earache—will be easily detected by physical examination, and easily corrected by removing the physical defect.

Preventable nervousness due to "habit" can be quite as serious in its effects upon the mind and health as the other two forms of nervousness. Twitching the face, biting the nails, wetting the lips, blinking the eyelids, continually toying with something, being in perpetual motion and never relaxing, always changing from one thing to the next, being forever on the rush, never accomplishing anything, are common faults of both teacher and pupil. We call them mannerisms or tricks of personality. They are readily imitated by children. I once knew a young lawyer who had started life as an oyster dealer, whose power of imitation helped to make him responsive to both helpful and harmful influences. After [112]being at the same table for two weeks with a talented man whom he admired, he acquired the latter's habit of constantly twitching his shoulder and making certain gestures. These habits in turn quickly produced a nervousness that interfered with his power to reason straight.

Nervousness is often confused with aggressiveness, initiative, confidence. "Think twice before you jump, and perhaps you won't want to jump" is a very difficult rule to follow for any one whose bodily movements are not under perfect control.

It is said that the confusion of city life causes habits of nervousness. Unfortunately no one knows whether the city children or the country children have the highest percentage of nervousness. There is a general feeling that city life causes an unwholesome degree of activity, yet one finds that those people in the city who least notice the elevated railway are those whose windows it passes. City noises irritate those who come from the country, or the city man on returning to the city from the country, but a similar irritation is felt by the city-bred man on coming to the country. Mr. Dooley's description of a night in the country with the crickets and the mosquitoes and the early birds shows that it is the unusual noise rather than the volume or variety of noises that wreck nerves. At the time of the opening of the New York schools in 1907 a newspaper published an editorial on "Where can the city child study?" showing that in New York the curriculum, the schoolhouse, and the tenements are so crowded and so noisy that study is practically impossible. Lack of sleep, lack of a quiet place in which to study at school and at home, are causes for nervousness, whether these conditions are in the city or in the country. What evidence is there that the country curriculum is less crowded or country work better adjusted to the psychological and physiological age of the country pupil? The index is there; it should be read.

[113]In breaking habits of nervousness the first step is to explain how easily habits are formed, why their effects may be serious, and how a little attention will correct them. When a habit loses its mystery it becomes unattractive. Children will take an interest in coöperating with each other and with the teacher in curing habits acquired either at home or at school. My pupils greatly enjoyed overcoming the habit of jumping or screaming after some sudden noise. I told them how, when a boy, my imagination had been very much impressed by one of Thackeray's characters, the last remnant of aristocratic traditions, almost a pauper, but possessing one attribute of nobility,—absolute self-control. When his house burned he stood with his ankles crossed, leaning on his cane, the only onlooker who was not excited. For months I imitated that pose, using sticks and rakes and fork handles. The result was that when I taught school, a scream, a broken desk, or unusual noise outside reminded me of my old aristocrat in time to prevent my muscles from jumping. In a very short time several fidgety and nervous girls and boys had learned to think twice and to relax before jumping.

One test of thorough relaxation in a dentist's chair proves the folly of tightening one's muscles. When in school or out the remedy for nervousness is relaxation. The discipline that prohibits a pupil from stretching or changing his posture or seat is as much to be condemned as that which flourishes the rod. It has been said of our schools that children are not worked to death but bored to death. Wherever a room must be stripped of all beauty and interest to induce concentration, wherever the greater part of the teacher's time must be spent in keeping order, there is confession either of inappropriateness of the present curriculum or of the failure of teacher and text-book to present subjects attractive to the pupils. Nervous habits will be inevitable until the pupil's attention is obtained through interest. [114]Sustained interest will be impossible until teacher and pupil alike practice relaxation, not once a morning or twice a day, not during recess or lunch hour, but whenever relaxation is needed.

In overcoming nervousness of teacher and pupil, both must be interested in home causes as well as school causes of that nervousness. Time must be found to ask questions about those causes and to discuss means for removing them. Naturally it will be embarrassing for a very nervous teacher to discuss nervousness with children, — until after she has overcome her own lack of nerve stability. To help her or to compel her to learn the art of relaxation of bodily and of mental control is the duty and the privilege of the school physician, of her doctor, and of superintendent and trustees. The outside point of view is necessary, because of the peculiar fact that almost every nervous person believes that he has unusually good control over his nerves, just as a man in the midst of his anger will declare that he is cool and self-controlled. Had Robert Burns been thinking of the habit of nervousness he could not have thought of a better cure than when he wrote:

> Oh wad some power the giftie gie us
> To see oursel's as ithers see us;
> It wad frae mony a blunder free us,
> And foolish notion.

FOOTNOTES:

[6]*The Unconscious Mind* by Schofield, *The Study of Children and their School Training* by Dr. Frances Warner, and *The Development of the Child* by Nathan Oppenheimer show clearly the physical and mental limitations and possibilities of children.

[115]

HEALTH VALUE OF "UNBOSSED" PLAY AND PHYSICAL TRAINING

A boy without play means a father without a job. A boy without physical training means a father who drinks. When people have wholesome, well-disciplined bodies there will be less demand for narcotics as well as for medicines. On these three propositions enthusiasm has built arguments for city parks and playgrounds, for school gymnastics, and for temperance instruction. We have tried the remedies and now realize that too much was expected of them. Neither movement appreciated the mental and physical education of spontaneous games and play.

Like hygiene instruction, physical training was made compulsory by law in many states, and, like hygiene instruction, physical training had to yield to the pressure of subjects in which children are examined. At the outset both were based upon distorted psychology and physiology. Of late physical training has been revived "to correct defects of the school desk and to relieve the strain of too prolonged study periods." In New York grammar schools ten minutes a day for the lower grades, and thirty minutes a week for the higher grades, are set aside for physical training. With the exception of eighteen schools where apparatus is used, the exercise has been in the class rooms. It consists of what are known as "setting-up exercises," — deep breathing and arm movements for two minutes between each study period, often forgotten until it is time to go home, when the children are tired and need it least. Many teachers so conduct these exercises that children keenly enjoy them.

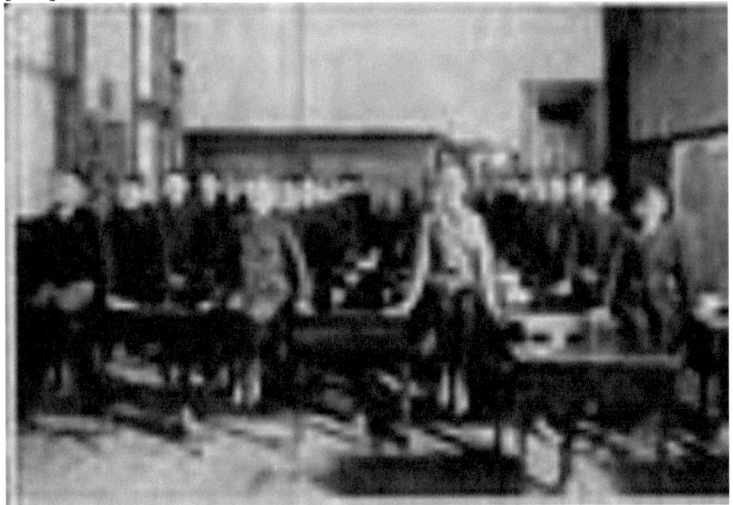

SERVICEABLE RELIEF FROM SCHOOL STRAIN, BUT A POOR SUBSTITUTE FOR OUTDOOR PLAY

Like hygiene instruction, physical training preceded physical examination. Generally speaking, it has not yet, either in schools or in colleges, been related to physical needs of the individual pupil. In fact, there is no guarantee that it is not in many schools working a positive injury on defective children or imposing a defective environment on healthy children. Formal exercises in cramped space, in ill-ventilated rooms, with tight belts and heavy shoes, are conceded to be pernicious. Formal exercises should never be given to any child without examination and prescription by a physician. Children with heart weakness, enlarged tonsils, adenoid growths, spinal curvature, uneven shoulders, are frequently seen doing exercises for which they are physically unfit, and which but serve to deplete further their already low vitality. Attention might be called to many a class engaged in breathing exercises when by actual count over half the boys were holding their mouths open. Special exercises are needed by children who show some marked [117]defect like flat foot, flat chest, weak abdominal muscles, habitual constipation, uneven shoulders, spinal trouble, etc.

That no physical training should be provided for normal children is the belief of many leading trainers. This special training is useful to develop athletes or to correct defects. Like massage, osteopathy, or medicine, it should follow careful diagnosis. The time is coming when formal indoor gymnasium exercises for normal pupils or normal students will be considered an anomaly. There is all the difference in the world between physical development and what is called physical training. The test of physical development is not the hours spent upon a prescribed course of training, but the physical condition determined by examination. To be refused permission to substitute an hour's walk for an hour's indoor apparatus work is often an outrage upon health laws. Given a normal healthy body, plenty of space, and plenty of playtime, the spontaneous exercise which a child naturally chooses is what is really health sustaining and health giving.

Mere muscular development artificially obtained through the devices of a gymnasium is inferior to the mental and moral development produced by games and play in the open air. Eustace Miles, M.D., amateur tennis player of England, says:

I do not consider a mere athlete to be a really healthy man. He has no more right to be called a really healthy man than the foundations or scaffolding of a house have a right to be called a house. They become a good house, and, indeed, they are indispensable to a good house, but at present the good house exists only in potentiality.

The "healthy-mindedness" and "physical morality" which play and games foster rarely result from physical training as a business, at stated times, indoors, under class direction. It is too much like taking medicine. A certain breakfast food is said to have lost much of its [118]popularity since advertised as a health food. When the National Playground Association was organized President Roosevelt cautioned its officers against too frequent use of the word "supervision" on the ground that supervision and direction were apt to defeat the very purpose of games and to stultify the play spirit. Is the little girl on the street who springs into a hornpipe or a jig to the tune of a hurdy-gurdy, or even the boy who runs before automobiles or trolley cars or under horses' noses, getting less physical education than those who play a round game in silence under the supervision of a teacher in the school basement, or who stretch their arms up and down to the tune of one, two, three, four, five, six? Who can doubt that the much-pitied child of the tenement playing with the contents of the ash can in the clothes yard or with baby brother on the fire escape is developing more originality, more lung power, and better arteries than the child of fortune who is led by the hand of a governess up and down Fifth Avenue.

Children have not forgotten how to play, but adults have forgotten to leave space in cities, and time out of school, home work, and factory work in which children may play. Again, the child — whether a city child or a country child — rarely needs to be taught how to play. Teaching him games will not produce vitality. Games are the spontaneous product of a healthy body, active mind, and a joy in living. Give the children parks and piers, roof gardens and playgrounds in which they may play, and leave the rest to them. Give them time away from school and housework, and leave the rest to them. Instead of lamenting the necessity for playing in the streets, let us reserve more streets for children's play. There are too many students of child welfare whose reasoning about play and games is like that of a lady of Cincinnati, who, upon reading the notice of a child-labor meeting, said: "Well, I am glad to see there is going to be a meeting here for child labor. It is high time [119]some measure was taken to keep the children off the streets." Physical examinations would prove that streets are safer and better than indoor gymnasiums for growing children. Intelligent physical training will train children to go out of doors during recess; will train pupils and teachers not to use recess for study, discipline, or eating lunch.

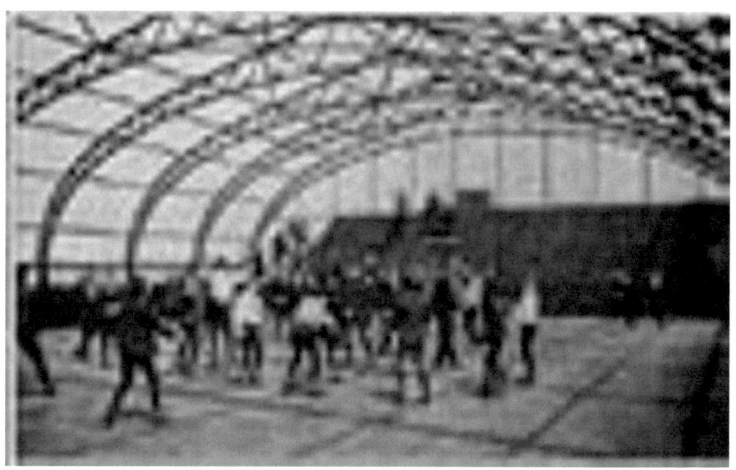

SPONTANEOUS PLAY ON ONE OF NEW YORK CITY'S SCHOOL ROOF PLAYGROUNDS

"After-school" conditions are quite as important as physical training and gymnastics at school. Not long ago a nurse was visiting a sick tenement mother with a young baby. She found a little girl of twelve standing on a stool over a washtub. This child did all the housework, took care of the mother and two younger children, got all the meals except supper, which her father got on his return from work. As the nurse removed the infant's clothes to give it a bath, the little girl seized them and dashed them into the tub. "Yes, I am pretty tired when night comes," she confessed. This child has prototypes in the country as well as the city, and she did not need physical training. She did not lack initiative or originality. She did need playmates, open air, a run in the park, and "fun."

[120]The educational value of games and outdoor play should be weighed against the advantages of lowering the compulsory school age, and of bridging over the period from four to seven with indoor kindergarten training. Neither physical training nor education is synonymous with confinement in school. The whole tendency of Nature's processes in children is nutritional; it is not until adolescence that she makes much effort to develop the brain. Overuse of the young mind results, therefore, in diverting natural energy from nutritive processes to hurried growth of the overstimulated brain.

The result is a type of child with a puny body and an excitable brain,—the neurotic. The young eye, for example, is too flat (hypermetropic)—made to focus only on objects at a distance. Close application to print, or even to weaving mats or folding bits of paper accurately, causes an overstrain on the eye, which not only results in the chronic condition known as myopia,—short-sightedness,—so common to school children, but which acts unfavorably on the constitution and on the whole development of the child. At the recent International Congress of School Hygiene in London, Dr. Arthur Newsholme, medical officer of health of Brighton, made a plea for the exclusion of children under five years of age from schools. "During the time the child is in the infant department it has chiefly to grow. Nutrition and sleep are its chief functions. Paints, pencils, paper, pins, and needles should not be handled in school by children below six." Luther Burbank, in an article on "The Training of the Human Plant," says:

The curse of modern child life in America is overeducation, overconfinement, overrestraint. The injury wrought to the race by keeping too young children in school is beyond the power of any one to estimate. The work of breaking down the nervous systems of the children of the United States is now well under way. Every child should have mud pies, grasshoppers, and tad-poles, wild strawberries, acorns, and pine cones, trees to climb [121]and brooks to wade in, sand, snakes, huckleberries, and hornets, and any child who has been deprived of these has been deprived of the best part of his education.

Not every child can have these blessings of the country, but every child can be protected from the stifling of the nature instinct of play by formal indoor "bossed" exercises, whether called games, physical training, gymnastics, or Delsarte.

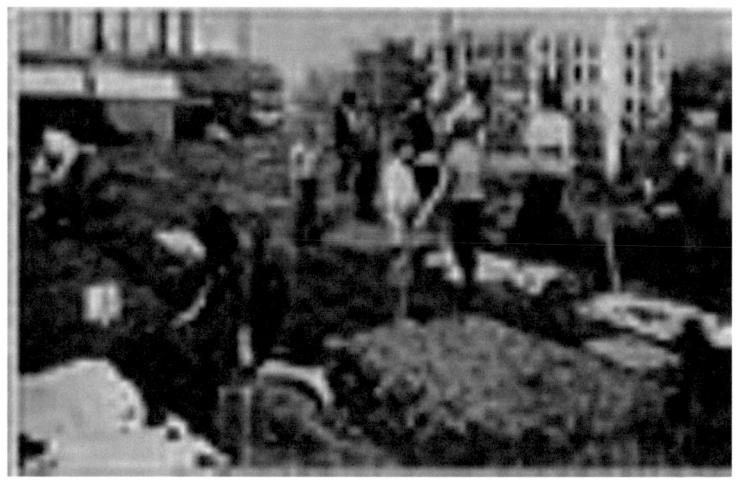

NEW YORK CITY'S SCHOOL FARM DOES NOT STIFLE NATURE INSTINCT

The answer to the protest against too early and too constant confinement in school has always been: "Where will the child be if out of school? Will its environment at home not work a worse injury to its health? Will not the street injure its morals?" Because we have not yet worked out a method of supervising the health of those children who are not in school, it does not follow that such supervision is impossible. Perhaps the time will come when there will be state supervision over the health of children from birth, parents being expected to present them once a year at school for examination by the school physician. In this way defects can be corrected and health measures [122]devised to build up a physique that should not break down under the strain of school life. For children whose mothers work during the day, and for those whose home environment is worse than school, it might be cheaper in the long run to assign teachers to protect them from injury while they play in a park, roof garden, or out-of-door gymnasium. If parks and playgrounds come too slowly, why not adopt the plan advocated by Alida S. Williams, a New York principal, of reserving certain streets for children between the hours of three and five, and of diverting traffic to other streets less suitable for children's play? So great is the value—mentally, morally, and physically—of out-of-door play that it has even been suggested that the substitution of such play for school for all children up to the age of ten would insure better minds and sounder physiques at fifteen. It is generally admitted that the child who enters school at eight rather than at six will be the gainer at twelve. What a travesty upon education to insist upon schooling for children because they are apt to be run over on the street, or to be neglected at home, to shoot craps, or belong to a gang and develop bad morals.

Educators will some day be ashamed to have made the schools the catch-all or the court-plaster for the evils of modern industry. Instead of pupils and mothers going to the school, enough hygiene teachers, and play teachers, and district physicians could be employed with the money now spent on indoor instruction to do the house-to-house visiting urged in many chapters of this book. Such a course of action would have an incalculable effect on the reduction of tuberculosis, not only in making healthier physiques but by inculcating habits of outdoor life and love of fresh air. The danger of those contagious diseases which ravish childhood would be greatly reduced. An ambition for physical integrity would make unnatural living unpopular. Competition in games with children *of the same [123]physical class* develops accuracy, concentration, dispatch, resourcefulness, as much as does instruction in arithmetic. Smoking can easily be discredited among boys trying to hit the bull's-eye. A boy would sooner give up a glass of beer than the championship in rifle shooting or a "home run."

The influence of the "spirit of the game" on practical life has been described thus by New York's director of physical training, Dr. Luther H. Gulick:

Play is the spontaneous enlistment of the entire personality in the pursuit of some coveted end. We do not have to pursue the goal; we wish to—it is our main desire. This is the way in which greatest discoveries, fortunes, and poems are made. It is the way in which we take the responsibilities and problems of life that makes it either a deadly bore—a mere dull round of routine and drudgery—or the most interesting and absorbing game, capable of enlisting all the energy and enthusiasm we have to put into it. The people who accomplish things are the people who play the game. They let themselves go; they are not afraid. Under the stimulus and enthusiasm of play muscles contract more powerfully and longer than under other conditions. Blood pressure is higher in play. It is far more interesting to play the game than to work at it. When you work you are being driven, when you play you are doing the driving yourself. We play not by jumping the traces of life's responsibilities, but by going so far beyond life's compulsions as to lose sight of the compulsion element. Play up, play up, and play the game.

[124]

VITALITY TESTS AND VITAL STATISTICS

Two things will disclose the strength or weakness of a bank and the soundness or unsoundness of a nation's banking policy, namely, a financial crisis or an expert audit. A searching audit that analyzes each debit and each credit frequently shows that a bank is solvent only because it is not asked to pay its debts. It continues to do business so long as no obvious weaknesses appear, analogous to measles, adenoids, or paralysis. A frequent disorder of banking results from doing too big a business on too little capital, in making too many loans for the amount of cash held ready to pay depositors upon demand. This disorder always comes to light in a crisis—too late. It can be discovered if looked for in advance of a crisis. Many individuals and communities are likewise physically solvent only because their physical resources are not put to the test. Weaknesses that lie near the surface can be discovered before a crisis by physical examination for individuals and sanitary supervision for communities. Whether individuals or communities are trying to do too much business for their health capital, whether the health reserves will pay debts that arise in a crisis, whether we are ill or well prepared to stand a run on our vitality, can be learned only by carefully analyzing our health reserves. Health debits are compared with health credits for individuals by vitality tests, for communities by vital statistics.

Of the many vitality tests none is practicable for use in the ordinary class room. Scientific training is just as necessary for such tests as for discovering the quality of [125]the blood, the presence or absence of tubercle bacilli in the sputum, diphtheria germs in throat mucus, or typhoid germs in milk. But scientific truth, the results of scientific tests, can be made of everyday use in all class rooms. State and national headquarters for educators, and all large cities, can afford to engage scientists to apply vitality tests to school children for the sake of discovering, in advance of physical breakdown and before outward symptoms are obvious, what curriculum, what exercise, what study, recreation, and play periods are best suited to child development. It will cost infinitely less to proceed this way than to neglect children or to fit school methods to the loudest, most persistent theory.

The ergograph is an interesting strength tester. It takes a picture (1) of the energy exerted, and (2) of the regularity or fitfulness of the manner in which energy is exerted. Perhaps the time will come when science and commerce will supply every tintype photographer with an ergograph and the knowledge to use it. Then we shall hear at summer resorts and fairs, "Your ergograph on a postal card, three for a quarter." We can step inside, harness our middle finger to the ergograph, lift it up and down forty-five times in ninety seconds, and lo! a photograph of our vitality! If we have strong muscles or good control, the picture will be like this:

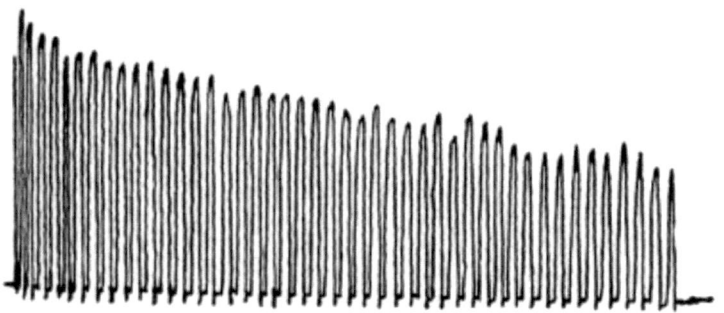

Fig. 1. Ergogram of T.R., a strong, healthy girl, before taking 40 minutes' work in the gymnasium. Weight used, 3.5 kg. Distance lifted, 151 cm. Work done, 528.5 kg.-cm.

[126]If weak and nervous, we shall look like this before taking exercise:

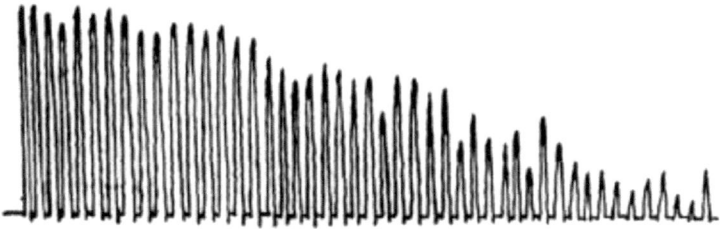

Fig. 2. Ergogram of C.E., a weak and somewhat nervous girl, before taking 40 minutes' work in the gymnasium. Weight used, 3.5 kg. Distance lifted, 89 cm. Work done, 311.5 kg.-cm.

And like this after gymnasium exercise:

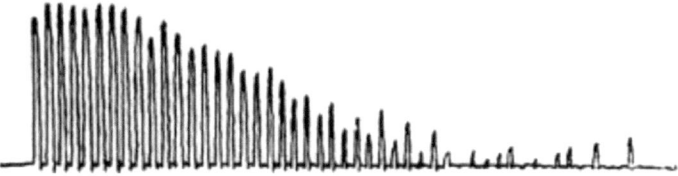

Fig. 3. Ergogram of C.E. after taking 40 minutes' work in the gymnasium, showing that the exercise proved very exhausting. Weight used, 3.5 kg. Distance lifted, 55 cm.

In Chicago, two of whose girls are above photographed, the physician was surprised to have four pupils show more strength late in the day than in the morning. "Upon investigation it was found that the teacher of the four pupils had been called from school, and that they had no regular work, but had been sent to another room and employed themselves, as they said, in having a good time." The chart on page 127 shows the effect of the noon recess and of the good time after three o'clock.

Chicago's child-study experts concluded after examining a large number of children:

1. In general there is a distinct relationship in children between physical condition and intellectual capacity, the latter varying directly as the former.

[127]2. The endurance (ergographic work) of boys is greater than that of girls at all ages, and the difference seems to increase after the age of nine.

3. There are certain anthropometric (body measurements) indications which warrant a careful and thorough investigation into the subject of coeducation in the upper grammar grades.

4. Physical condition should be made a factor in the grading of children for school work, and especially for entrance into the first grade.

5. The great extremes in the physical condition of pupils in the upper grammar grades make it desirable to introduce great elasticity into the work of these grades.

6. The classes in physical culture should be graded on a physical instead of an intellectual basis.

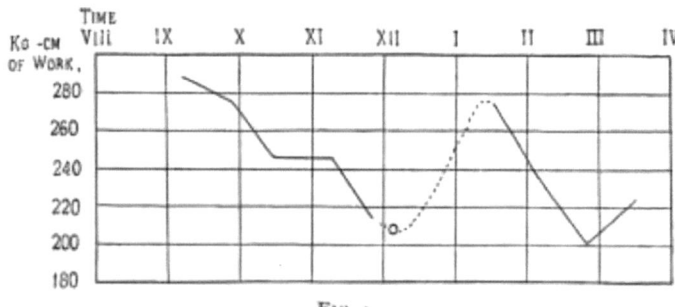

Fig. 4

| Average time of test | | 9:15 | 9:55 | 10:32 | 11:15 | 11:51 | 1:30 | 2:11 | 2:49 | 3:30 |
| Average work done (kilograms) | | 289 | 275 | 248 | 245 | 215 | 275 | 237 | 201 | 224 |

Fig. 4.

To these conclusions certain others should be added, not as settled beyond any possibility of modification, but as being fairly indicated by these tests.

1. The pubescent period is characterized by great and rapid changes in height, weight, strength of grip, vital capacity, and endurance. There seems to accompany this physical activity a corresponding intellectual and emotional activity. It therefore is a period when broad educational influences are most needed. From the pedagogic standpoint it is preëminently a time for character building.

[128]2. The pubescent period is characterized by extensive range of all physical features of the individuals in it. Hence, although a period fit for great activity of the mass of children, it is also one of numerous individual exceptions to this general law. During this period a greater per cent of individuals than usual pass beyond the range of normal limits set by the mass. It is a time, therefore, when the weak fail and the able forge to the front, and hence calls for a higher degree than usual of individualization of educational work and influence.

3. Unidexterity is a normal condition. Rapid and marked accentuation of unidexterity is a pubescent change. On the whole, there is a direct relationship between the degree of unidexterity and the intellectual progress of the pupil. At any given age of school life bright or advanced pupils tend toward accentuated unidexterity, and dull or backward pupils tend toward ambidexterity.... Training in ambidexterity is training contrary to a law of child life.

4. Boys of school age at the Bridewell (reform school) are inferior in all physical measurements to boys in the ordinary schools, and this inferiority seems to increase with age.

5. Defects of sight and hearing are more numerous among the dull and backward pupils. These defects should be taken into consideration in the seating of pupils. Only by removing the defects can the best advancement be secured.

6. The number of eye and ear defects increases during the first years of school life. The causes of this increase should be investigated, and, as far as possible, removed.

7. There are certain parts of the school day when pupils, on the average, have a higher storage of energy than at other periods. These periods should be utilized for the highest forms of educational work.

8. The stature of boys is greater than that of girls up to the age of eleven, when the girls surpass the boys and remain greater in stature up to the age of fourteen. After fourteen, girls increase in stature very slowly and very slightly, while boys continue to increase rapidly until eighteen.

9. The weight of the girl surpasses that of the boy about a year later than her stature surpasses his, and she maintains her [129]superiority in weight to a later period of time than she maintains her superiority in height.

10. In height, sitting, girls surpass boys at the same age as in stature, namely, eleven years, but they maintain their superiority in this measurement for one year longer than they do in stature, which indicates that the more rapid growth of the boy at this age is in the lower extremities rather than in the trunk.

11. Commencing at the age of thirteen, strength of grip in boys shows a marked accentuation in its rate of increase, and this increase continues as far as our observations extend, namely, to the age of twenty. In girls no such great acceleration in muscular strength at puberty occurs, and after sixteen there is little increase in strength of grip. The well-known muscular differentiation of the sexes practically begins at thirteen.

12. As with strength of grip, so with endurance as measured by the ergograph; boys surpass girls at all ages, and this differentiation becomes very marked after the age of fourteen, after which age girls increase in strength and endurance but very slightly, while after fourteen boys acquire almost exactly half of the total power in these two features which they acquire in the first twenty years of life.

13. The development of vital capacity bears a striking resemblance to that of endurance, the curves representing the two being almost identical.

Physiological age, according to studies made in New York City, should be considered in grading, not only for physical culture classes but for all high school or continuation classes. Dr. C. Ward Crampton, assistant physical director, while examining boys in the first grade of the High School of Commerce, noticed a greater variation in physical advancement than in years. He kept careful watch of the educational progress and discovered three clear divisions: (1) boys arrived at puberty,—postpubescent; (2) boys approaching maturity,—pubescent; (3) boys not yet approaching maturity,—prepubescent.

The work in lower grades they had all passed satisfactorily, but in high school only the most advanced class [130]did well. Practically none of the not-yet-maturing boys survived and few of the almost mature. In other words, the high school course was fitted to only one of the three classes of boys turned out of the grammar schools. The others succumbed like hothouse azaleas at Christmas time, forced beyond their season. Physiological age, not calendar years or grammar school months, should determine the studies and the companions of children after the tenth year. Physiological strength and vitality, not ability to spell or to remember dates, should be the basis of grading for play and study and companionship among younger children. Vitality, power to endure physically, should be the test of work and recreation for adults. Physicians may be so trained to follow directions issued by experts that physical examinations will disclose the chief enemies of vitality and the approximate limits of endurance.

Teachers may train themselves to recognize signs of fatigue in school children and to adapt each day's, each hour's work to the endurance of each pupil. One woman principal has written:

School programmes, after they have been based upon the laws of a child's development, should provide for frequent change of subject, alternating studies requiring mental concentration with studies permitting motor activity, and arranging for very short periods of the former. Anæmic children should be relieved of all anxiety as to the results of their efforts, and only short hours of daylight work required of them. The disastrous consequences of eye strain should be understood by all in charge of children who are naturally hypermetropic. The ventilation of a class room is far more important than its decoration or even than a high average percentage in mathematics, and the lack of pure air is one of the auxiliary causes of nervous exhaustion in both pupils and teachers. Deficient motor control is a most trustworthy indication of fatigue in children, and teachers may safely use it as a rough index of the amount of effort to be reasonably expected of their pupils. Facial pallor or feverish flushes are [131]both evidences of overtasking, and either hints that fatigue has already begun. As to unfavorable atmospheric conditions, the teacher herself will undoubtedly realize them as soon as the children, but she should remember that effort carried to the point of exhaustion, injurious as it is in an adult, is yet less harmful than it is to the developing nerve centers of the child.

Because adults at work and at play reluctantly submit themselves to vitality tests, because few scientists are beseeching individuals to be tested, because almost no one yearns to be tested, the promotion of adult vitality and of community vitality can best be hastened by demanding complete vital statistics. Industrial insurance companies and mutual benefit societies are doing much to educate laborers regarding the effect upon vitality of certain dangerous and unsanitary trades, and of certain unhygienic habits, such as alcoholism and nicotinism. Progress is slower than it need be because state boards of health are not gathering sufficiently complete information about causes of sickness and death. American health and factory inspection is not even profiting, as it should, from British, German, and French statistics. Statistics are in ill repute because the truth is not generally known that our boasted sanitary improvements are due chiefly to the efficient use of vital statistics by statesmen sanitarians.[7]

The vital statistics of greatest consequence are not the number of deaths or the number of births, not even the number of deaths from preventable diseases, but rather the number of cases of sickness from transmissible diseases. The cost and danger to society from preventable diseases, such as typhoid, diphtheria, scarlet fever, measles, are imperfectly represented by the number of deaths. Medical skill could gradually reduce death rates in the face of [132]increasing prevalence of infectious disease. With few exceptions, only those patients who refuse to follow instructions will die of measles, diphtheria, or smallpox. The scarlet-fever patient who recovers and goes to church or school while "peeling" can cause vastly more sickness from scarlet fever than a patient who dies. Dr. W. Leslie Mackenzie, who has recently written *The Health of the School Child*, said ten years ago, while health officer of Leith:

Death is the ultimate and most severe injury that any disease can inflict, but short of death there may be disablement, permanent or temporary, loss of wages, loss of employment, loss of education, increase of home labor, increase of sickness outlays, increase of worry, anxiety and annoyance, disorganization of the household, general impairment of social efficiency.

The best guarantee against such loss, the best protection of health, and the most essential element of vital statistics is prompt, complete record of cases of sickness. Statistics of sickness are confined to sickness from transmissible diseases, because we have not yet arrived at the point where we recognize the state's right to require information, except when the sick person is a menace to the health of other persons.

The annual report of a board of health should give as clear a picture of a community's health during the past week or past quarter as the ergograph gives of the pupils mentioned on page 126. As ragged, rapidly shortening lines show nervousness and depleted vitality, so charts and diagrams can be made to show the needless waste of infant life during the summer months, the price paid for bad ventilation in winter time, when closed windows cause the sickness-and-death line from diphtheria and scarlet fever to shoot up from the summer level. In cities it is now customary for health boards to report weekly the number of deaths from transmissible diseases. Health officers will [133]gladly furnish facts as to cases of sickness, if citizens request them. Newspapers will gladly publish such information if any one will take the pains to supply it. Wherever newspapers have published this information, it quickly takes its place with the weather reports among the news necessities. Marked changes are commented on editorially. Children can easily be interested, as can adults, in filling out week by week a table that will show increases and decreases in preventable sickness due to transmissible diseases.

Table X

Cases of Infectious and Contagious Diseases Reported

	WEEK ENDING												
	Oct. 26	Nov. 2	Nov. 9	Nov. 16	Nov. 23	Nov. 30	Dec. 7	Dec. 14	Dec. 21	Dec. 28	Jan. 4	Jan. 11	Jan. 18
Tuberculosis pulmonalis	350	350	317	364	345	337	422	360	354	308	344	432	402
Diphtheria and croup	313	264	283	331	282	343	326	369	338	347	308	370	406
Measles	142	212	203	261	293	323	472	471	517	346	581	691	803
Scarlet fever	208	228	231	252	278	323	372	397	417	426	478	562	585
Smallpox	–	1	–	1	–	–	2	4	3	2	–	2	–
Varicella	40	83	91	162	136	115	167	160	198	123	98	199	169
Typhoid fever	106	105	107	123	86	77	71	62	35	42	37	55	36
Whooping cough	6	13	15	14	27	9	8	12	19	3	25	24	14
Cerebro-spinal meningitis	6	11	3	4	4	8	15	13	7	6	11	16	13
Total	1171	1267	1250	1512	1451	1535	1855	1844	1888	1603	1882	2351	242

In cities where physicians are not compelled to notify the health board of danger centers,—that is, of patients sick from measles, smallpox, or diphtheria,—and in smaller communities where notices are sent only to state boards of health, parents will find it difficult to take a keen interest in vital statistics. But if teachers would start at the beginning of the year to record in such a table the days of absence from school because of transmissible disease, both they and their pupils would discover a new interest in efficient health administration. After a national board of [134]health is organized we may reasonably expect that either state boards of education or state boards of health will regularly supply teachers with reports that will lead them to compare the vitality photographs of their own schools and communities with the vitality photographs of other schools and other communities working under similar conditions. Then children old enough to study physiology and hygiene will be made to see the happiness-giving possibilities of vitality tests and vital statistics.

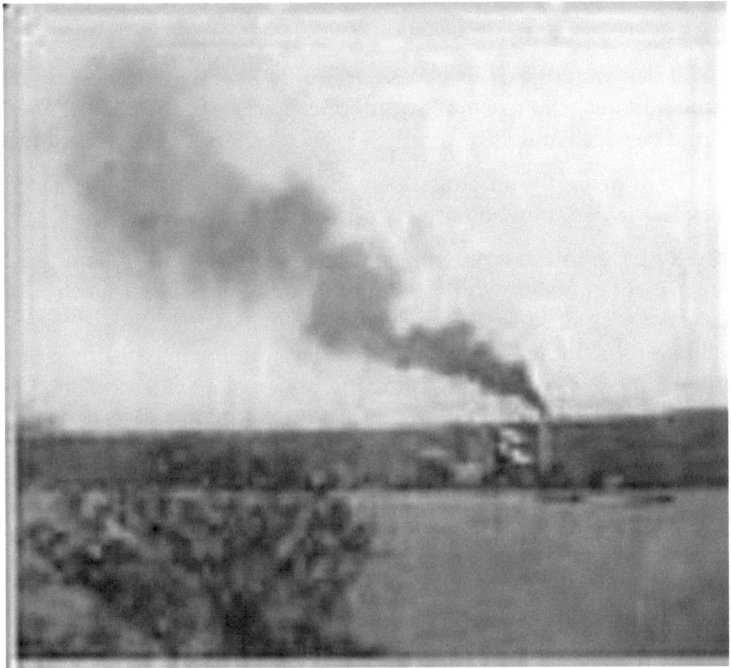

VITAL STATISTICS CAN MAKE DISEASE CENTERS AS OBVIOUS AND AS OFFENSIVE AS THE SMOKE NUISANCE

Instead of discussing the theory of vital statistics, or the extent to which statistics are now satisfactory, it would be better for us at this point to make clear the significance of the movement for a national fact center for matters pertaining to personal, industrial, and community vitality. [135]Five economic reasons are assigned for establishing a national department of health:

1. To enable society to increase the percentage of exceptional men of each degree, many of whom are now lost through preventable accidents, and also to increase the total population.

2. To lessen the burden of unproductive years by increasing the average age at death.

3. To decrease the burden of death on the productive years by increasing the age at death.

4. To lessen the cost of sickness. It is estimated that if illness in the United States could be reduced one third, nearly $500,000,000 would be saved annually.

5. To decrease the amounts spent on criminality that can be traced to overcrowded, unwholesome, and unhygienic environment.

In addition to the economic gain, the establishment of a national department of health would gradually but surely diminish much of the misery and suffering that cannot be measured by statistics. Sickness is a radiating center of anxiety; and often death in the prime of life closes the gates of happiness on more than one life. Let us not forget that the "bitter cry of the children" still goes up to heaven, and that civilization must hear, until at last it heeds, the imprecations of forever wasted years of millions of lives.

If progress is to be real and lasting, it must provide whatever bulwarks it can against death, sickness, misery, and ignorance; and in an organization such as a national department of health, adequately equipped,—a vast preventive machine working ceaselessly,—an attempt at least would be made to stanch those prodigal wastes of an old yet wastrel world.

Among the branches of the work proposed for the national bureau are the following: infant hygiene; health education in schools; sanitation; pure food; registration of physicians and surgeons; registration of drugs, druggists, and drug manufacturers; registration of institutions of public and private relief, correction, detention and residence; organic diseases; quarantine; immigration; labor conditions; [136]disseminating health information; research libraries and equipment; statistical clearing house for information.

Given such a national center for health facts or vital statistics, there will be a continuing pressure upon state, county, and city health officers, upon physicians, hospitals, schools, and industries to report promptly facts of birth, sickness, and death to national and state centers able and eager to interpret the meaning of these facts in such simple language, and with such convincing illustrations, that the reading public will demand the prompt correction of preventable evils.

Our tardiness in establishing a national board of health that shall do this great educational work is due in part to the fact that American sanitarians have frequently chosen to *do things* when they should have chosen to *get things done*. Almost every state has its board of health, with authority to require registration of births, deaths, and sickness due to transmissible disease; with few exceptions the heads of these state boards have spent their energies in abating nuisances. In a short time they have degenerated into local scavengers, because they have shown the public neither the meaning of the vital statistics gathered nor its duty to support efficient health administration.

The state reports of vital statistics have not been accurate; therefore in many states we have the anomalous situation of an aggressive veterinary board arousing the farmer and the consumer of milk to the necessity of protecting the health of cattle, and an inactive, uninformed state board of health failing to protect the health of the farmer and the consumer.

Vital statistics presume efficient health administration. An inefficient health officer will not take the initiative in gathering health statistics. If some one else compels him to collect vital statistics, or furnishes him with statistics, they are as a lantern to a blind man. Unless some one [137]also compels him to make use of them, unless we remove the causes of transmissible or infectious diseases and check an epidemic when we first hear of it, the collection of information is of little social value. "Statistics" is of the same derivation as "states" and "statesmen." Statistics have always been distinguished from mere facts, in that statistics are instruments in the hands of the statesman. Wherever the term "statistics" is applied to social facts it suggests action, social control of future contingencies, mastery of the facts whose action they chronicle. The object of gathering social facts for analysis is not to furnish material for future historians. They are to be used in shaping future history. They are facts collected with a view to improving social vitality, to raising the standard of life, and to eliminating permanently those forces known to be destructive to health. Unless they are to be used this way, they are of interest only to the historical grub. No city or state can afford to erect a statistical office to serve as a curiosity shop. Unless something is to be done to prevent the recurrence of preventable diseases annually experienced by your community or your school, it is not reasonable to ask the public printer to make tables which indicate the great cost of this preventable sickness. A tax collector cannot discharge his duties unless he knows the address of every debtor. The police bureau cannot protect society unless it knows the character and haunts of offenders. A health officer cannot execute the law for the protection of society's health unless he knows the haunts and habits of diseases. For this he must look to vital statistics.

But the greatest service of vital statistics is the educational influence. Health administration cannot rise far above the hygienic standards of those who provide the means for administering sanitary law. The taxpaying public must believe in the economy, utility, and necessity of efficient health administration. Power and funds come [138]from town councils and state legislatures. To convince and move these keepers of the purse, trustworthy vital statistics are indispensable. Information will be used for the benefit of all as soon as it is possessed by all.

Fortunately the gathering of vital statistics is not beyond the power of the kind of health officer that is found in small cities and in rural communities. If years of study of mathematics and of the statistical method were required, we should despair of obtaining light within a century. But the facts we want are, for the most part, common, everyday facts, easily recognizable even by laymen; for example, births, deaths, age at death, causes of death, cases of transmissible diseases, conditions found upon examination of children applying for work certificates, etc. Where expert skill is required, as at state and national headquarters, it can be found. Every layman can train himself to use skillfully the seven ingredients of the statistical method which it is his duty to employ, and to know when to pay for expert analysis and advice. We can all learn to base judgment of health needs upon the seven pillars,—desire to know, unit of inquiry, count, comparison, percentages, classification, and summary.

FOOTNOTES:

[7] Dr. Arthur Newsholme's *Vital Statistics* should be in public libraries and on the shelves of health officers, public-spirited physicians, and school superintendents.

[139]

IS YOUR SCHOOL MANUFACTURING PHYSICAL DEFECTS?

Last year a conference on the physical welfare of school children was told by a woman principal: "Of course we need physicians to examine our children and to teach the parents, but many of us principals believe that our school curriculum and our school environment manufacture more physical defects in a month than all your physicians and nurses will correct in a year." At the same meeting the physical director of schools of New York City appealed eloquently for "biological engineers" at school, who would test the child's strength as building engineers are employed to test the strength of beams and foundations.[8] As explanation for the need of the then recently organized National School Hygiene Association, he elaborated the proposition that school requirements and school environment damage child health. "Ocular defects are in direct ratio to the length of time the pupil has attended school.... A desk that is too high may easily be the indirect agent for causing scoliosis, producing myopia or astigmatism.... Physically examine school children by all means, but do not fail to examine school desks."

Fifty schools in different parts of New York City were examined last year with especial reference to the factors likely to cause or to aggravate physical defects.[9] The results, [140]tabulated and analyzed, prove that the woman principal was right; many schools are so built or so conducted, many school courses are so devised or so executed, that children are inevitably injured by the environment in which the compulsory education law forces them to spend their formative years.

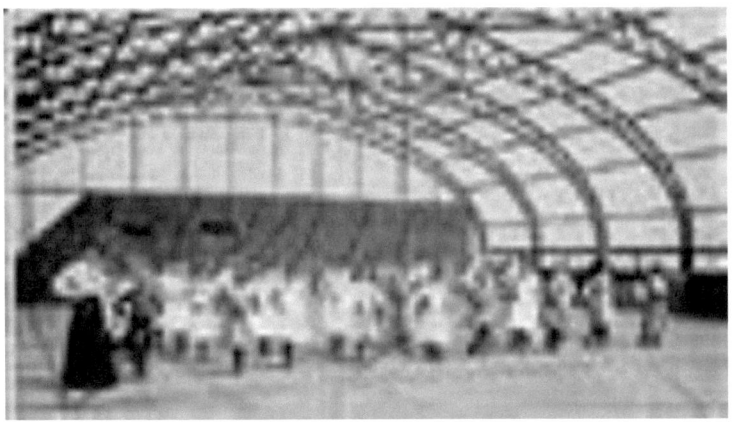

ONE OF NEW YORK CITY'S ROOF PLAYGROUNDS

Recently I noticed that our little office girl, so anæmic and nervous when she left school that we hesitated to employ her, was becoming rosy and spirited. The child herself explained the change: "I like it better. I have more money to spend. I get more outdoor exercise, and then, oh, the room is so much sunnier and there is more air and the people are all so nice!" And these were just the necessities which were lacking in the school from which she came. Moreover, it is a fair commentary on the school work and the school hygiene in too many of our towns and cities to-day. "I like it better" means that school work is not adapted to the dominant interests of the child, that the curriculum includes subjects remote from the needs and ambitions of the modern school child, and fails to include certain other subjects which it recognizes as useful and necessary, and [141]therefore finds interesting. "I have more money to spend" means that this little girl was able to have certain things, like a warm, pretty dress, rubbers, or an occasional trolley ride, which she longed for and needed. "I get more outdoor exercise" means that there was no open-air playground for her school, that "setting up" exercises were forgotten, that recess was taken up in rushing home, eating lunch, and rushing back again, and that "after school" was filled up with "helping mother with the housework." "The office is so much sunnier and I get more air" accounts for the increase in vitality; and "the people are all so nice," for the happy expression and initiative which the undiscriminating discipline at school had crushed out.

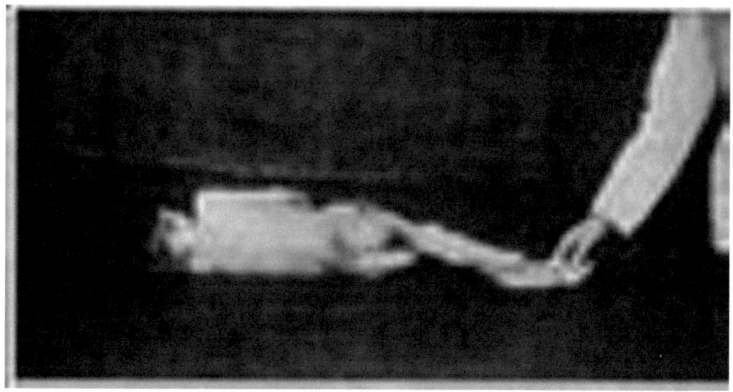

BONE TUBERCULOSIS IS ONE OF THE PENALTIES FOR DRY SWEEPING AND FEATHER DUSTERS

For such unsanitary conditions crowded sections of great cities have no apologies to make to rural districts. A wealthy suburb recently learned that there was overcrowding in every class room, and that one school building was so unsanitary as to be a menace to the community. Unadjustable desks, dry sweeping, feather dusters, shiny blackboards, harassing discipline that wrecks nerves, excessive home study and subjects that bore, are not peculiar to great [142]cities. In a little western town a competition between two self-governing brigades for merit points was determined by the amount of home study; looking back fifteen years, I can see that I was encouraging anæmic and overambitious children to rob themselves of play, sleep, and vitality. Many a rural school violates with impunity more laws of health than city factories are now permitted to transgress.

After child labor is stopped, national and state child labor committees will learn that their real interest all the time has been child welfare, not child age, and will be able to use much of the old literature, simply substituting for "factory" the word "school" when condemning "hazardous occupations likely to sap [children's] nervous energy, stunt their physical growth, blight their minds, destroy their moral fiber, and fit them for the moral scrap heap."

Many of the evils of school environment the teacher can avert, others the school trustee should be expected to correct. So far as unsanitary conditions are permitted, the school accentuates home evils, whereas it should counteract them by instilling proper health habits that will be taken home and practiced. Questions such as were asked in Miss North's study will prove serviceable to any one desiring to know the probable effect of a particular school environment upon children subject to it. Especially should principals, superintendents, directors, and volunteer committeemen apply such tests to the public, parochial, or private school, orphanage or reformatory for which they may be responsible.

I. Neighborhood Health Resources

1. Is the district congested?

2. Is congestion growing?

3. How far away is the nearest public park?

a. Is it large enough?
b. Has it a playground or beauty spot?
c. Has it swings and games?
[143]*d.* Is play supervised?
e. Have children of different ages equal opportunities, or do the large children monopolize the ground?
f. Are children encouraged by teachers and parents to use this park?

4. Are the streets suitable for play?

a. Does the sun reach them?
b. Are they broad?
c. Are they crowded with traffic?

5. How far away is the nearest public bath?

a. Has it a swimming pool?
b. Has it showers?
c. Is it used as an annex to the school?

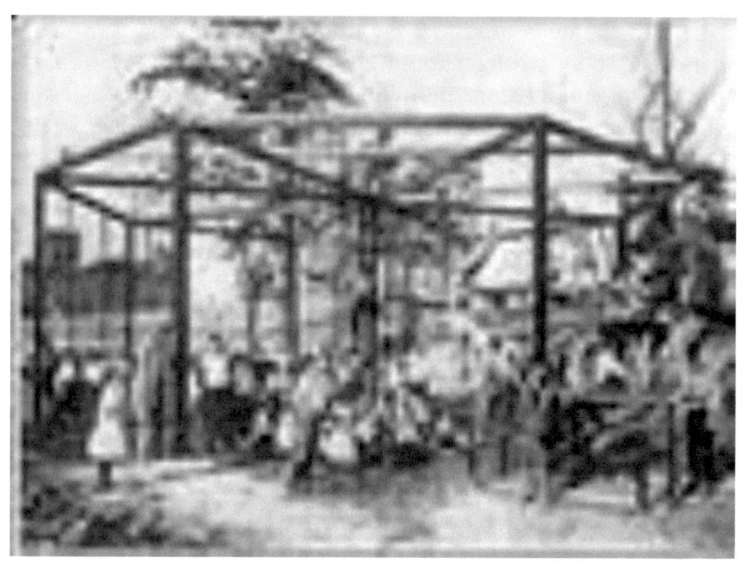

VACATION-SCHOOL PLAY CLINIC ON A "VACANT" CITY LOT OWNED BY THE ROCKEFELLER INSTITUTE FOR MEDICAL RESEARCH

II. Effect of School Equipment upon Health

1. Is there an indoor yard?

a. Is the area adequate or inadequate?
b. Is the floor wood, cement, or dirt?
[144]*c.* Is the heat adequate or deficient?
d. Is the ventilation adequate or deficient?
e. Is the daylight adequate, deficient, or almost lacking?
f. Is there equipment for light gymnastics and games?
g. Is it used out of school hours; by special classes, athletic teams, etc., or by pupils generally?

2. Is there an outdoor yard?

a. Is the area ample or inadequate?
b. Is the area mainly occupied by toilets?
c. Is the daylight sufficient or deficient?
d. For how many hours does the sun reach it?
e. Is it equipped for games?

f. How much larger ought it to be?

g. Is it used out of school hours; by special classes, athletic teams, etc., or by pupils generally?

   3. Is there a gymnasium?

a. Is it large enough?

b. Is it used for a gymnasium?

c. Is it cut up into class rooms?

d. Is it used out of school hours; by special classes, athletic teams, etc., or by pupils generally?

   4. Is there a roof playground?

a. Is there open ventilation?

b. Is it used in the daytime?

c. Is it used at night?

d. Is it used during the summer?

e. Is it monopolized by the larger children?

f. Is it used out of school hours; by special classes, athletic teams, etc., or by pupils generally?

   5. Are washing facilities adequate?

a. How many pupils per washbasin?

b. Are there individual towels?

c. Have eye troubles been spread by roller towels?

d. Are only clean towels permitted?

e. Are there bathing facilities; are these adequate?

f. Are swimming pools used for games, contests, etc.?

[145]*g.* Are bathing facilities used out of school hours?

h. Who is responsible for cleanliness of towels, washbasins, and swimming pools?

i. How often is water changed in swimming pool, or is it constantly changing?

   6. Is adequate provision made for clean drinking water?

a. Are sanitary fountains used that prevent contamination of faucet or water?

b. How often are cups or faucets cleaned?

   7. Is provision made for airing outer clothing?

a. Are children permitted to pile their clothing in the class room?
b. Are there hooks for each child?
c. Are lockers provided with wire netting to permit ventilation?
d. Are lockers or hooks in the halls or in the basement?
e. Have you ever thought of the disciplinary and social value of cheap coat hangers to prevent wrinkling and tearing?

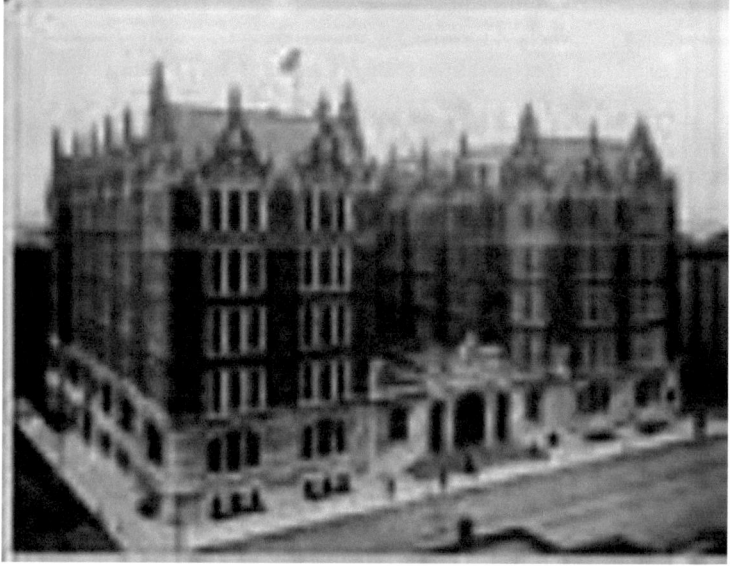

AN ATTEMPT TO OVERCOME THE DISADVANTAGES OF CONGESTION — A BOYS' HIGH SCHOOL, NEW YORK CITY

[146]III. The Class Room as a Place of Confinement

1. How many sittings are provided?

a. How many pupils are there?

2. What is the total floor area?

a. What proportion is not occupied by desks?

3. Are the seats adjustable?

a. Are the seats adjusted to pupils?
b. Where desks are adjustable, are short children seated in low desks, or are children seated according to class or according to dis-

cipline exigencies without regard to size of desk?

c. Are seats placed properly with reference to light?

4. Is the light ample and proper?

a. For how many hours must artificial light be used in the daytime?

b. Is artificial light adequate for night work?

c. Does the reflection of light from blackboard and walls injure the eye?

d. Are the blackboards black enough?

e. Are the walls too dark?

f. Is the woodwork too dark?

g. Are window panes kept clean?

5. Is the air always fresh?

a. Is ventilation by open windows?

b. Is ventilation artificial?

c. Does the ventilating apparatus work satisfactorily?

d. Are the windows thrown open during recess, and after and before school?

e. Do unclean clothes vitiate the atmosphere?

f. Do unclean persons vitiate the atmosphere?

g. Does bad breath vitiate the atmosphere?

h. Are pupils and parents taught that unclean clothes, unclean persons, and bad breath may decrease the benefits of otherwise adequate ventilation and seriously aggravate the evils of inadequate ventilation?

[147]6. Is the temperature properly regulated?

a. Has every class room a thermometer?

b. Are teachers required to record the thermometer's story three or more times daily?

c. Is excess or deficiency at once reported to the janitor?

7. Are the floors, walls, desks, and windows always clean?

a. How often are they washed?

b. Is twice a year often enough?

c. Do the floors and walls contain the dust of years?

d. Is dry sweeping prohibited?

e. Has wet sawdust or even wet sand been tried?

f. Has oil ever been used to keep down surface dust on floors?

g. Are feather dusters prohibited?

h. Are dust rags moist or dry?

i. Is an odorless disinfectant used?

8. Does overheating prevail?

a. Do you know teachers and principals who protest against insufficient ventilation, particularly against mechanical ventilation, while they themselves are "in heavy winter clothing in a small room closely sealed, the thermometer at 80 degrees"?

IV. Exercise and Recreation

1. How much time and at what periods is exercise provided for in the school schedule?

a. Indoors?

b. Outdoors?

2. How much exercise indoors and outdoors is actually given?

3. Are the windows open during exercise?

4. Is exercise suited to each child by the school physician after physical examination, or are all children compelled to take the same exercise?

5. Whose business is it to see that rules regarding exercise are strictly enforced?

[148]6. Do clouds of dust rise from the floor during exercise and play?

7. Are children deprived of exercise as a penalty?

8. Should hygiene talks be considered as exercise?

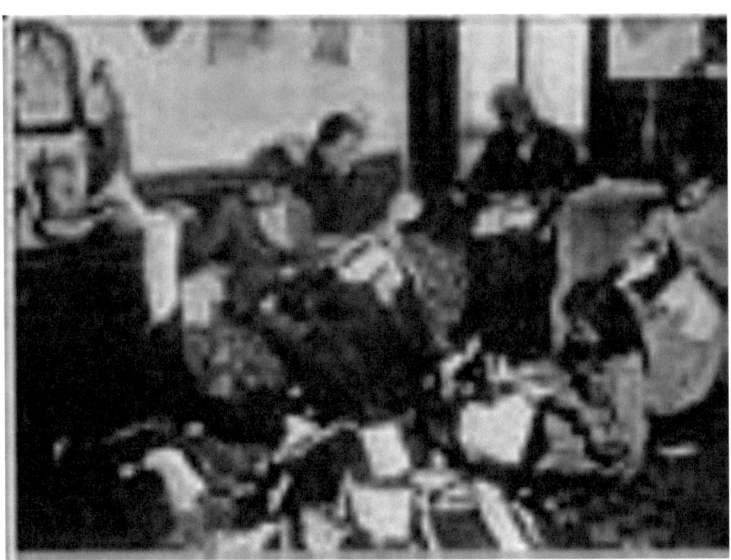

HOME WORKSHOPS NEED FRESH AIR

V. The School Janitor and Cleaners

1. Do they understand the relation of cleanliness to vitality?

2. Is their aim to do the least possible amount of work, or to attain the highest possible standard of cleanliness?

3. Will the teacher's complaint of uncleanliness be heeded by trustees? If so, is the teacher not responsible for uncleanliness?

4. Have you ever tried to stimulate the pride of janitors and cleaners for social service?

a. Have you ever tried to show them how much work they save themselves by thorough cleansing?
b. Have you ever shown them the danger, to their own health, of dust and dirt that may harbor infection and reduce their own vitality?

[149]5. What effort is made to instruct janitors and cleaners by your school trustees or by your community?

6. Have you explained to pupils the important responsibility of janitors for the health of those in the tenements, office buildings, or schools?

a. Do you see in this an opportunity to emphasize indirectly the mother's responsibility for cleanliness of home?

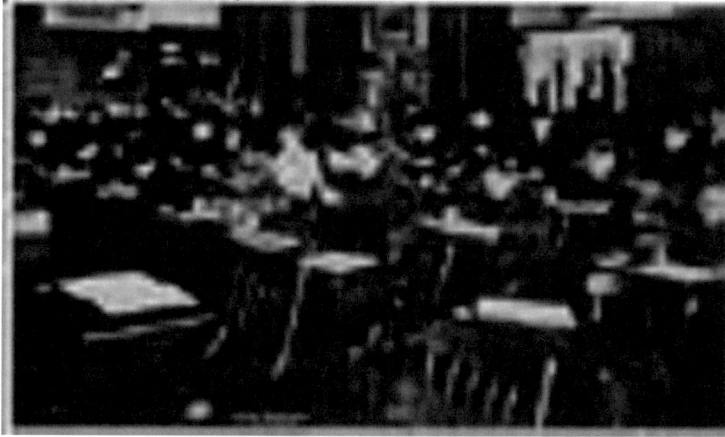

SCHOOL WORKSHOPS ALSO NEED FRESH AIR

VI. Requirements of Curriculum

1. How much home study is there?

a. How much is required?
b. What steps are taken to prevent excessive home study?
c. Are light and ventilation conditions at home considered when deciding upon amount of home study?

2. Is the child fitted to the curriculum, or is the curriculum fitted to the child?

a. Does failure or backwardness in studies lead to additional study hours or to regrading?
b. Are there too many subjects?
c. Are the recitation periods too long?
d. Are the exercise periods too short and too few?
e. Is there too much close-range work?
[150]*f.* Is it possible to give individual attention to individual needs so as to awaken individual interest?

3. Is follow-up work organized to enlist interest of parents, or, if necessary, of outside agencies in fitting a child to do that for which, if normal, he would be physically adapted?

By reducing the harm done by old buildings and by the traditions of curriculum and discipline, teachers can do a great deal. Perhaps they cannot move the windows or the desks, but they can move the children. If they cannot insure sanitary conditions for home study, they can cut down the home study. If the directors do not provide proper blackboards, they can do less blackboard work. They can make children as conscious, as afraid, and as resentful of dirty air as of dirty teeth. They can make janitors believe that "dry sweeping" or "feather dusting" may give them consumption, and leave most of the dirt in the room to make work for the next day; that adjustable desks are made to fit the child's legs and back, not the monkey wrench; that the thermometer in the schoolroom is a safer guide to heat needed than a boiler gauge in the basement; that fresh air heated by coal is cheaper for the school fund than stale air heated by bodies and by bad breath. Finally, they can make known to pupils, to parents, to principals and superintendents, to health officials and to the public, the extent to which school environment violates the precepts of school hygiene.

If the state requires the attendance of all children between the ages of five and fourteen at school for five hours a day, for five days in the week, for ten months in the year, then it should undertake to see that the machinery it provides for the education of those children for the greater part of the time for nine years of their lives—the formative years of their lives—is neither injuring their health nor retarding their full development.

If the amount of "close-range" work is rapidly manufacturing myopic eyes; if bad ventilation, whether due to [151]faulty construction or to faulty management, is preparing soil for the tubercle bacillus; if children with contagious diseases are not found and segregated; if desks are so ill adapted to children's sizes and physical needs that they are forming crooked spines; if too many children are crowded into one room; if lack of air and light is producing strained eyes and malnutrition; if neither open air, space, nor time is provided for exercise, games, and physical training; if school discipline is adapted neither to the psychology nor the physiology of child or teacher, then the state is depriving the child of a greater right than the compulsory education law forces it to endure. Not only is the right to health sacrificed to the right to education, but education and health are both sacrificed.

In undertaking to enforce the compulsory education law, to put all truants and child laborers in school, the state should be very sure for its own sake that it is not depriving the child of the health on which depends his future usefulness to the state as well as to himself.

Table XI

Effects of a Child Labor Law

Increase in Chicago Attendance

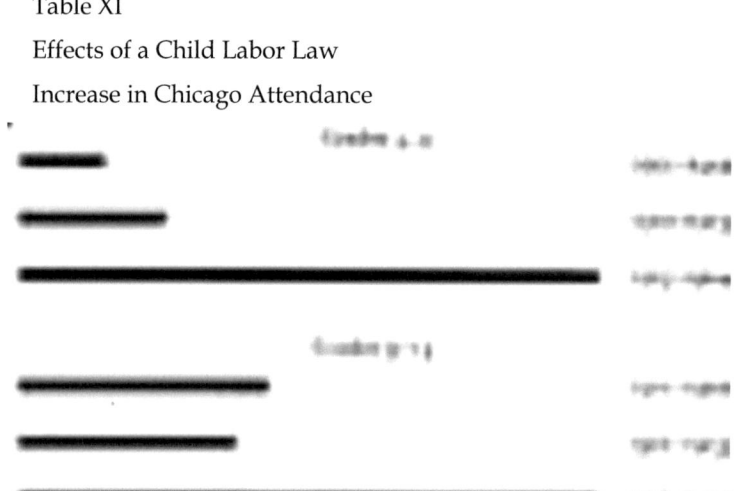

FOOTNOTES:

[8]*The Sanitation of Public Buildings*, by William Paul Gerhard, contains a valuable discussion of how the school may avoid manufacturing physical defects.

[9] By Professor Lila V. North, Baltimore College for Women, for the New York Committee on the Physical Welfare of School Children, 105 East 22d Street, New York City.

[152]

CHAPTER XVToC

THE TEACHER'S HEALTH

"Teachers, gentlemen, no less than pupils, have a heaven-ordained right to work so adjusted that the highest possible physical condition shall be maintained automatically." This declaration thundered out by an indignant physician startled a well-meaning board of school directors. The teacher's right to health was, of course, obvious when once mentioned, and the directors concluded:

1. School conditions that injure child health also injure teacher health.

2. Poor health of teacher causes poor health of pupil.

3. Poor health of pupil often causes poor health of teacher.

4. Adequate protection of children requires adequate protection of their teachers.

5. Teachers have a right to health protection for their own sake as well as for their children's sake.

Too little concern has hitherto been shown for the vitality of teachers in private or public schools and colleges. Without protest, and without notice until too late, teachers often neglect their own health at home and at school,—recklessly overwork, undersleep, and undernourish; ruin their eyes, their digestion, and their nerves. School-teachers are frequently "sweated" as mercilessly as factory operatives. The time has come to admit that a school environment which destroys the health of the teacher is as unnecessary and reprehensible as an army camp that spreads typhoid among a nation's defenders. A school curriculum or a college tradition that breaks down teachers is as inexcusable as a gun that kills the gunner when discharged. [153]Experience everywhere else proves that periodic physical examinations and health precautions, not essays about "happy teachers—happy pupils," are indispensable if teachers' health rights are to be protected.

Physical tests are imposed upon applicants for teachers' licenses by many boards of education. In New York City about three per cent of those examined are excluded for defects of vision, of hearing, of probable endurance. Once a teacher, however, there is no further physical examination,—no way of discovering physical incapacity, nothing to prevent a teacher from exposing class after class to pulmonary tuberculosis contracted because of overwork and underventilation. The certainty of salary increase year by year and of a pension after the twentieth year will bribe many a teacher to overtax her own strength and to jeopardize her pupils' health.

Seldom do training schools apply physical tests to students who intend to become teachers. One young girl says that before starting her normal course she is going to the physician of the board of education for examination, so as to avoid the experience of one of her friends, who, after preparing to be a teacher, was rejected because of pulmonary tuberculosis. During her normal course no examination will be necessary. Overwork during the first year may cause pulmonary tuberculosis, and in spite of her foresight she, too, may be rejected four years hence.

The advantages of physical examination upon beginning and during the courses that prepare one for a teacher are so obvious that but little opposition will be given by prospective teachers. The disadvantages to teacher and pupil alike of suffering from physical defects are so obvious that every school which prepares men and women for teachers should make registration and certification dependent upon passing a satisfactory physical test. No school should engage a teacher who has not good proof that she can do the [154]required work without injury to her own or her pupils' health. Long before physicians can discover pulmonary tuberculosis they can find depleted vitality which invites this disease. Headaches due to eye trouble, undernourishment due to mouth breathing, preventable indigestion, are insidious enemies that cannot escape the physical test.

Three objections to physical tests for teachers will be urged, but each loses its force when considered in the light of general experience.

1. *A sickly teacher is often the most efficient teacher in a school or a county.* It is true that some sickly teachers exert a powerful influence over their pupils, but in most instances their influence and their efficiency are due to powers that exist in spite of devitalizing elements. Rarely does sickness itself bring power. It must be admitted that many a man is teaching who would be practicing law had his health permitted it. Many a woman's soul is shorn of its self-consciousness by suffering. But even in these exceptional instances it is probable that children are paying too dearly for benefits directly or indirectly traceable to defects that physical tests would exclude.

2. *There are not enough healthy candidates to supply our schools.* This is begging the question. In fact, no one knows it is true. On the contrary, it is probable that the teacher's opportunity will make even a stronger appeal to competent men and women after physical soundness and vitality are made conditions of teaching,—after we all believe what leading educators now believe, that the highest fulfillment of human possibilities requires a normal, sound body, abounding in vitality.

3. *Examination by a physician, especially if a social acquaintance, is an unnecessary embarrassment.* The false modesty that makes physical examination unwelcome to many adults, men as well as women, is easily overcome when the advantages of such examination are understood. [155]It is likewise easy to prove to a teacher that the loss of time required in having the examination is infinitesimal compared with the loss of time due to ignoring physical needs. The programme for school hygiene outlined in Chapter XXVII, Part IV, assumes that state and county superintendents will provide for the examination of teachers as well as of pupils.

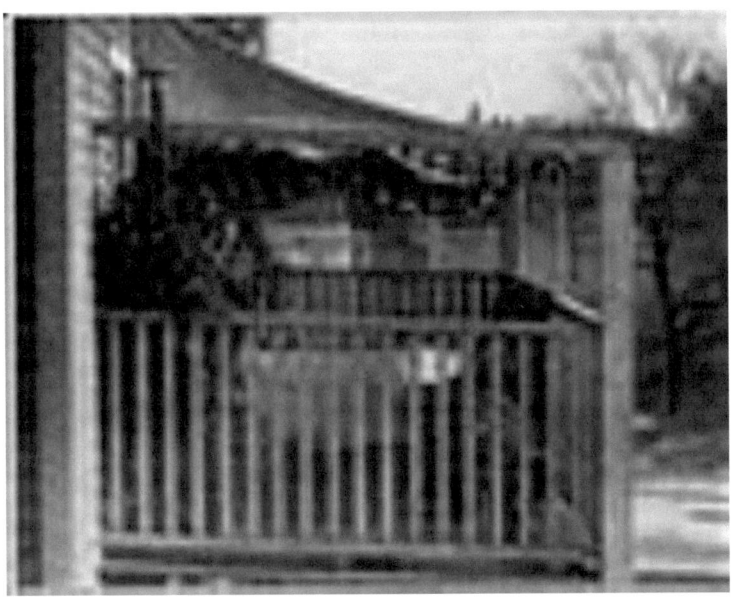

TEACHERS WILL PREFER PHYSICAL EXAMINATIONS TO FORCED VACATIONS
Boston Society for Relief and Study of Tuberculosis

Because the health of others furnishes a stronger motive for preventive hygiene than our own health, it is probable that the general examination of teachers will come first as the result of a general conviction that unhealthy teachers positively injure the health of pupils and retard their mental development. Children at school age are so susceptible and imitative that their future habits of body and mind, their dispositions, their very voices and expressions, are influenced by those of their teachers. Experts in child [156]study say that a child's vocal chords respond to the voices and noise about him before he is able to speak, so that the tones of his voice are determined before he is able to express them. This influence is also marked when the child begins to talk. Babies and young children instinctively do what adults learn not to do only by study,—follow the pitch of others' voices. Can we then overestimate the effect upon pupils' character of teachers who radiate vitality?

The character and fitness, aside from scholarship, of applicants for teachers' licenses are now subjected by the board of examiners of New York City to the following tests:

1. Moral character as indicated in the record of the applicant as a student or teacher or in other occupation, or as a participant in an examination.

2. Physical fitness for the position sought, reference being had here to all questions of physical fitness other than those covered in a physician's report as to "sound health."

3. Satisfactory quality and use of voice.

4. Personal bearing, cleanliness, appearance, manners.

5. Self-command and power to win and hold the respect of teachers, school authorities, and the community.

6. Capacity for school discipline, power to maintain order and to secure the willing obedience and the friendship of pupils.

7. Business or executive ability, — power to comprehend and carry out and to accomplish prescribed work, school management as relating to adjustment of desks, lighting, heating, ventilation, cleanliness, and attractiveness of schoolroom.

8. Capacity for supervision, for organization and administration of a school, and for the instructing, assisting, and inspiring of teachers.

These tests probably exclude few applicants who should be admitted. Experience proves that they include many who, for their own sake and for children's sake, should be rejected. The moral character, physical fitness, quality of voice, personal bearing, self-command, executive ability, [157]capacity for supervision, are qualities that are modified by conditions. The voice that is satisfactory in conference with an examiner may be strident and irritating when the teacher is impatient or is trying to overcome street noises. On parade applicants are equally cleanly; this cannot be said of teachers in the service, coming from different home environments. Self-command is much easier in one school than in another. Physical fitness in a girl of twenty may, during one short year of teaching, give way to physical unfitness. Therefore the need for *periodic tests* by principal, superintendent, and school board, *to determine the continuing fitness* of a teacher to do the special task assigned to her, based upon physical evidence of her own vitality and of her favorable influence upon her pupils' health and enjoyment of school life. Shattered nerves due to overwork may explain a teacher's shouting: "You are a dirty boy. Your mother is a dirty woman and keeps a dirty store where no decent people will go to buy." A physical examination of that unfortunate teacher would probably show that she ought to be on leave of absence, rather than, by her overwork and loss of control, to cause the boys of her class to feel what one of them expressed: "Grandmother, if she spoke so of my mother I would strike her."

Just as there should be a central bureau to count and correct the open mouths and closed minds that clog the little old red schoolhouse of the country, so a central bureau should discover in the city teacher as well as in the country teacher the ailments more serious than tuberculosis that pass from teacher to pupil; slovenliness, ugly temper, frowning, crossness, lack of ambition, cynicism,—these should be blackballed as well as consumption, contagious morphine habit, and contagious skin disease. Crooked thinking by teacher leads to crooked thinking by pupil. Disregard of health laws by teacher encourages unhygienic living by pupils. A man whose fingers are yellow, nerves [158]shaky, eyes unsteady, and mind alternately sleepy and hilarious from cigarettes, cannot convey pictures of normal, healthy physical living, nor can he successfully teach the moral and social evils of nicotinism. Both teacher and pupil have a right to the periodic physical examination of teachers that will give timely warning of attention needed. Until there is some system for giving this right to all teachers in private, parochial, charitable, and public schools, we shall produce many nervous, acrid, and physically threadbare teachers, where we should have only teachers who inspire their pupils with a passion for health by the example of a good complexion, sprightly step, bounding vitality, and forceful personality born of hygienic living.

[159]

CHAPTER XVIToC

EUROPEAN REMEDIES: DOING THINGS AT SCHOOL

Recently I traveled five hundred miles to address an audience on methods of fitting health remedies to local health needs. I told of certain dangers to be avoided, of results that had always followed certain remedies, of motives to be sought and used, of community ends to seek. Not knowing the local situation, I could not tell them exactly what to do next, or how or with whom to do it; not seeing the patient or his symptoms, I did not diagnose the disease or prescribe medicine. Several members of the audience who were particularly anxious to start a new organization on a metropolitan model were disappointed because they were told, not just how to organize, but rather how to find out what sort of organization their town needed. They were right in believing that it was easier to copy on paper a plan tried somewhere else, than to think out a plan for themselves. They had forgotten for the time being their many previous disappointments due to copying without question some plan of social work, just as they copy Paris or New York fashions. They had not expected to leave this meeting with the conviction that while the *ends* of sanitary administration may be the same in ten communities, health *machinery* should fit a particular community like a tailor-made suit.

[160]American-like, they had a mania for organization. I once heard an aged kindergartner—the savant of an isolated German village—describe my fellow-Americans as follows: "Every American belongs to some organization. The total abstainers are organized, the brewers are organized, the teachers are organized, the parents are organized, the young people and even the juniors are organized.

Finally, those who belong to no organization go off by themselves and organize a society of the unorganized." Love of organization and love of copying have given us Americans a feverish desire for what we see or read about in Europe. When we talk about our European remedies we try to make ourselves believe that we are broad-minded and want to learn from others' experience. In a large number of cases our impatient demand for European remedies is similar to the schoolboy's desire to show off the manners, the slang, or the clothes picked up on his first visit away from home. With many travelers and readers European remedies or European ways are souvenirs of a pleasant visit, to be described like a collection of postal cards, a curious umbrella, a cane associated with Alpine climbing, or a stolen hymnal from an historic cathedral.

Experience proves, however, that just as Roman walls and Norman castles look out of place in New York and Kansas, so European laws and European remedies are too frequently misfits when tried by American schools, hospitals, or city governments. Yesterday a Canadian clergyman, after preaching an eloquent sermon, met a professional beggar on the street in New York City and emptied his purse—of Canadian money! Quite like this is the enthusiastic demand of the tourist who has seen or read about "the way it's done in Germany." The trouble is that European remedies are valued like ruins, by their power to interest, by their antiquity or picturesqueness, or, like the beggar, by their power to stimulate temporary emotion. [161]But we do not sleep in ruins, go to church regularly in thirteenth-century abbeys, or live under the remedies that fire our imagination. We do not therefore see their everyday, practical-result side.

The souvenir value of European remedies is due to the assumption that no better way was open to the European, and that the remedy actually does what it is intended to do. Because free meals are given at school to cure and prevent undernourishment, it is taken for granted that undernourishment stops when free meals are introduced; therefore America must have free meals. Because it is made compulsory in a charming Italian village for every child to eat the free school meal, it is taken for granted that the children of that village have no physical defects; therefore let Kansas City, Seattle, and Boston introduce compulsory free meals. But when one goes to

Europe to see exactly how those much-advertised, eulogized remedies operate from day to day, it is often necessary to write, as did a great American sanitarian recently, of health administration in foreign cities continually held up as models to American cities: "In spite of the rules and theories over here, the patient has better care in New York City."

We have been asked of late to copy several very attractive European remedies for the physiological ills of school children, and for the physical deficiencies of the next generation of adults: breakfasts or lunches, or both, at school for all children, rich as well as poor, whether they want school nourishment or not; school meals for the poor only; school meals to be given the poor, but to be bought by those who can afford the small sum required; free eyeglasses for the poor, for poor and well-to-do, for those who wish them, for those who need them whether they want to wear eyeglasses or not; free dental care; free surgical treatment; free rides and outings during summer and winter; country children to visit the metropolis, city children to visit country [162]and village; free treatment in the country of all children whose parents are consumptives; free rides on street cars to and from school; city-owned street railways that will prevent congestion by making the country accessible; city-built tenements to prevent overcrowding, dark rooms, insufficient air and light; free coal, free clothes, free rent for those whose parents are unable to protect them properly against hunger and cold. Every one of these remedies is attractive. Every one is being tried somewhere, and can be justified on emotional, economic, and educational grounds, if we think only of its purpose. Let us view them with the eyes of their advocates.

Would it not be nice for country children to know that toward the end of the school year they would be given an excursion to the largest city of their state, to its slums, its factories, parks, and art galleries? They would grow up more intelligent about geography. They would read history, politics, sociology, and civil government with greater interest. They would have less contracted sympathies. They might even decide that they would rather live their life in the spacious country than in the crowded, rushing city.

City children, on the other hand, would reap worlds of physical benefit and untold inspiration from periods of recreation and study in the country, with its quiet, its greens and bronzes and yellows, its birds and animals, its sky that sits like a dome on the earth, its hopefulness. Winter sleigh rides and coasting would give new vigor and ambition. Why spend so much on teaching physiology, geography, and nature study, if in the end we fail to send the child where alone nature and hygiene tell their story? Why tax ourselves to teach history and sociology and commercial geography out of books when excursions to the city and country will paint pictures on the mind that can never be erased? What more attractive or more reasonable than appetizing, warm meals, or cool salads and drinks for [163]the boys and girls who carry their little dinner pails and baskets down the long road where everything runs together in summer and everything freezes in winter? One needs little imagination to see the "smile that won't come off," health, punctuality, and school interest resulting from the school meal.

Again, if children must have teeth filled and pulled, eyes tested and fitted for glasses, adenoids and enlarged tonsils removed, surely the school environment offers the least affrighting spot for the tragedy. Thence goblins long ago fled. There courage, real or feigned, is brought to the surface by the anxious, critical, competitive interest of one's peers.

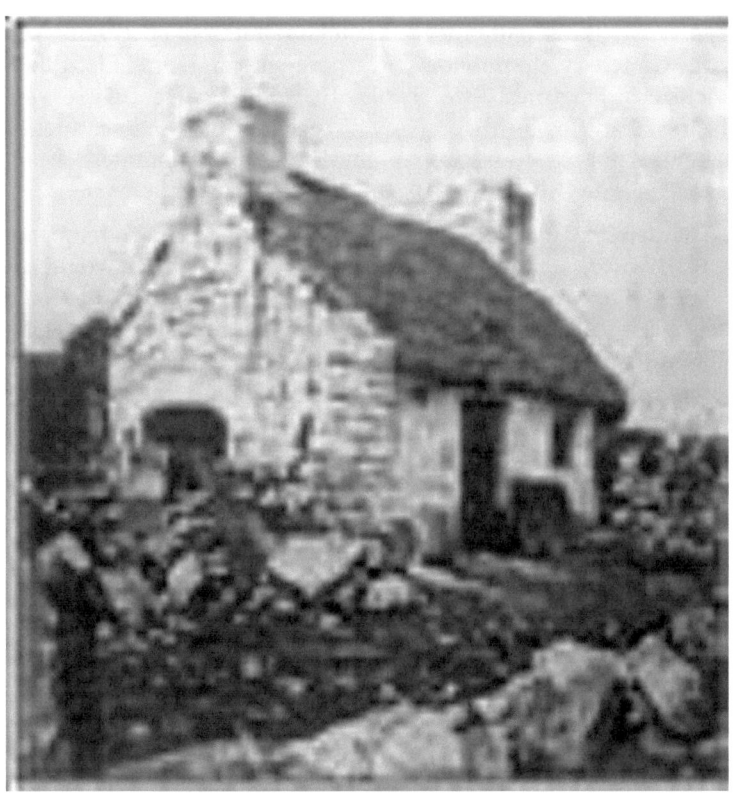

A SOUTH IRELAND ARGUMENT FOR "DOING THINGS"

The economic defense of these remedies is many-sided. An English drummer once instructed me during a railroad journey from southern to northern Ireland. As we entered the fertile fields of Lord Dunraven's estate near Athlone, I expressed sympathy for other countries impoverished of soil, of wealth, and of thrift. My instructor replied: "It would pay the government to bring them all to this land free once a year, just to show them what they are missing." That his idea of an investment is sound has been proved by railroads and land companies and even by states, who give away excursions to entice settlers and buyers. Ambition at almost any cost is cheaper than indifference to opportunity. It would be cheaper for our American taxpayer to send school children to city and country than to pay the penalty for having a large number of citizens with narrow interests, unconscious of the struggles and joys of [164]their co-citizens. Free meals, free books, free rides, free eyeglasses, are cheaper than free instruction for the second, third, and sixth terms in studies not passed because of physical defects, — infinitely cheaper than jails and almshouses, truant officers and courthouses.

The demoralizing results of giving "something for nothing" did not follow free schooling or free text-books. Perhaps they would not follow the free remedies that we are asked to copy from Europe. In fact, the word "free" is the wrong word. These remedies rather require coöperation of parent with parent. It has demoralized nobody because the streets are cleaned by all of us, country roads made by the township, police paid for by taxes and not by volunteer subscription.

The man whose children do not need glasses or nourishment or operation for adenoids would find it cheaper to pay for European remedies than for the useless schooling of boys unable to get along in school because of removable defects. An unruly, uninterested boy sitting beside your boy in public school, a pampered, overfed, undisciplined child sitting beside yours at private school, is taxing you without your consent and doing your child injury that may prove irreparable.

It costs $2.50 to furnish a child with eyeglasses. It costs $25 to $50 to give that child a year's schooling. If the child cannot see right and fails in his studies, we have lost a good investment and, after one year so lost, we are out $22.50. In two years we have lost $47.50. But, what is more serious, we have discouraged that boy. Used to failure in school, his mind turns to other things. He is made to think that it is useless for him to try for first place. Perhaps he can play ball, and excels. He chooses a career of ball playing. Valuable years are lost.

Initiative and competition are not interrupted any more by free eyeglasses and free operation for adenoids than by [165]free schooling. There is only one place in the world where there is less competition or less struggle than among the ignorant, and that is among the ignorant and unwell. The boy who can't see the blackboard, who can't learn to spell, who can't breathe through his nose, and can't be interested, doesn't compete at all with the bright, healthy boy. Remove the adenoids, give glasses, make interest possible, and fitness to survive takes a higher level because larger numbers become fit to survive.

Professor Patten says that it is easier to support in the almshouse than in competitive industry a man who cannot earn more than $1.50 a day. The question, therefore, regarding European remedies is not, To what general theory do they belong? but, What will they accomplish? How do they compare with other remedies of which we know?

[166]

AMERICAN REMEDIES: GETTING THINGS DONE

In New York City there is a committee called the Committee on the Physical Welfare of School Children. The word "welfare" was used rather than "condition" because the committee proposed to use whatever facts it could gather for the improvement of home and school conditions prejudicial to child welfare. The following programme was adopted:

1. *Study of the physical welfare of school children.*

a. Examination of board of health records of children needing medical, dental, or ocular care, and better nourishment.

b. Home visitation of such children, in order to ascertain whether their need arises from deficient income or from other causes.

c. Effort to secure proper treatment, either from parents or from free clinics or other established agencies.

d. Effort to secure proper physical surroundings of children while at school — playgrounds, baths, etc.

2. *Effort to secure establishment of such a system of school records and reports* as will disclose automatically significant school facts, — e.g. regarding backward pupils, truancy, regularity of attendance, registered children not attending, sickness, physical defects, etc.

3. *Effort to utilize available information regarding school needs* so as to stimulate public interest and thus aid in securing adequate appropriations to meet school needs.

The committee grew out of the discussion, in the year 1905, of the following proposition: *To insure a race physically able to receive our vaunted free education, we must provide at school free meals, free eyeglasses, free medical [167]and dental care.* Thanks to the superintendent of schools of New York City, to Robert Hunter's *Poverty*, to John Spargo's *Bitter Cry of the Children*, hundreds of thousands of American citizens were made to realize for the first time that a large proportion of our school children are in serious need of medical, dental, or ocular attention, or of better nourishment.

Because physicians, dentists, oculists, hospitals, dispensaries, relief agencies, had seemingly been unconscious of this serious state of affairs, they had no definite, constructive remedy to propose. Their unpreparedness served to strengthen the arguments for the European method of *doing things*. France, Germany, Italy, England, had found it necessary to do things at school. Arguing from their experience, it was only a matter of time when American cities must follow their example. Why not, therefore, begin at once to deal radically with the situation and give school meals, school eyeglasses, etc.? Those who organized the Committee on the Physical Welfare of School Children realized the danger of trying to settle so great a question with the little definite information then available. If *doing things at school* were to be adopted as a principle and logically carried out, vast sums must be added to the present cost of the public school system. Complications would arise with private and parochial schools, whose children might have quite as serious physical defects, even though not educated by public funds. It would be difficult to obtain proper rooms for medical and dental treatment and meals, and perhaps still more difficult to insure proper food, skilled oculists, dentists, surgeons, and physicians. No one was clear as to how the problem was to be solved by small cities and rural districts, whose needy children are no less entitled to public aid simply because their numbers are smaller. Great as were the difficulties, however, the committee saw that difficulties are in themselves no reason for not doing the right thing. On the [168]other hand, if doing things at school is wrong, if school meals fail to correct and remove physical defects, great social and educational wrong would result from New York's setting an example that would not only misdirect funds and attention in that city, but would undoubtedly lead other cities to move in the wrong direction. Right could be hastened, wrong could be prevented more effectually by facts than by any amount of theory. School meals had been made a political issue in England. The arguments supporting them were stronger than any possible arguments against them, except proof that they would be less effective in helping children than other means that might be proposed. If the American people must choose between sickly, unteachable, dull children without school meals, on the one hand, and bright, teachable, healthy children plus school meals, on the other hand, they will not hesitate because of expense or eighteenth-century objections to "socialism."

During one year of investigation and of *getting things done* the committee has prepared three studies for publication: (1) a report on the home conditions of fourteen hundred school children of different nationalities, found by school physicians to have defects of vision, breathing, hearing, teeth, and nourishment; (2) an examination of fifty schools—curriculum, buildings, home-study requirements, play space and playtime, physical culture—in an attempt to answer the question, How far does school environment directly cause or aggravate physical defects of school children; (3) a comparative study of methods now employed in a hundred cities to record, classify, and make public significant school facts.

The results of the first year's work prove conclusively that physical defects are not caused solely by the inability of parents to pay for proper food. Among the twenty significant facts reported by the committee are the following:

1. Physical defects found in public schools are, for the most[169] part, such as frequently occur in wealthy families and do not of themselves presume as the cause insufficient income. Of 145 reported for malnutrition, 44 were from families having over $20 weekly.

2. Few of the defects can be corrected by nourishment alone; plenty of fresh air, outside nourishment at school, or extra nourishment at home will not entirely counteract the influences of bad ventilation and bad light in school buildings. Country children have adenoids, bad teeth, and malnutrition. Plenty of food will not prevent

bad teeth and bad ventilation from causing adenoids, enlarged tonsils, and malnutrition.

3. Children whose parents have long lived in the United States need attention quite as much as the recent immigrant.

4. A large part of the defects reported could be produced by conditions due directly to neglect of teeth.

From twenty such statements of fact and from its experience in *getting things done* for one year, the committee drew fifteen practical conclusions, among which the following deserve emphasis here:

1. The only new thing about the physical defects of school children is not their existence, but our recent awakening to their existence, their prevalence, their seriousness if neglected, and their cost to individual children, to school progress, to industry, and to social welfare.

2. *Physical deterioration*, applied to America's school children, is a misnomer. No evidence whatever has been given that the percentage of children suffering from physical defects in 1907 is greater than the percentage of children suffering from such defects in 1857. On the contrary, the small proportion of defects that are not easily removable, as well as a vast amount of evidence from medical experience and vital statistics, indicates that, if a comparison were possible, the children of 1907 would be found to have sounder bodies and fewer defects than their predecessors of fifty years ago. If there is an exception to this statement, it is probably defects of vision, with regard to which school authorities and oculists seem to agree that confinement in school for longer [170]hours and more constant application under unfavorable lighting conditions have caused a marked increase. Positive evidence as to tendencies will be easily obtained after thorough physical examination has been carried on for a generation.

3. The effect of massing facts as to physical defects of school children should not be to cause alarm, but to stimulate remedial and preventive measures, to invoke congratulations and aggressive

optimism, not doleful pessimism and palliative measures born of despair.

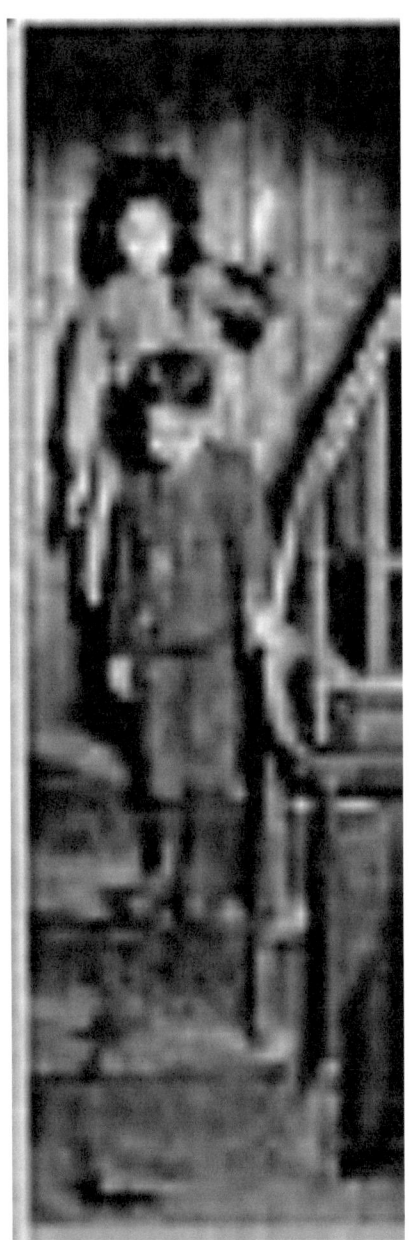

4. The causes of physical defects are not confined to "marginal" incomes, but, while more apt to be present in families having small incomes, are found among all incomes wherever there exist bad ventilation, insufficient outdoor exercise, improper light, irregular eating, overeating, improper as well as insufficient food, lack of medical, dental, and ocular attention.

5. Whatever may be said of free meals at school as a means of insuring punctual attendance or better attention, they are inadequate to correct physical conditions that home and street environment produce.

6. *To remove physical defects, causal conditions among all income classes should be treated, and not merely symptoms revealed at school by children of the so-called poor.*

7. Parents can and will correct the greater part of the defects discovered by the physical examination of school children, if shown what steps to take. Where parents refuse to do what can be proved to be within their power, and where existing laws are nonenforced or inadequate, the segregation of children having physical defects in special classes might prove an effective stimulus to obstinate parents.

8. Where parents are unable to pay for medical, dental, and ocular care and proper nourishment, private philanthropy must either provide adequately or expect the state to step in and assume the duty.

9. Private dispensaries and hospitals must either arrange themselves to treat cases and to educate communities as to the importance of detecting and correcting physical defects, or must expect the state to provide hospital and dispensary care. Until private hospitals and dispensaries take steps to prevent people [171]with adequate incomes from imposing upon them for free treatment, it is difficult to make out a case against free eyeglasses and free meals for school children.

10. Either private philanthropy or the state must take steps to procure more dental clinics and an educational policy on the part of

the dental profession that will prevent the exploitation of the poor when dental care is needed.

11. The United States Bureau of Education is the only agency with authority and equipment adequate to secure from all sections of the country proper attention to the subject. Nothing in the world can prevent free meals, free eyeglasses, free medical care, free material relief at school, unless educational use is made by each community of the facts learned through physical examination to correct home, school, and street conditions that produce and aggravate physical defects. The national bureau can mass information in such a way as to convince budget makers in city, county, and state to vote gladly the funds necessary to promote the physical welfare of school children.

How the committee got things done is often referred to. There is something about a request for coöperation, whether by schools or by any other agency, that enlists the interest of those whose help is asked. The reason is not that people are flattered by requests to serve on committees, or that human nature finds it difficult to be unfriendly or unkind. On the contrary, men and women are by nature social; there is more joy in giving than in withholding, in working with others than in working alone. Men and women, official and volunteer agencies, will coöperate with school-teachers when invited, for the same reason and [172]with the same readiness that ninety-nine farmers out of a hundred, on the prairie or in the mountain, will welcome a request for food and lodging.

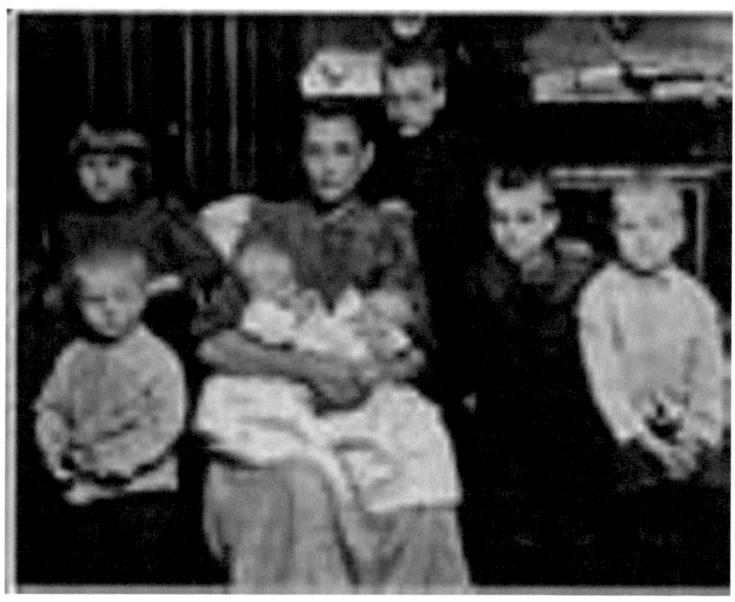

WHERE "GETTING THINGS DONE" IS POSSIBLE BUT "DOING THINGS" INEFFECTIVE

Mothers will naturally take a greater interest in the welfare of their children if held responsible for proper food and proper home surroundings than if not reminded of their responsibility. In New York City a woman district superintendent of schools, Miss Julia Richman, has organized a unique "social settlement." She and several school-teachers occupy a house, known as "The Teachers' House." This is their residence. Here they are subject to neither intrusion nor importunity; no clubs or classes are held here; visitors are treated as guests, not as beneficiaries. The purpose these teachers have in living together is to work out the methods of interesting private and official leaders in community needs disclosed at school.

[173]Where clubs and social gatherings are held in school buildings, it is not unusual for a thousand mothers, recent immigrants, to meet together in one hall to hear talks on the care of children. Thus, instead of principals, teachers, and physicians taking the place of mothers (which they nowhere have succeeded in doing), they do succeed in harnessing mothers to the school programme. It may

take two, three, or ten visits to get a particular mother to do the necessary thing for her child, but when once convinced and once inspired to do that thing, she will go on day in and day out doing the right thing for that child and for all others in her home. It may take a year to convert a police magistrate whose sympathy for delinquent parents and truant children is an active promoter of disorder; but a magistrate convinced, efficient, and interested is worth a hundred volunteer visitors. To get things done in this way for a hundred thousand children costs less in time and money than to do the necessary things for one thousand children.

[174]

COÖPERATION WITH DISPENSARIES AND CHILD-SAVING AGENCIES

Scientists agree that the human brain is superior to the animal brain, not because it is heavier, but because it is finer and better supplied with nerves. As one writer has said, the human brain is better "wired," has better organized "centrals." A poor system of centrals will spoil a telephone service, no matter how many wires it provides. An independent wire is of little use, because it will not reach the person desired at the other end. The ideal system is that which almost instantly connects two persons, no matter how far away or how many other people are talking at the same time on other wires.

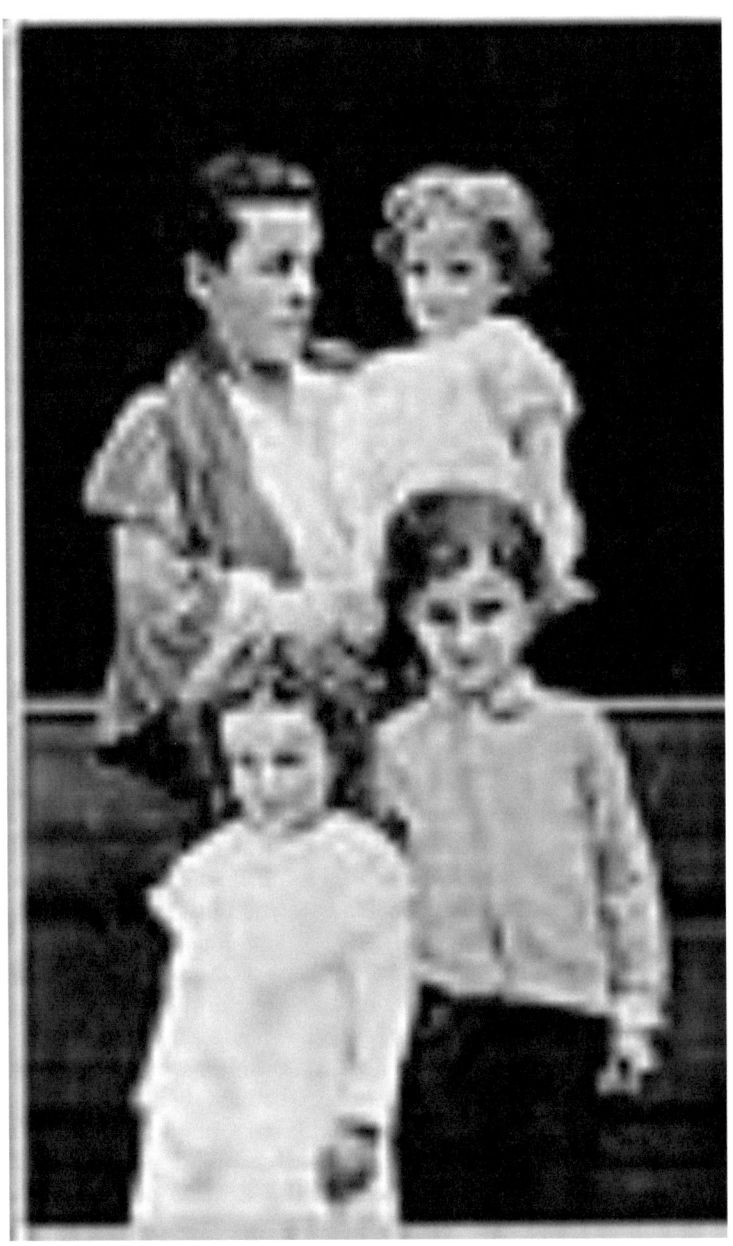

ADEQUATE RELIEF RECOGNIZES THE FAMILY AS THE UNIT

The school that tries to do everything for its pupils without using other existing agencies for helping children[10] will be like the man who refuses to connect his telephone with a central switch board, or like a bank that will not use the central clearing house. As one telephone center can enable scores of people to talk at once, and as one clearing house can make one check pay fifty debts, so hospital and relief agencies enable a teacher who employs "central" to help several times as many children as she alone can help.

It seems easier for a teacher to give twenty-five cents to a child in distress than to see that the cause of the misery is removed. In New York City there are over five hundred school principals, under them are over fifteen thousand [175]teachers, and the average attendance of children is about six hundred thousand, representing one hundred and fifty thousand homes. If teachers give only to those children who ask for help, many will be neglected. In certain sections of the city principals have combined to establish a relief fund to be given out to children who need food, clothes, shoes, etc. One principal had to stop replacing stolen overcoats because, when it was known that he had a fund, an astonishingly large number of overcoats disappeared. At Poughkeepsie school children get up parties, amateur vaudeville, minstrel shows, basket picnics, to obtain food and clothing for children in distress. They are, of course, unable to help parents or children not in school. Of this method a district superintendent in New York said to his teachers and principals: "For thirty-two years I have been working in the schools of this district. I have given food and shoes to thousands of children. I know that however great our interest in a particular child when it comes to us with trouble at home, our duty as teachers prevents us from following our gift into the home and learning the cause of the child's trouble. This last winter we have made an experiment in using a central society, which makes it a business to find out what the family needs, to supply necessaries, country board, medicine, etc. We now know that we can put a slip of paper with the [176]name and address of the child into a general hopper and it will come out eyeglasses, food, rent, vacation parties, as the need may be."

Relief at home through existing agencies was brought about by the distribution of cards like those on opposite page, which offer winter and summer coöperation.

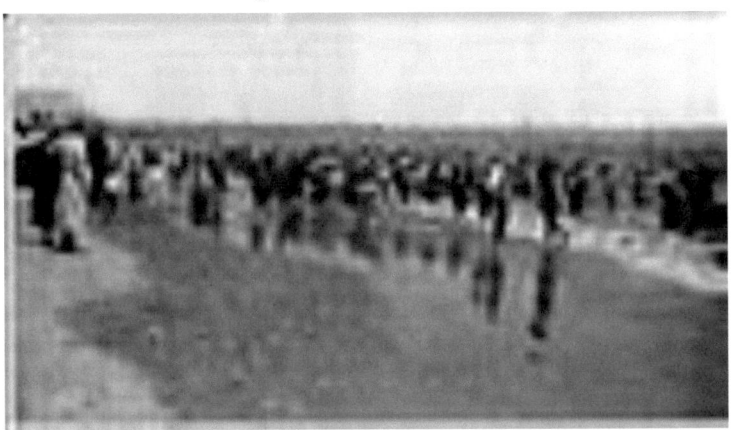

FRESH-AIR AGENCIES LIKE SEA BREEZE PREFER TO AID CHILDREN IN ORDER OF NEED

When these cards were first distributed several teachers went from room to room, asking children who needed help to raise the hand. In many cases parents were very angry that their children should have asked for help. But help given in instances like the following soon proved to teachers that they could afford the time necessary to notice children who appeared neglected, when so much good would ensue:

The father is sick and unable to work. They cannot get clothes for the children, who are not attending school on that account. Children were provided with shoes and clothes.

November 30, 1907, a school principal reported that six children in one family needed underwear. A visitor discovered that one of the boys who had the reputation of being unruly and light-fingered also had adenoids. He was taken to a hospital for operation, and was later interested in his school work.

For School Children

COMPULSORY education implies the ability of all families, even the poorest, to take advantage of school benefits. This means that children should be fed properly, clad comfortably, and healthfully housed.

The New York Association for Improving the Condition of the Poor aims to coöperate with school-teachers in every part of Manhattan and The Bronx to insure comfort and prevent suffering among school children, their parents, and younger brothers and sisters. On one day last winter we received appeals from school principals and teachers in behalf of twenty-nine families. Within six hours every family was visited, emergent aid in food and coal provided for many, and orders given for shoes and dresses and coats required by the children of school age. During the winter we gave not only clothing, groceries, food, and rent, but found work for older boys and parents, taught mothers to prepare food properly, and sent a visiting cleaner to make sick mothers comfortable and to get the children ready for school.

In a word, we followed that need, the surface evidence of which comes to the attention of the teacher, back into the home and its conditions, aiding throughout the period when the family was unable to do justice by the school child.

In many instances the home income was sufficient, but the home management inefficient. Probably such homes could be more effectively benefited through educational work emanating directly from the school.

We can be reached by telephone (348, 349, and 1873 Gramercy) from 9 A. M. to 12 M. Letters or postal cards should be addressed to Mrs. H. Ingram, Superintendent, 105 East 22d Street. Reference slips will be gladly furnished upon application.

The New York Association for Improving
1843 · the Condition of the Poor · 1905

Teachers of Manhattan and The Bronx

Do you know of such children as these:

1. Convalescent children now out of school, who would be benefited by a stay at the seashore in May or June?

2. Children in school whose anæmic condition would be greatly improved by a week at Sea Breeze during July or August?

3. Small brothers and sisters (and tired mothers) who may need outings or special help?

The New York Association for Improving the Condition of the Poor will act promptly. Write or telephone (348 Gramercy).

[177]

[178]A little girl was unruly and truant. No attempt was made to keep her at school, but she was reported to the Committee on the Physical Welfare of School Children. The parents could not control her. The girl was taken for examination by a specialist and found to be feeble-minded. Later she was sent to a custodial institute.

Another little girl was nine years old, but could not talk. A University Extension Society worker found that she was not kept at school because it was too much trouble. The child was taken to a physician who operated and corrected the tongue-tie.

A girl of twelve said she must stay home to "help mother." The mother was found to be a janitress, temporarily incapacitated by rheumatism. A substitute was provided until the mother was well, and all the children were properly clad for school.

After the adenoid operations in a New York school that occasioned the East Side riots of 1906, the physicians and principals who had persuaded parents to permit the operations were fearful lest the summer in unsanitary surroundings might make the demonstration less complete. Over forty children in three parties were sent away for the summer, where they had wholesome food and all the milk they could drink and fresh air day and night. When they returned in the fall the principal wrote: "The improvement in each individual is simply marvelous. We shall try to continue this condition and shall constantly urge the parents to keep up the good work by means of proper food and fresh air."

In none of these instances could the teachers have accomplished equal results for the individual children or for the families without neglecting school duties. By informing other agencies as to children's needs, teachers started movements that have since helped practically every school child in New York City. Dispensaries are setting aside separate hours for school children; fresh-air agencies are giving preference to children found by teachers or school physicians to be in physical need; relief agencies are making "rush orders" of every note from teachers; the health board is more active because volunteer agencies [179]have added their voice to that of teacher and health officer in demanding adequate funds for physical examination of school children.

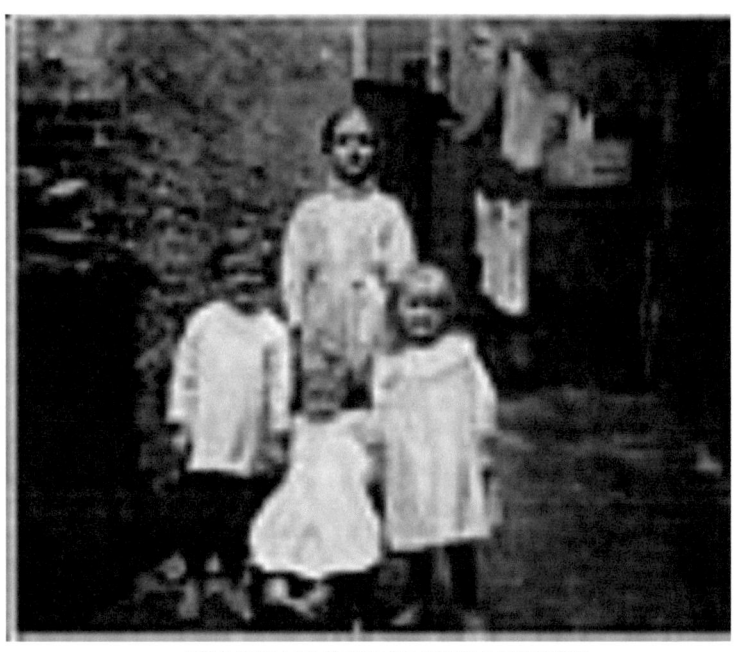

"CENTRAL" FOUND THE MOTHER
SICK IN A HOSPITAL, THE FATHER
KILLED—THE CHILDREN WERE
BOARDED IN THE COUNTRY UNTIL
THE MOTHER RECOVERED

Coöperation is at present easier in New York than in any other city. Charitable societies, hospitals, dispensaries, are probably more keenly alive to their responsibilities and are at least more apt to have acquired the habit of coöperation when asked. Yet even here I have been told repeatedly by teachers: "If we have to wait for that hospital or that charitable society, our children will go barefoot." In small communities where hospital and relief agencies are for emergencies only and generally inactive, it seems that the first thing to do is to ask some friends to establish a small relief fund, just as it is easier to give a child a five-cent [180]meal than to teach its mother how to prepare its food. But the school-teacher will find that it takes very much less energy to arouse the relief society than to maintain her own relief work. In fact, in many cities nothing could do more to strengthen hospitals and charitable societies than to put them in touch with the needs of school children. For a principal to make known the fact that school children are neglected will help the charitable society and hospital to get the funds necessary to do their part better than they are now doing it and better than the school could ever do it. Finally, one reason for a breakdown of charitable societies is not their own inadequacy, but rather the failure of the [181]school and church to make use of an agency better equipped than themselves to give material relief. The teacher sees the child every day, while the relief society will never see it and has no reason to see it until some one calls attention to it. The very first step, and an indispensable one in relief policy, is for teachers to be on the lookout for children not adequately provided for, and then have the physical evidence discovered at school followed to the home for the cause of the child's distress.

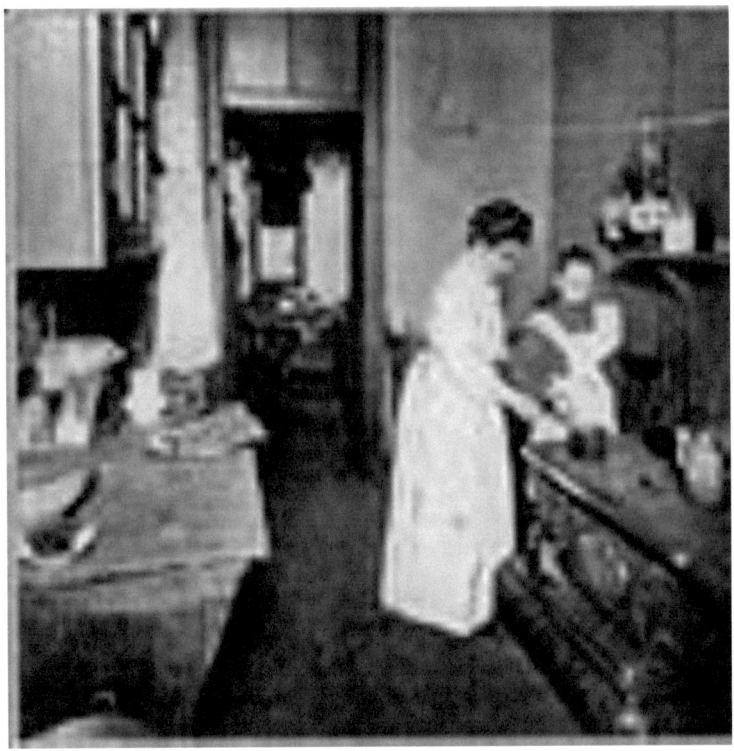

HOME-TO-HOME INSTRUCTION IN COOKING
Anæmic condition of child due to bad cooking, not to lack of income

Coöperation removes the cause of distress; *doing* may aggravate it. Teachers would do well to draw up for themselves a chart which will show exactly what part of the community's work can be best done by their school. On the following page is charted the social work now being conducted at the Massachusetts General Hospital, Boston. So far as agencies exist to deal with any individual or family problem coming into the social-work square, the hospital aims to utilize that agency. Its own direct dealing with neurasthenics, with hygiene education, with sexual deviates, is primarily for the purpose of giving adequate treatment to the needy, and secondarily to demonstrate how adequate treatment should be organized for the community. Please to note that governmental agencies are not mentioned in Dr. Cabot's chart. This does not mean that he would not emphasize the importance of those agencies, but that up to the present time, for the particular cases dealt with in his clinics, governmental agencies can be reached most effectively through the private charitable agencies in the reference square. So the teacher will frequently find that the relief bureau, children's society, public education association, or church can get better results for her pupils from public health and correctional agencies than can she by writing directly.

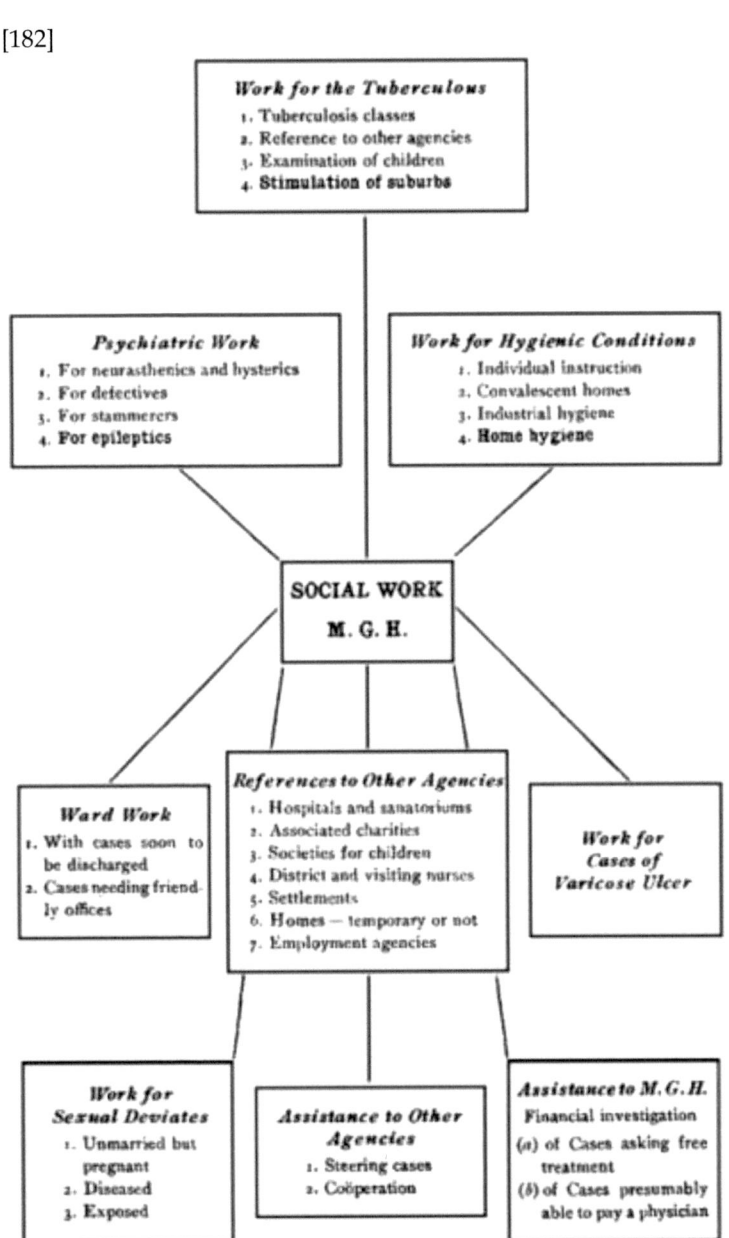

Work for the Tuberculous
1. Tuberculosis classes
2. Reference to other agencies
3. Examination of children
4. Stimulation of suburbs

Psychiatric Work
1. For neurasthenics and hysterics
2. For defectives
3. For stammerers
4. For epileptics

Work for Hygienic Conditions
1. Individual instruction
2. Convalescent homes
3. Industrial hygiene
4. Home hygiene

SOCIAL WORK
M. G. H.

Ward Work
1. With cases soon to be discharged
2. Cases needing friendly offices

References to Other Agencies
1. Hospitals and sanatoriums
2. Associated charities
3. Societies for children
4. District and visiting nurses
5. Settlements
6. Homes — temporary or not
7. Employment agencies

Work for Cases of Varicose Ulcer

Work for Sexual Deviates
1. Unmarried but pregnant
2. Diseased
3. Exposed

Assistance to Other Agencies
1. Steering cases
2. Coöperation

Assistance to M. G. H.
Financial investigation
(a) of Cases asking free treatment
(b) of Cases presumably able to pay a physician

[183]In country districts no plan has yet been worked out for adequate relief. Fortunately, however, the distress is generally of such a kind, and the teacher so well acquainted with all the parents of her district, that it will not be difficult to procure such attention as is necessary. Country schools should be furnished by county and state superintendents with clear directions for getting the treatment afforded in the immediate vicinity. Where teachers are alone in seeing the need for coöperation they can quickly interest young and old, physicians, dentists, pastors, health officers, in home visiting, street cleaning, nursing, helping truants, needed changes of curriculum, etc. *Getting things done* is easy because it is human to love the *doing*; getting things done is *doing* of the highest order.

FOOTNOTES:

[10] The importance of recognizing the family as the unit of social treatment is presented in Edward T. Devine's *Principles of Relief,* and in Homer Folks's *Care of Dependent, Defective, and Delinquent Children.*

[184]

CHAPTER XIXToC

SCHOOL SURGERY AND RELIEF OBJEC-
TIONABLE, IF AVOIDABLE

The popular arguments for free meals, free relief, free medical treatment at school, are based upon the assumption that there are but two ways to travel, one leading to a physically sound, moral, teachable child, the other to an undernourished, subnormal, backward child. They tell us we must choose either school meals or malnutrition, school eyeglasses or defective vision, free coal or freezing poor, free rent or people sleeping on the streets, free dental clinics at school or indigestion and undernourishment, free operation at school for adenoids or backward, discouraged pupils. If there is no other alternative than neglect of the child, if we must either waste fifty dollars in giving a child education that he is physically unable to take, or pay two, three, four, or even fifty dollars to fit him for that education, the American people will not hesitate. Whether there are other roads to healthy children, whether it is cheaper and better for the school to see that outside agencies prepare the child for education rather than itself to take the place of those outside agencies, is a question of fact, not of theory.

Facts prove, as we have seen, that there is more than one way to prevent malnutrition. Parents can be taught to attend to their children; hospitals and dispensaries will furnish eyeglasses where parents are unable to pay for them; charitable societies will go back of the need for eyeglasses to the conditions that produce that need and will do vastly more for the child than can eyeglasses alone. If [185]parents, hospitals, dispensaries, and charitable societies will attend to children's needs, then relief at school is unnecessary, even though it may seem desirable.

The objection to school surgery should be clearly before us, so that we can judge of the two methods that are open to us,— *treatment at school* vs. *treatment away from school.*

Society is so organized that the treatment of serious physical defects and social needs at school would upset the machinery a very great deal. For the school to do for its children whatever they may need during their school years will require the setting up of a miniature society in every school building or under every school board. Unless schools are to equip themselves to take the place of all existing facilities for relief and surgery, children would not be so well taken care of as at present. It should not be forgotten that the physical welfare of the school child is the most accurate index to the physical needs of the community. After all, the child lives for six important years before coming to the school and leaves at the early age of fourteen or fifteen; even while attending school it sleeps at home and is influenced more by home and street standards of ventilation, cleanliness, and morality than by conditions at school. It would seem, therefore, the wider use of the school's influence to use the child's appeal to strengthen every agency having to do with community health, rather than to concentrate upon the child himself. If babies were properly cared for up to the sixth year, the protection of the school child's health would be infinitely easier. To take our eyes from the child not yet in school and from the child just out of school is to make the mistake that so many advocates of the child labor movement have made of going whither and only so far as our interest leads us and of not continuing until our work is accomplished.

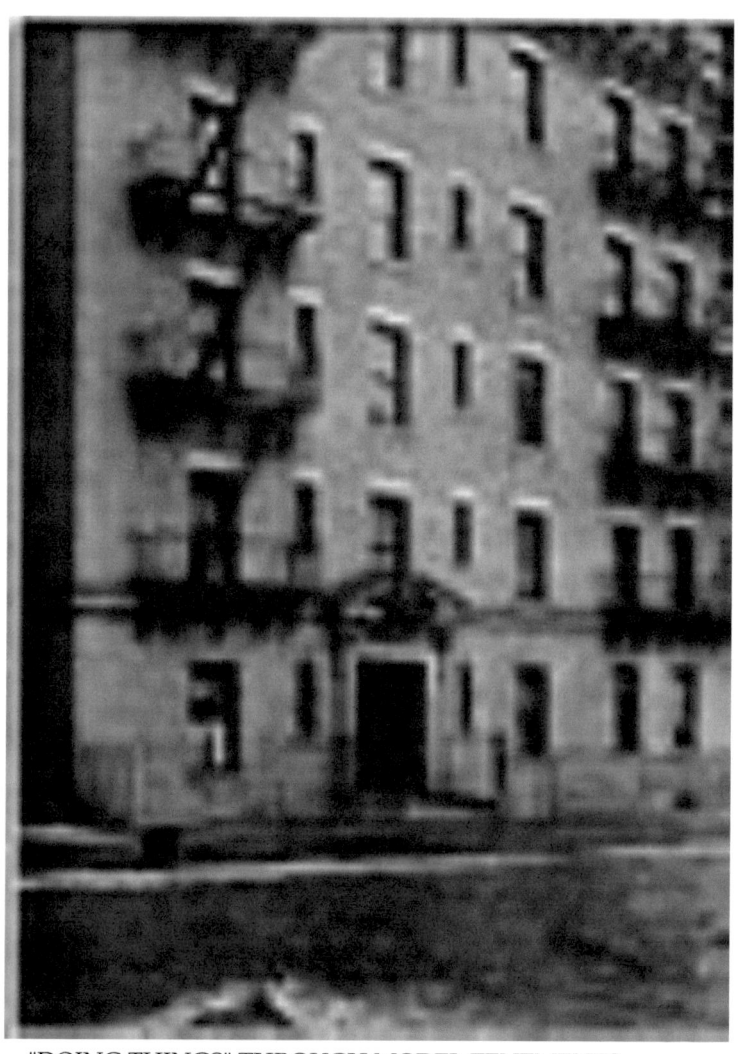

"DOING THINGS" THROUGH MODEL TENEMENTS

Do we want to make of our schools miniature hospitals, dispensaries, relief bureaus, parks? Or shall we use the [186]momentum of society's interest in the school child to put within the reach of every school building adequate hospitals, dispensaries, relief centers, and parks for school child and adult? Shall every little school have its library, or shall the child be taught at school how to use the same library that [187]is available to his parents and older brothers and sisters? If the library is to be under the school roof, if dispensary and relief hospital are to be conducted on the same site as the school, shall they be known as dispensary, library, relief bureau, each under separate management, or shall [188]they be known as school under the management of school principal and superintendent? So complicated and many-sided is the problem of working together with one's neighbor for mutual benefit that it is a safe rule for the schools to adopt: *We shall do nothing that is unnecessary or extravagant. We shall have done our part if we do well what no one else can do. Whatever any agency can do better than we, we shall leave to that agency. Work that another agency ought to have done and has left undone, we shall try to have done by that agency.*

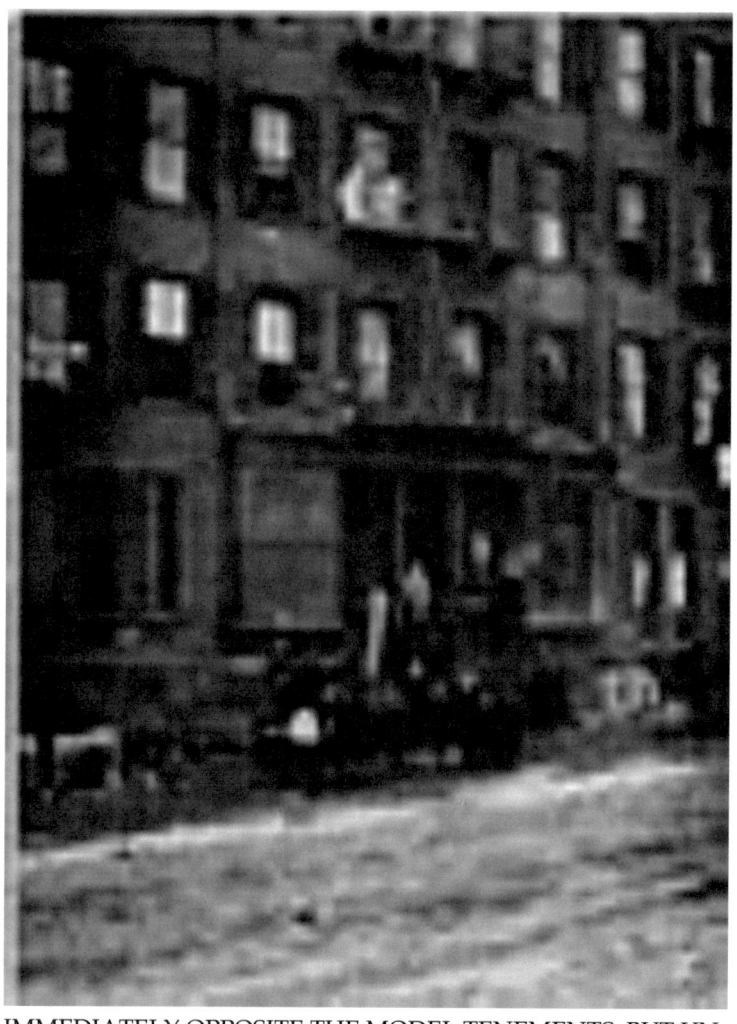

IMMEDIATELY OPPOSITE THE MODEL TENEMENTS, BUT UN-INFLUENCED
"Getting things done" by the Tenement House Department their special need

I know a hospital where a welfare nurse was recently employed. Within a few blocks were three different relief agencies and two visiting-nurse's associations, having among them over one hundred visitors and nurses going to all sections of Manhattan. This nurse had the choice of telephoning to one of these agencies and asking it to call at the needy home of one of her hospital patients, or of going to the home herself. Had she chosen to use another agency, she could have been the means of furnishing the kind of help needed in every needy home discovered in her hospital rounds, but she chose to do the running about herself and thus of helping ten families where she ought to have helped five hundred. Much the same condition confronts the school that tries to do all extra work for its child instead of seeing that the work is done. Illustration is afforded by the New York tenement department. Whereas European cities have built a few model tenements, New York City secured a law declaring that everybody who built a tenement and everybody who owned a tenement should provide sanitary surroundings. At the present time a philanthropist, by spending two million dollars, could give sanitary surroundings to thirty-five families; by spending each year the interest on one tenth that sum he could insure the enforcement of the tenement laws affecting every tenement resident in New York City.

[189]If schools are to perform surgical operations, they are in danger of being sued for malpractice; discipline will be interfered with. Finally, let us not forget that we are dealing with buildings, teachers, and school institutions as they exist. Where education is made compulsory, the unpleasant and the controversial should be kept out of school. Because a democratic institution, the American school should represent at all times a maximum of general agreement.

To take *palliative measures to public schools* not only *leaves undone remedial* work necessary for the health of public school children but *neglects entirely the still large numbers who go to parochial, private pay, and private free schools*; no one has had the temerity to suggest that the public shall force upon nonpublic schools a system of free operations, free eyeglasses, free meals.

Civilization has painstakingly developed a large number of agencies for the education and protection of mankind. Of these agencies the school is but one. Its first and peculiar function is *to teach and to train.* This it can do better than any other agency or combination of agencies. In attempting to "bring all life under the school roof," we use but a small part of our resources. Instead of persuading each of the agencies for the promotion of health to do its part for school children, we set up the school in competition with them. Thus in trying to *do things* for school children we are in danger of crippling agencies equipped to do things for both school children and their parents, for babies before they come to school, and for wage earners after they leave school.

Getting things done will lead schools to study underlying causes; *doing things* has heretofore caused schools to confine themselves to symptoms. *Getting things done* will leave the school free to concentrate its attention upon school problems; *doing things* will lead it afield into the problem of medicine, surgery, restaurant keeping, and practical charity.

[190]

PHYSICAL EXAMINATION FOR WORKING PAPERS

There is no sacred right to work when our work involves injury to ourselves and to our neighbor. Work at the expense of health is an unjustifiable tax upon the state. It is the duty of society to protect itself against such depletion of national efficiency.

Three classes of workmen need special attention: (1) those who are physically unfit to work; (2) those who are physically unfitted for the work they are doing; (3) those who are subjected to unhealthful surroundings while at work. Viewing these three classes from the standpoint of their neighbors, we have three social rights that should be enforced by law: (1) the right to freedom from unhealthy work; (2) the right to work fitted to the body; (3) the right to healthy surroundings at work.

It is undoubtedly true that just as the sick child may be found at the head of his class, so unhealthy men and women are often good business managers, good salesmen, good typewriters, successful capitalists. They excel, however, not because of their ill health, but in spite of it, excepting of course those instances where men and women, because of ill health, have devoted to business an attention that would have been given to recreation if bad health had not deprived recreation of its pleasure. As statistics in school have proved that the majority of mentally superior children are also physically superior, so statistics will probably prove that the number of the "sick superior" among the working classes is very small, while the danger of inefficiency that comes from physical defect is very great.

[191]There is one time in the individual's working life when the state may properly step in and demand an inventory of physical resources, and that is when the child asks the state for permission to go to work. Strategically, this is probably the most important of all

contact as yet provided between society and the future wage earner. Here at the threshold of his industrial career the boy may be told for what work he is physically fitted, what physical defects need to be remedied, what physical precautions he needs to take, in order to do justice to himself and his opportunity.

Every year from two to three million children leave the public schools of this country to join the army of workers. The percentage of those recruits who have physical defects needing attention is undoubtedly great; how great we shall never know until the benefits of physical examination are given to all of them. What steps is your state taking to ascertain the physical fitness of the children who present themselves each year for working papers? How does it insure itself against the risk of their defective eyesight, chorea, deafness, or general debility? Does it inform children of their defects, or tell them how they may increase their earning power by correcting these defects? What effort does it make to induce children to avoid dangerous trades, or trades that are particularly dangerous for their physiques?

At the close of school last spring I had my secretary look in upon the New York board of health and see what demands that city makes upon its boys and girls before allowing them to drive its machinery, to run its elevators, to match its colors, to sew on its buttons, to set its type, to carry its checks to the bank. The officer at the door of the room where the children were being examined, greeted her as follows: "You must bring your child with you; bring his birth certificate or swear that he is fourteen years old, and bring a signed statement from his teacher that he has been in school for one hundred and thirty consecutive days [192]within twelve months." "Is there no physical examination or test?" she asked. "No, no," he answered impatiently. Yet the board of health certifies that "said child has in our opinion reached the normal development of a child of its age, and is in sound health and is physically able to perform the work which it intends to do." In addition the blank calls for place and date of birth, color of hair and of eyes, height, weight, and facial marks. Volunteer societies in practically every state in the Union have been working for years to have it made a criminal offense to employ a child who has not been in school a minimum of days after a stated age (12, 13, 14, 15). Even in New York, however, the center of this agitation, no strong demand was made upon the board of health to apply a physical-fitness test as well as an age test until 1908 when examination for working papers was added to the programme for child hygiene. Yet who does not know girls and boys of sixteen less fit for factory or shop work than other boys and girls of twelve? It is the fetich of age which has made possible the "democracy" that permits a child of fourteen to work all day on condition that he go to school at night!

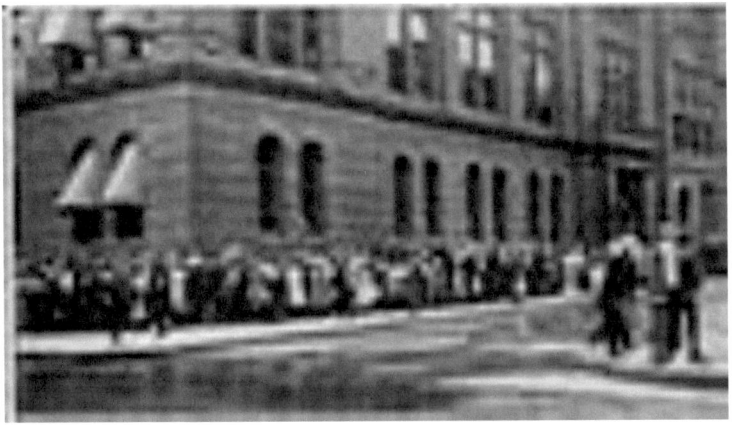

CHILDREN ENLISTING IN THE INDUSTRIAL ARMY

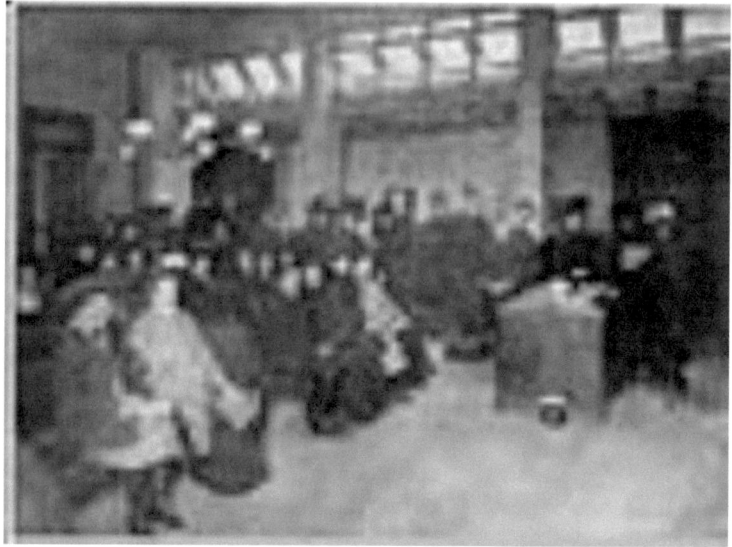

WAITING TO BE EXAMINED FOR WORKING PAPERS
An excellent opportunity for physical-fitness tests

So great is the risk of defective, sickly, or intemperate employees, that in some trades employers take every precaution to exclude them. One man with defective eyesight or unsteady nerves may cost a railroad thousands of dollars. As insurance companies rank trades as first-, second-, or third-class risks, so many factories, from long experience, debar men with certain characteristics which have been found detrimental to business. The Interborough Rapid Transit Company of New York City examines all applicants for employment, as to age, weight, height, keenness of vision, hearing, color perception, lungs, hearts, arteries, alcoholism, and nicotinism. Those who fall below the standard are rejected, but in each case the physical condition is explained to the applicant. Where defects are removable or correctable, the applicant is told what to do and invited to take another test after treatment. Moreover, accepted employees are periodically reëxamined. While designed to [194]increase company profits and to reduce company losses, this examination obviously decreases the employees' losses also, and increases the certainty of work and prospect of promotion.

Our states, and many of our industries, still have the attitude of a certain manufacturer who employs several hundred boys and girls. I asked him what tests he employed. "I look over a long line of the applicants and say," pointing his finger, "I want you, and you, and you; the rest may go." I asked him if he made a point of picking out those who looked strong. "No. The work is easy, sitting down all day long and picking over things. I select those whose faces I like. Yes, there is one question we now ask of all the girls. One day a girl in the workroom had an epileptic fit and it frightened everybody and upset the work so that the foreman always asks, 'Do you have fits? Because if you do, you can't work here.'" He makes no attempt to determine the physical fitness and endurance of the children employed, because when the strength of one is spent there is always another to step into her place.

Because the apprentice's future is of no value to the manufacturer, the state must restrict the manufacturer's freedom to spend like water society's capital, — the health of the coming generation. Could there be a grosser mis-management of society's business than to permit trade to waste children on whose education society spends so many millions yearly? The most effective and most timely remedy is physical examination as a condition of the work certificate. A simple, easily applied, inexpensive measure that imposes only a legitimate restriction upon individual freedom, it is absolutely necessary in order to get to the bottom of the child labor problem. If thoroughly applied, children of the nation will no longer be exploited by unscrupulous or indifferent employers, nor will their health be hazarded by lack of discriminating examination that rejects the obviously sick and favors the apparently robust. Furthermore, knowledge [195]that this test will be applied when work certificates are required, will be an incentive to the school boy and girl to keep well. Tell a boy that adenoids or weak lungs will keep him from getting a job, and you will make him a strong advocate of operation and of fresh air. Show him that his employers will not wish his services when his week is out if he is physically below par, and he will gladly submit to a [196]board of health examination and ask to be told what his defects are and how to correct them.

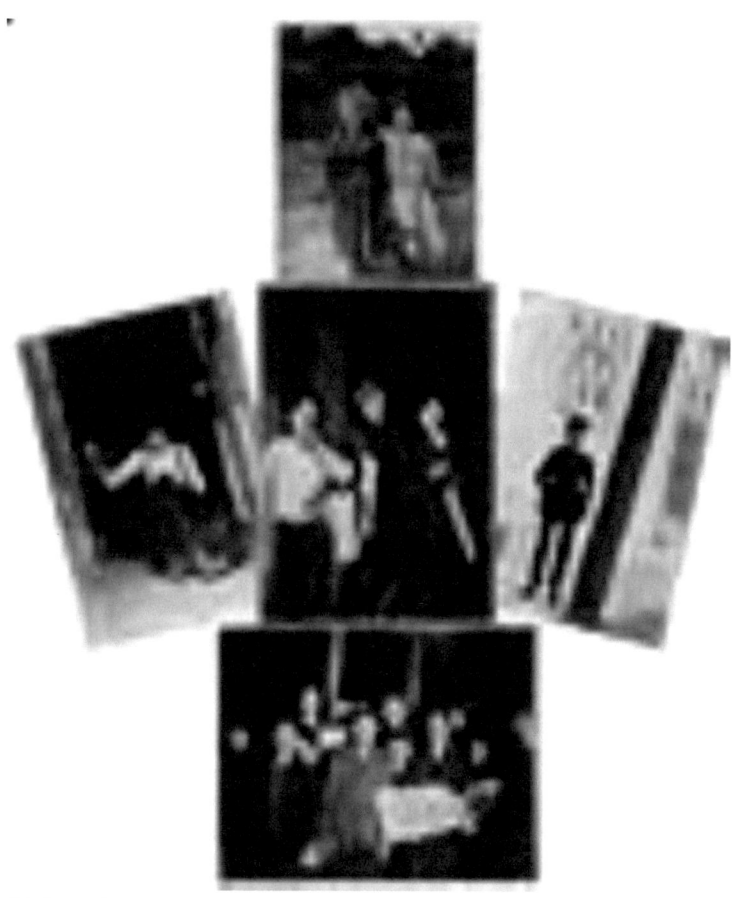

CHILDREN AT WORK BELOW BOTH AGE LIMIT AND VITALI-TY LIMIT

National Child Labor Committee

Some there are who will object to this appeal to the child's economic instinct. This objection does not remove the instinct. The normal child is greedy for a job. His greed, as well as that of the manufacturer and parent, is responsible for much of the child labor; his greed for activity, for association, for money, and so for work. A little boy came into my office and wanted to hire as an office boy. I looked at him and said: "My little fellow, you ought to be in school.

What do you want to hire out here for?" He said, "I am tired of school; nothing doing." He doesn't care about work for its own sake; he doesn't care about wealth for its own sake; he wants to get into life; to be where there is "something doing." In this lies one potent argument for vocational training. To tell a boy of his physical needs just before he has taken his first business step is to put him everlastingly in our debt. Then he is responsive, and, fortunately for the extreme cases, necessarily dependent, for he knows that his refusal would stand between himself and his ambition.

When boys and girls go for work certificates to Dr. Goler, medical officer of health at Rochester, he requires not merely evidence of age and of schooling, but examines their eyes for defective vision and for disease, their teeth for cavities and unhealthy gums, and their noses and throats for adenoids and enlarged tonsils. If a boy has sixteen decayed teeth, Dr. Goler explains to him that teeth are meant to be not only ornaments and conveniences, but money getters as well. The boy learns that decayed teeth breed disease, contaminate food, interfere with digestion, make him a disagreeable companion and a less efficient worker. If he will go and have them put into proper condition he will enjoy life better and earn good wages sooner. After the teeth are attended to the boy secures his work [197]certificate. If the boy's mother protests in tears or in anger that her boy does not work with his teeth, she learns what she never learned at school, that sound teeth help pay the rent. If a girl applicant for working papers has adenoids, she is asked to look in the mirror and to notice how her lips fail to meet, how the lower jaw drops, how much better she looks with her jaws and lips together. She is told that other people breathe through the nose, and that perhaps the reason she dislikes school and does not feel as she used to about play is that she cannot breathe through her nose as she used to. She is shown that her nose is stopped up by a spongy substance, as big as the end of her little finger, which obstruction can be easily removed. She is shown adenoids and enlarged tonsils that have been removed from some other girl, and is so impressed with the before-operation and after-operation contrast and by the story of the other girl's rapid increase in wages, that she and her mother both decide not to wait for the adenoids to disappear by absorption. After the operation they come back with proof that the trouble is gone, and get the "papers." Similar instruction is given when defects of vision seriously interfere with a child's prospects of getting ahead in his work, or when evidence of incipient tuberculosis makes it criminal to put a child in a store or factory.

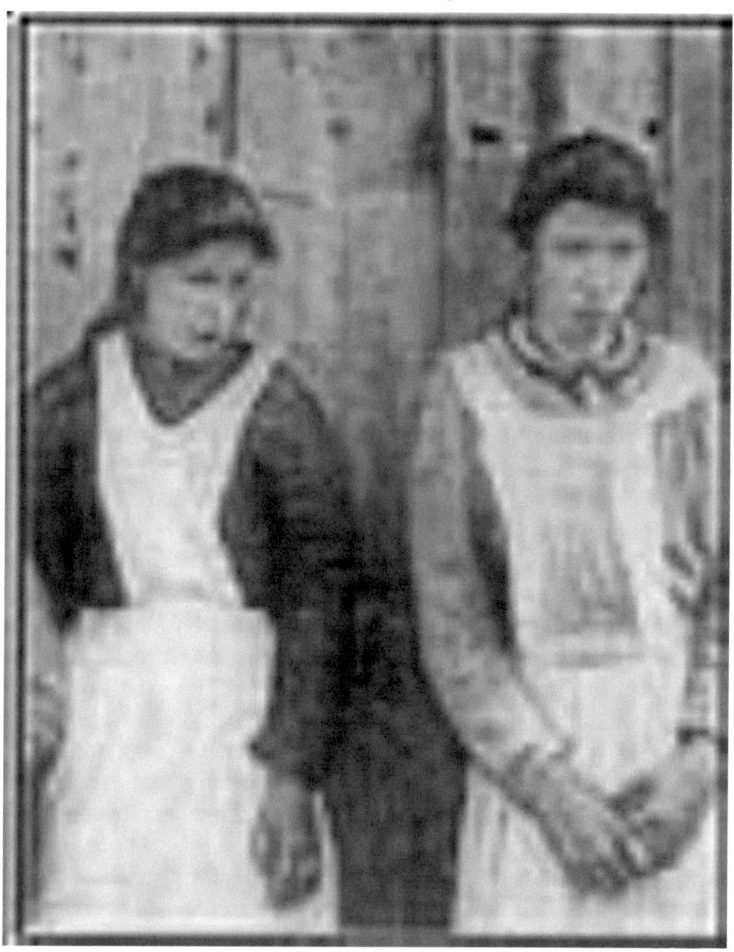

THE GRENFELL ASSOCIATION FINDS MOUTH
BREATHERS AT WORK IN LABRADOR

No law as yet authorizes the health officer of Rochester to refuse work certificates to children physically unfit to become wage earners. A higher law than that which any legislature can pass or revoke, has given Dr. Goler power [198]over children and parents, namely, interest in children and knowledge of the industrial handicap that results from physical defects. This higher law authorizes every health officer in the United States to examine the school child before issuing a work certificate, to tell the child and his parents what defects need to be removed, for what trades he is physically unfitted, what trades will not increase his physical weakness, and to what trade he is physically adapted.

We should not forget that a large proportion of our children never apply for work certificates; some because they never intend to work; some because they expect to remain in school until sixteen or later; some because they live on farms, in small towns, or in cities and states where prohibition of child labor is not enforced. Because there is no reason for this large proportion of children to visit a board of health, some substitute must be found. This substitute has been already suggested by principals and district superintendents in New York City, who claim that the natural place for the examination of children is the school and not health headquarters. Developing the idea that the school should pronounce the child's fitness to leave school and to engage in work, we are led to the suggestion that the state, which compels evidence that every child, rich or poor, is being taught during the compulsory school age, shall also at the age of fourteen or sixteen require evidence that the child is physically fit to use his education, and that it shall not, because of preventable ill health, prove a losing investment.

Parochial and private schools, the ultra-religious and ultra-rich, may resent for a time public supervision of the physical condition of children who do not ask for work certificates. This position will be short-lived, because however much we may disagree about society's right to control a child's act after his physical defects are discovered, few of us will question the state's duty to tell that child and his [199]parents the truth about his physical needs before it accepts his labor or permits him to go to college, to "come out," to "enter society," or to live on an income provided by others. Thus an invaluable commencement present can be given by the state to children in country schools and to those compelled to drop out of fourth or fifth grades of city schools.

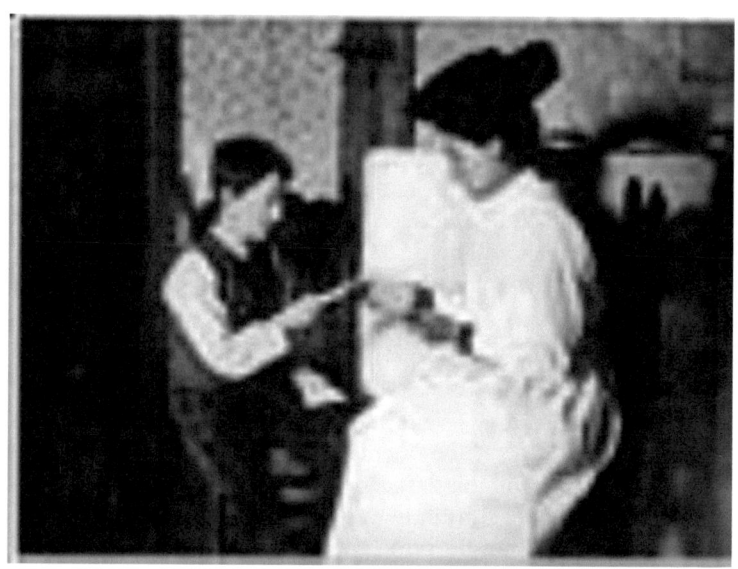

THE HEALTH DEPARTMENT'S CLINICAL CARE AND HOME IN- STRUCTION COME AFTER WAGE LOSSES, WHILE WORK CERTIFI- CATES PRECEDE BREAKDOWNS FROM TUBERCULOSIS

A brief test of this method of helping children, such as is now be- ing made by several boards of health at the instance of the National Bureau of Labor, will prove conclusively that parents are grateful for the timely discovery of these defects which handicap because of their existence, not because of their discovery. Of the cadets prepar- ing for war at West Point, it has recently been decided that those "who in the physical examinations are found to have deteriorated below the prescribed physical standard will be dropped from the rolls of the academy." Shall not cadets preparing [200]for an indus- trial life and citizenship be given at least a knowledge of an ade- quate physical standard? To allow the school child to deteriorate whether before or after going to work is only to waste potential citizenship. Citizens who use themselves up in the mere getting of a living have no surplus strength or interest for overcoming incompetence in civic business, or for achieving the highest aim of citizenship, — the art of self-government for the benefit of all the governed.

[201]

PERIODICAL PHYSICAL EXAMINATION AFTER SCHOOL AGE

Governor Hughes, in his address to the students in Gettysburg College, pleaded for such lives that strength would be left for the years of achievement. How many men and women can you count who are squandering their health bank account? How many do you know who are now physically bankrupt? The man who is prodigal of his health may work along all right for years, never realizing until the test comes that he is running behind in his vitality. The test may be hard times, promotion, exposure to cold, heat, fever, or a sudden call for all his control in avoiding accident. If his vitality fails to stand the test, his career may be ruined, "all for the want of a horseshoe nail": because of no health bank account to draw upon in time of need, — failure; because of vitality depleted by alcohol, tobacco, overeating, underexercise, or too little sleep, — no power to resist contagious diseases; because of ignorance of existing lung trouble, — a year or more of idleness, perhaps poverty for his family; or there is neglected ear or eye trouble, — and thousands of lives may be lost because the engineer failed to read the signals.

Adults are now examined when applying for insurance or accident policies, for work on railroads, for service in the army and on the police and fire forces of cities that provide pensions. It is somewhat surprising that the hundreds of thousands who carry life insurance policies have not realized that a test which is rigorously imposed for business reasons by insurance companies can be applied by individuals for [202]business reasons. Generations hence the state will probably require of every person periodic physical examination after school age. Decades hence business enterprises will undoubtedly require evidence of health and vitality from employees before and during employment, just as schools will require such evidence from teachers. It is, after all, but a step from the police passport to the health passport. Why should we not protect ourselves against enemies to health and efficiency as well as against enemies to order? But for the present we must rely upon the intelligence of individuals to recognize the advantage to themselves, their families, and their employers, of knowing that their bodies do not harbor hidden enemies of vitality and efficiency. From a semi-annual examination of teeth to a semi-annual physical examination is but a short step when once its effectiveness is seen by a few in each community.

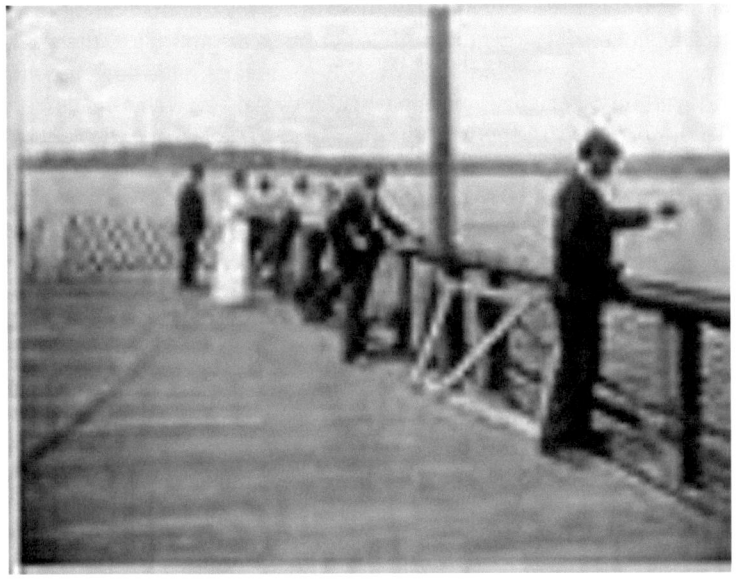

THE OLD SOUTHFIELD, NOW ANCHORED AT BELLEVUE HOSPITAL'S DOCK, NEW YORK CITY, GIVES DAILY LESSONS IN THE PREVENTABLE TAX LEVIED BY TUBERCULOSIS

[203]Ignorance of one's physical condition is a luxury no one can afford. No society is rich enough to afford members ignorant of physical weaknesses prejudicial to others' health and efficiency. Every one of us, even though to all appearances physically normal, needs the biological engineer. New conditions come upon us with

235

terrific rapidity. The rush of work, noise, dust, heat, and overcrowding of modern industry make it important to have positive evidence that we have successfully adapted ourselves to these new conditions. Only by measuring the effects of these environmental forces upon our bodies can we prevent some trifling physical flaw from developing into a chronic or acute condition. As labor becomes more and more highly specialized, the body of the laborer is forced to readapt itself. The kind of work a man does determines which organs shall claim more than their share of blood and energy. The man who sets type develops keenness of vision and manual dexterity. The stoker develops the muscles of his arms and back, the engineer alertness of eye and ear. All sorts of devices have been invented to aid this specialization of particular organs, as well as to correct their imperfections: the magnifying glass, the telescope, the microscope, extend the powers of the eye; the spectacle or an operation on the eye muscles enables the defective eye to do normal work. A man with astigmatism might be a policeman all his life, win promotion, and die ignorant of his defect; whereas if the same man had become a chauffeur, he might have killed himself and his employer the first year, or, if an accountant, he might have been a chronic dyspeptic from long-continued eye strain. It is a soul tragedy for a man to attempt a career for which he is physically unadapted.[11] It is a social tragedy when men and women squander their health. A great deal of the success attributed to luck and opportunity, or unusual [204]mental endowment, is in reality due to a chance compatibility of work with physique. To secure such compatibility is the purpose of physical examination after school age.

If the periodic visit to the doctor is the first law of adult health, still more imperative is the law that competent physicians should be seen at the first indication of ill health. Even when competent physicians are at hand, parents and teachers should be taught what warning signs may mean and what steps should be taken. In Germany insurance companies find that it saves money to provide free medical and dental care for the insured. Department stores, many factories and railroads, have learned from experience that they save money by inducing their employees to consult skilled physicians at the first sign of physical disorder. Many colleges, schools, and "homes" have a resident physician. Wherever any large number of people are assembled together,—in a hotel, factory, store, ship, college, or school,—there should be an efficient consulting physician at hand. If people are needlessly alarmed, it is of the utmost importance to show them that there is nothing seriously wrong. Therefore visits to the consulting physician should be encouraged.

The reader's observation will suggest numerous illustrations of pain, prolonged sickness, loss of life, that could have been prevented had the physician been semi-annually visited. A strong man, well educated, with large income, personally acquainted with several of the foremost physicians of New York City, after suffering two weeks from pains "that would pass away," was hurriedly taken to a hospital at three o'clock in the morning, operated upon immediately, and died at nine. A business man of means put off going to a physician for fifteen years, for fear he would be told that his throat trouble was tobacco cancer, or incipient tuberculosis, or asthma; a physical examination showed that a difficulty of breathing and chronic throat [205]trouble were due to a growth in the nose, corrected in a few minutes by operation.

A celebrated economist was forced to give up academic work, and consecrated his life to painful and chronic dyspepsia because of eye trouble detected upon the first physical examination. A woman secretary suffered from alleged heart trouble; paralysis threatened, continuous headache and blurred vision forced her to give up work and income; a physical examination found the cause in nasal growths, whose removal restored normal conditions. A woman lecturer on children's health heard described last summer a friend's experience with receding gums: "'Why, I never heard of that disease.' she said. 'Don't you know you have it yourself'? I asked. She had never noticed that her gums were growing away in little points on her front teeth. I touched the uncovered portion and she winced. That ignorance has meant intense pain and ugly fillings. If it had gone longer, it might have meant the loss of her front teeth." A teacher lost a month from nervous prostration; physical examination would have discovered the eye trouble that deranged the stomach and produced the nerve-racking shingles which forced him to take a month's vacation. A journalist lost weeks each year because of strained ankles; since being told that he had flat foot, and that the arch of his foot could be strengthened by braces and specially made shoes, he has not lost a minute. A relief visitor, ardent advocate of the fresh-air, pure-milk treatment for tuberculosis, had a "little cough" and an occasional "cold sweat"; medical friends knew this, but humored her aversion to examination; when too late, she submitted to an examination and to the treatment which, if taken earlier, would most certainly have cured her. A mother's sickness cost a wage-earning daughter nearly $3000; softening of the brain was feared; after six years of suffering and unnecessary expense, physical examination disclosed an easily removable cause, [206]and for two years she has contributed to the family income instead of exhausting it. Untold suffering is saved many a mother by knowledge of her special physical need in advance [207]of her baby's birth. Untold suffering might be saved many a woman in business if she could be told in what respects she was transgressing Nature's law.

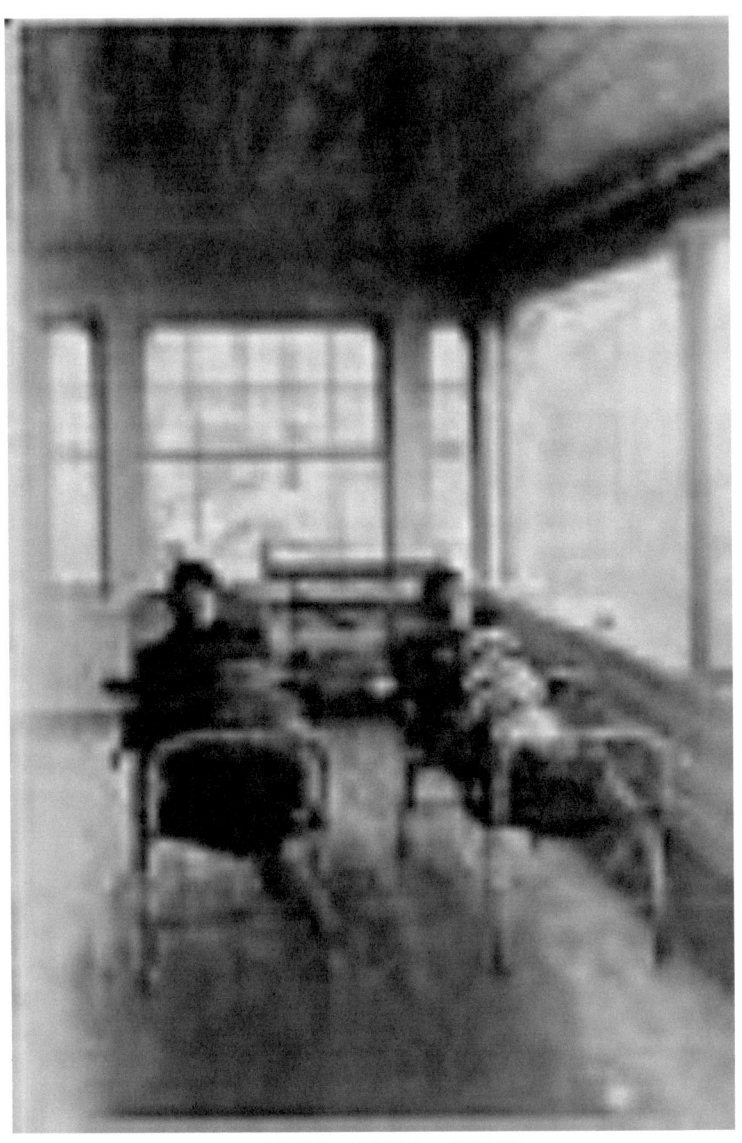

NEW YORK CITY'S
TUBERCULOSIS SANA-
TORIUM AT OTISVILLE

IS SENDING HOME
APOSTLES OF SEMI-
ANNUAL EXAMINA-
TIONS

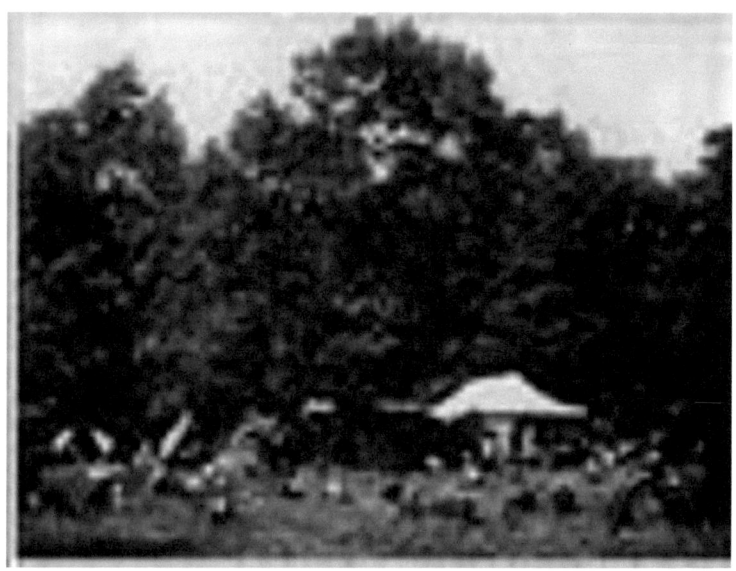

BOSTON'S PICTURESQUE DAY
CAMP FOR TUBERCULOSIS PA-
TIENTS IS TEACHING THE NEED
FOR A PERIODIC INVENTORY OF
PHYSICAL RESOURCES

To encourage periodic physical examination is not to encourage morbid thinking of disease. One reason for our tardiness in recognizing the need for thorough physical examination is the doctor's tradition of treating symptoms. After men and women are intelligent enough to demand an inventory of their physical resources, — a balance sheet of their physical assets and liabilities, — physicians will study the whole man and not the fraction of a man in which they happen to be specializing or about which the patient worries. By removing the mystery of bodily ailments and by familiarizing ourselves with the essentials to healthy living, we find protection against charlatans, quacks, faddists, and experimenters. By taking a periodic inventory of our physical resources we discharge a sacred obligation of citizenship.

FOOTNOTES:

[11] See *Dangerous Trades*, compiled by Thomas Oliver; also list of reports by the United States Bureau of Labor.

[208]

HABITS OF HEALTH PROMOTE INDUSTRI-
AL EFFICIENCY

Education's highest aim is to train us to do the right thing at the right moment without having to think. The technic of musician, stenographer, artist, electrician, surgeon, orator, is gained only from patient training of the body's reflex muscles to do brain work.[12] The lower nerve centers are storehouses for the brain energy, just as central power houses are used for storing electric energy to be spent upon demand. From habit, not from mental effort, we turn to the right, say "I beg pardon" when we step on another's foot, give our seats to ladies or to elderly persons, use acceptable table manners. No person seems "to the manner born" who has to think out each act necessary to "company manners." How numerous are the mental and physical processes essential to good manners no one ever recognizes but the very bashful or the uncouth person trying to cultivate habits of unconsciousness in polite society. The habit of living ethically enables us to go through life without being tempted to steal or lie or do physical violence. No person's morals can be relied upon who is tempted constantly to do immoral acts; ethical training seeks to incapacitate us for committing unethical deeds and to habituate us to ethical acts alone.

Eight different elements of industrial efficiency are concerned with the individual's health habits,—the industrial worker, his industrial product, his employer, his employer's [209]profit, his trade or profession, its product, his nation, national product. Obviously few men have so little to do that they have time to think out in detail how this act or that indulgence will affect each of these eight factors of industrial efficiency. Once convinced, however, that all of these elements are either helped or injured by the individual's method of living, each one of us has a strong reason for imposing habits of health upon all industries, upon employees and operatives, upon all who are a part of industrial efficiency. When these eight relations are seen, parents and teachers have particularly strong reasons for inculcating habits of health in their children.

That industrial inefficiency results from chronic habits of unhealthy living is generally recognized. The alcoholic furnishes the most vivid illustration. The penalties suffered by him and his family are grave enough, but because he has not full possession of his faculties he is unpunctual, wastes material, disobeys instructions, endangers others' lives, decreases the product of his trade and of his employer, lessens the profits of both, depresses wages, increases insurance and business risks. Because no one can foresee when the "drop too much" will be taken, industry finds it important to know that the habit of drinking alcoholics moderately has not been acquired by train dispatcher, engineer, switchman, chauffeur. Because the habit of drinking moderately is apt, among lower incomes, to go hand in hand with other habits injurious to business and fatal to integrity, positions of trust in industry seek men and women who have the habit of declining drink.

In the aggregate, milder forms of unhealthy living interfere with industrial efficiency even more than alcoholism. Many capable men and women, even those who have had thorough technical training, fail to win promotion because their persons are not clean, their breath offensive, their clothes suggestive of disorderly, uncleanly habits. Persons [210]of extraordinary capacity not infrequently achieve only mediocre results because they fail to cultivate habits of cleanliness and health. An employer can easily protect his business from loss due to alcoholism among his own employees; but loss through employees' constipation, headache, bad ventilation at home, irregular meals, improper diet, too many night parties, nicotinism, personal uncleanliness, is loss much harder to anticipate and avoid. Because evil results are less vivid, it is also hard to convince a clerk that intemperance in eating, sleeping, and playing will interfere with his earning capacity and his enjoyment capacity quite as surely as intemperance in the use of alcohol and nicotine. Where employees are paid by the piece, instead of by the hour, day, or week, the employer partially protects himself against uneven, sluggish, slipshod workmen; but, other things being equal, he awards promotion to those who are [211]most regular and who are most often at their best, for he finds that the man who does not "slump" earns best profits and deserves highest pay.

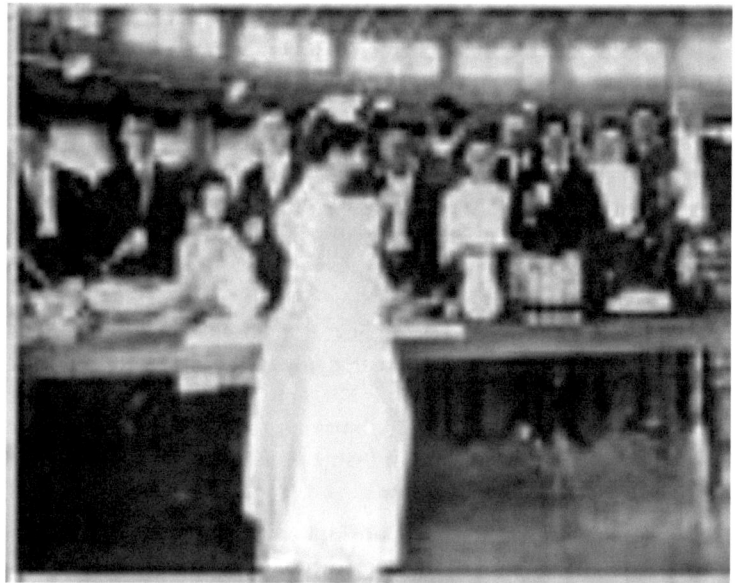

THESE PATIENTS ON THE OLD SOUTHFIELD ARE TAXING THEIR UNIONS AND THEIR TRADES AS WELL AS THEIR FAMILIES AND THE TUBERCULOSIS COMMITTEE

There are exceptions, it is true, where both industrial promotion and industrial efficiency are won by people who violate laws of health, — but at what cost to their efficiency? Your efficiency should be measured not by some other person's advancement, but by what you yourself ought to accomplish; while the effect of abusing your physical strength is shown not only in the shortening of your industrial life and in the diminishing returns from your labor, but by the decrease of national and trade efficiency. "Sweating" injures those who buy and those in the same trade who are not "sweated" just as truly as it injures the "sweated."

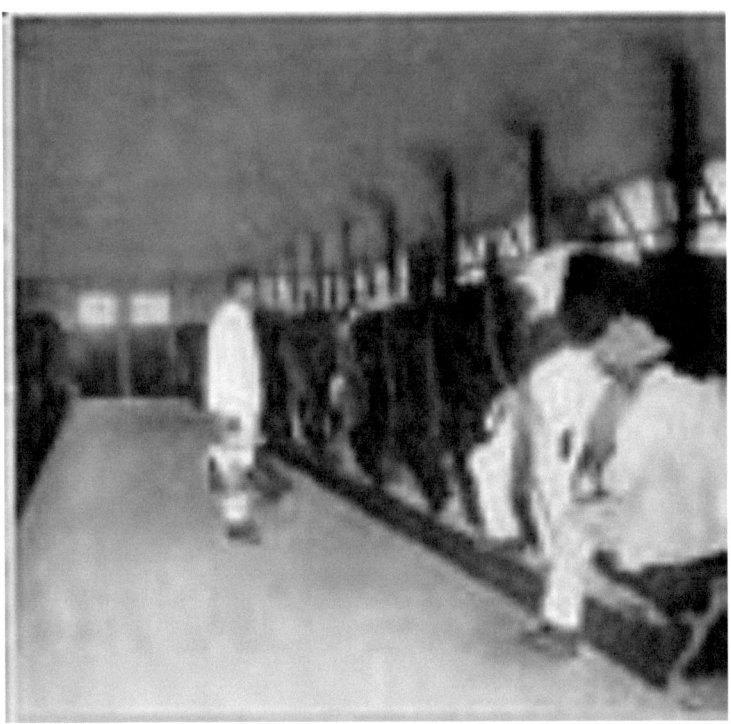

HABITS OF HEALTH AMONG DAIRYMEN MEAN SAFE MILK FOR BABIES

[212]What are the health habits that should become instinctive and effortless for every worker? What acts can we make our lower nerve centers—our subconscious selves—do for us or remind us to do? The following constitutes a daily routine that should be as involuntary as the process of digestion:

1. Throw the bedding over the foot of the bed.

2. Close the window that has been open during the night.

3. Drink a glass of water.

4. Bathe the face, neck, crotch, chest, armpits (finishing if not beginning with cold water), and particularly the eyes, ears, and nose. If time and conveniences permit, bathe all over.

5. Cleanse the finger nails.

6. Cleanse the teeth, especially the places that are out of sight and hard to reach.

7. Breakfast punctually at a regular hour. Eat lightly and only what agrees with you. If you read a morning paper, be interested in news items that have to do with personal and community vitality.

8. Visit the toilet; if impracticable at home, have a regular time at business.

9. Have several minutes in the open air, preferably walking.

10. Be punctual at work.

11. As your right by contract, insist upon a supply of fresh air for your workroom with the same emphasis you use in demanding sufficient heat in zero weather.

12. Eat punctually at noon intermission; enjoy your meal and its after effects.

13. Breathe air out of doors a few minutes, preferably walking.

14. Resume business punctually.

15. Stop work regularly.

16. Take out-of-door exercise—indoor only when fresh air is possible—that you enjoy and that agrees with you.

17. Be regular, temperate, and leisurely in eating the evening meal; eat nothing that disagrees with you.

18. Spend the evening profitably and pleasantly and in ways compatible with the foregoing habits.

[213]19. Retire regularly at a fixed hour, making up for irregularity by an earlier hour next night.

20, 21, 22. Repeat 4, 6, 8.

23. Turn underclothes wrong side out for ventilation.

24. Open windows.

25. Relax mind and body and go to sleep.

No man chronically neglects any one of the above rules without reducing his industrial efficiency. No man chronically neglects all of them without becoming, sooner or later, a health bankrupt.

In addition to this daily routine, there are certain other acts that should become habitual:

1. Bathing less frequently than once a week is almost as dangerous to health as it is to attractiveness.

2. Distaste for unclean linen or undergarments and for acts or foods that interfere with vitality should become instinctive.

3. Excesses in eating or playing should be automatically corrected the next day and the next. Parties we shall continue to have. It will be some time before reasonable hours and reasonable refreshments will prevail. Meanwhile it is probably better for an individual to sacrifice somewhat his own vitality for the sake of the union, the class, or the church. While trying to improve group habits, one can acquire the habit of not eating three meals in one, of eating less next day, of sleeping longer next night, of being particularly careful to have plenty of outdoor air.

4. Visits to the dentist twice a year at least, and whenever a cavity appears, even if only a week after the dentist has failed to find one; whenever the gums begin to recede; and whenever anything seems to be wrong with the teeth.

5. Periodic physical examination by a physician.

6. Examination by a competent physician whenever any disorder cannot be satisfactorily explained by violation of the daily routine or by interruption of business or domestic routine.

Health habits do not become instinctive until a continued, conscious effort is made to accustom the body to them. When this is once done, however, the body not only [214]attends to its primary health needs automatically, but it rebels at their omission, as surely as does the stomach at the omission of dinner. Witness the discomfort of the consumptive, trained to fresh air at a sanatorium, when he returns to his overheated and underventilated home, or the actual pain experienced in readjusting our own healthy bodies to the stuffy workroom or schoolroom after a summer vacation out of doors. I heard a consumptive say that he left a sanatorium for a day class after trying for three nights to sleep in an unventilated ward. For many people the regular morning bath is at first a trial, then a pleasure, and finally a need; if omitted, the body feels thirsty and dissatisfied, the eyes sleepy, and the spirit flags early in the day.

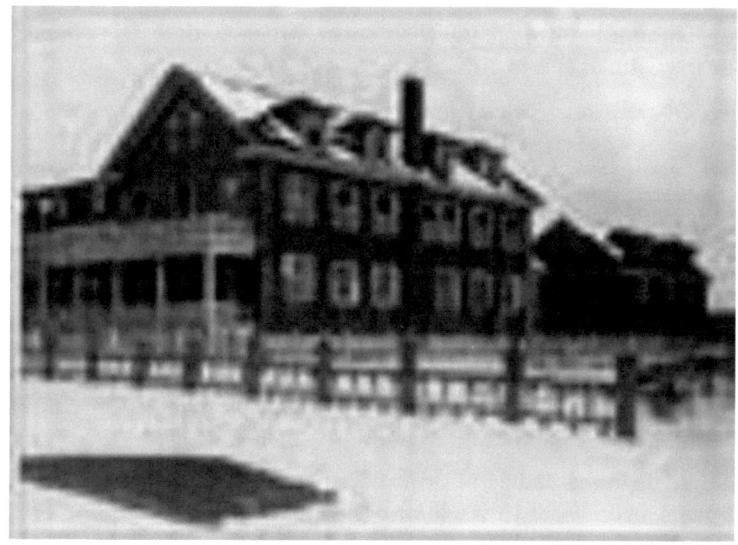

IMPROVISED SEASIDE HOSPITAL FOR NONPULMONARY TUBERCULOSIS AT SEA BREEZE TEACHES PASSERS-BY THE FRESH-AIR GOSPEL

Cold baths are not essential or even good for everybody. The same diet or the same amount of food or time for eating is not of equal value for all. The temperature of bath [215]water, the kind and quality of food, are influenced by one's work and one's cook. Set rules about these things do more harm than good. Such questions must be decided for each individual,—by his experience or by the advice of a physician,—but they must be decided and the decisions converted into health habits if he would attain the highest efficiency of which he is capable. Here again our old contrast between "doing things" and "getting things done" applies. Get your body to attend to the essential needs for you, and get it to remind you when you let the exigencies of life interfere. Don't burden your mind every day with work that your body will do for you if properly trained.

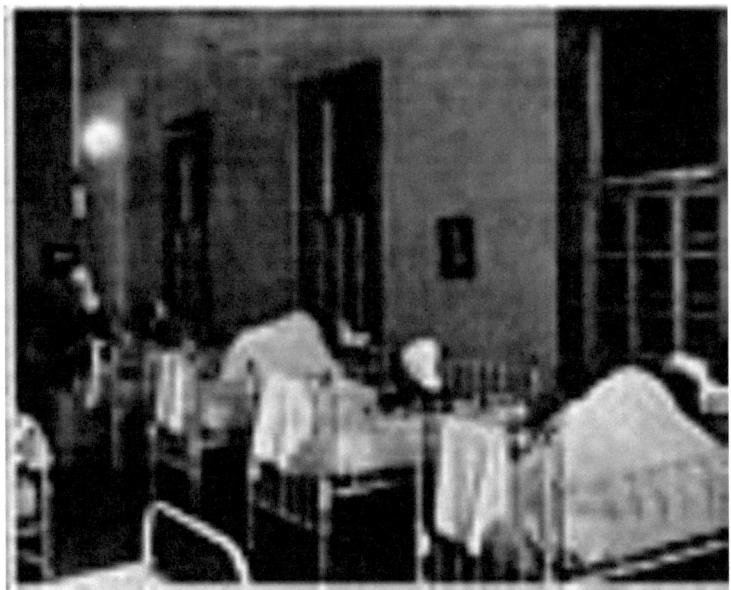

CRIPPLED CHILDREN LEAVING SEA BREEZE HOSPITAL FOR BONE TUBERCULOSIS FIND STALE AIR OFFENSIVE BY NIGHT OR BY DAY

Obstacles to habits of health are numerous; therefore the importance of correcting those habits of factory, family, trade, city, or nation that make health habits impracticable. [216]We must change others' prejudices before we can breathe clean air on street cars without riding outside. When one's co-workers are afraid of fresh air, ventilation of shop, store, and office is impossible. So long as parents fear night air, children cannot follow advice to sleep with windows open. Unless the family coöperates in making definite plans for the use of toilet and bath for each member, constipation and bad circulation are sure to result. Indigestion is inevitable if employees are not given lunch periods and closing hours that permit of regular, unhurried meals. Cleanliness of person costs more than it seems to be worth where cities fail either to compel bath tubs in rented apartments or to erect public baths. A temperate subsistence on adulterated, poisonous, or drugged foods might be better for one's health than gormandizing on pure foods. No recipe has ever been found for bringing up a healthy baby on unclean, infected milk; for avoiding tuberculosis among people who are [217]compelled to work with careless consumptives in unclean air; or for making a five-story leap as safe as a fire escape. Perfect habits of health on the part of an individual will not protect him against enervation or infection resulting from inefficient enforcement of sanitary codes by city, county, state, and national authorities.

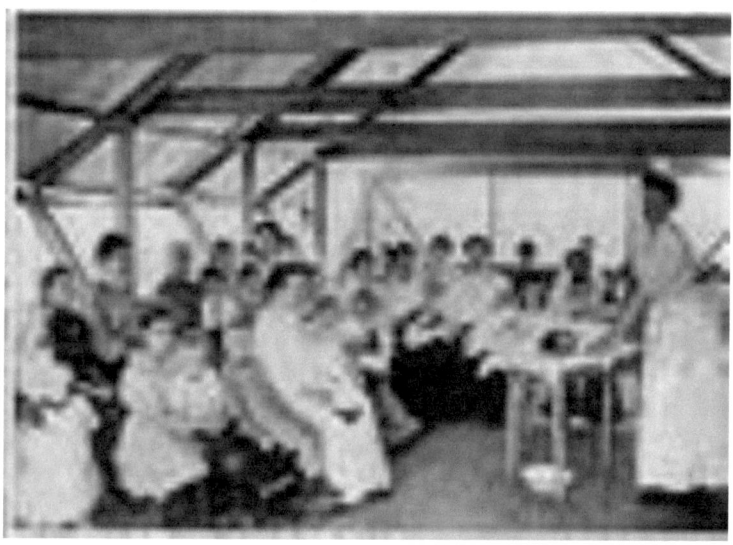

AT JUNIOR SEA BREEZE, TEACH-
ING MOTHERS THE HEALTH ROU-
TINE FOR BABIES

The "municipalization" or "public subsidy" of health habits is indispensable to protecting industrial efficiency. Public lavatories, above or below ground, have done much to reduce inefficiency due to alcoholism, constipation of the bowels, and congestion of the kidneys. Theaters, churches, and assembly rooms could be built so as to drill audiences in habits of health instead of fixing habits of uncleanly breathing. Street flushing, drinking fountains, parks and breathing spaces, playgrounds and outdoor gymnasiums, milk, food, and drug inspection, tenement, factory, and shop supervision, enforcement of anti-spitting penalties, restriction of hours of labor, prohibition of child labor,—these inculcate community habits of health that promote community efficiency. It is the duty of health boards to compel all citizens under their jurisdiction to cultivate habits of health and to punish all who persistently refuse to acquire these habits, so far as the evils of neglect become apparent to health authorities. The unlimited educational opportunity of health boards consists in their privilege to point out repeatedly and cumulatively the industrial and community benefits that result from habits of health, and the industrial and community losses that result from habits of unhealthy living.

FOOTNOTES:

[12] Serviceable guides to personal habits of health are *Aristocracy of Health* by Mary Foote Henderson, and *Efficient Life* by Dr. Luther H. Gulick.

[218]

INDUSTRIAL HYGIENE

To call the movement for better factory conditions the "humanizing of industry" implies that modern industry not influenced by that movement is brutalized. The brutalizing of industry was due chiefly to a general ignorance of health laws, — an ignorance that registers itself clearly and promptly in factory and mine. It is not that a man is expected to do too much, but that too little is expected of the human body. The present recognition of the body's right to vitality is not because the employer's heart is growing warmer, or because competition is less vicious, but because the precepts of hygiene are found to be practical. Where better ventilation used to mean more windows and repair bills, it now means greater output. Where formerly a comfortable place in which to eat lunch meant giving up a workroom and its profits, it now means 25 per cent more work done in all workrooms during the afternoon. The general enlightenment as to industrial hygiene has been accelerated by the awakening that always follows industrial catastrophes, by the splendid crusade against tuberculosis, and by compulsory notification and treatment of communicable diseases.

Catastrophes, however, have dominated the vocabulary that describes factory "welfare work." Because accidents such as gas in mines, fire in factories, fever in towns, and epidemics of diseases incident to certain trades were beyond the power of the workers themselves to control or prevent, wage earners have come to be looked upon as helpless victims of the cupidity and inhumanity of their employers. [219]This attitude has weakened the usefulness of many bodies organized to promote industrial hygiene. Although the term "industrial hygiene" is broad enough to include all sanitary and hygienic conditions that surround the worker while at work, it is restricted by some to the efforts made by altruistic or farsighted employers in the interest of employees; others think of prohibitions and mandates, in the name of the state, that either prevent certain evils or compel certain benefits; for too few it refers to what the wage earner does for himself.

Pity for the employee has caused the motive power of the employee to be wastefully allowed to atrophy. Yet when a man becomes an employee, he does not forfeit any right of citizenship, nor does being an employee relieve him from the duties of citizenship. In too many cases it has been overlooked that a worker's carelessness about habits of health, as well as about his machinery, causes accidents and increases industrial diseases. Too often the worker himself is responsible for uncleanliness and lack of ventilation and his own consequent lack of vitality. A study into the conditions of ventilation and cleanliness of workers' homes will prove this.

Knowing that a light, well-aired, clean, safe factory would not of itself insure healthy men, many employers have built and supplied houses for their workmen at low rents. Just as these employers failed to see that they could reach more people and secure more permanent results if they demanded that tenement laws and the sanitary code be enforced as well as the laws for the instruction of children in hygiene, so the employee has failed to see that he is a part of the public that passes laws and determines the efficiency of factory inspection. The enforcement of state legislation for working hours, proper water and milk supply, proper teaching of children, proper tenement conditions, efficient health administration, is dependent upon the interest and [220]activity of the public, of which the working class is no small or uninfluential part.

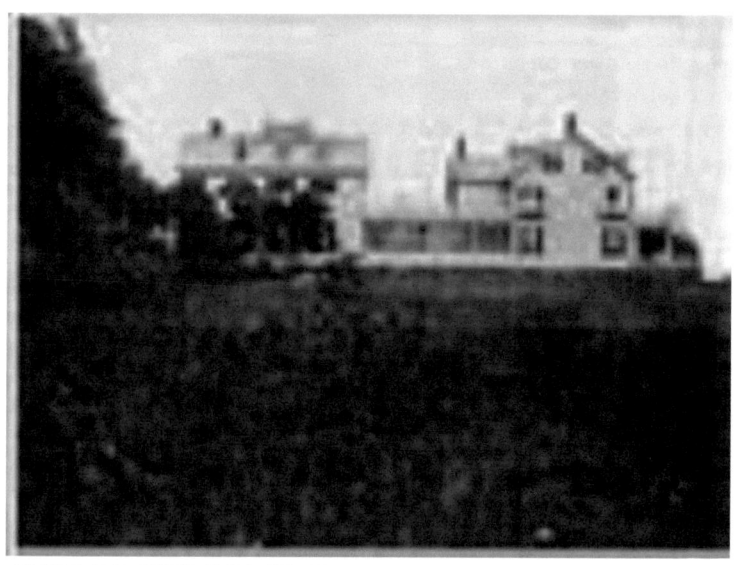

COUNTRY CLUB HOUSE FOR NEW YORK SOCIAL WORKERS
Given by the founder of Caroline Rest Educational Fund

The first and most important step in securing hygienic rights for workingmen is to make sure that they know the rights that the law already gives them. Men still throw out their chests when talking of their rights. The posting of the game laws in a club last summer, and the instruction of all the natives of the countryside in regard to their rights as against those of outsiders, meant that for the first time in their history the game laws were enforced. All the natives, instead of poaching as has been their wont, joined together in protecting club property from intruding outside sportsmen. Poachers were caught and served with the full penalties of the law. Over winter fires these people's heroism will grow, but their respect for law will grow also, and it is doubtful if the game laws can be violated in that section so long as the tradition of this summer's work [221]lives. And so it would be in a factory, if employees once realized that by uniting they could, as citizens, enforce health rights in the factory.

The hygiene of the workshop is not the same problem as the hygiene of the home and schoolhouse, because there are by-products of factory work that contaminate the air, overheat the room, and complicate the ordinary problems of ventilation. Certain trades are recognized as "dangerous trades." The problem of adequate government control of factories is one for a sanitary engineer. It has to do with disease-bearing raw material that comes to a factory, disease-producing processes of manufacture. There is need for revision of the dangerous-trade list. Many of the industries not so classed should be; many of the so-called dangerous trades can be made comparatively harmless by devices for exhausting harmful by-products. Industrial diseases should be made "notifiable," so that they can be controlled by the factory or health department. It is those trades that are dangerous because of remediable unsanitary and unhygienic conditions which demand the employer's attention. Complaints should be made by individuals when carelessness or danger becomes commonplace.

The manner in which many organizations have tried to better working conditions is similar to the manner in which Europeans are trying to help defective school children. Here, as there, is the difference between *doing things* and *getting things done*. Here more than there is the tendency to exaggerate legislation and to neglect enforcement of law. Instead of harnessing the whole army of workingmen to the crusade and strengthening civic agencies such as factory, health, and tenement departments, houses are built and given to men, clubs are formed to amuse factory girls, amateur theatricals are organized. All this is called "welfare work." "What is welfare work?" reads the pamphlet of a large national association. "It is especial consideration [222]on the part of the employer for the welfare of his employees." In the words of this pamphlet, the aim of this association "is to organize the best brains of the nation in an educational movement toward the solution of some of the great problems related to social and industrial progress." The membership is drawn from "practical men of affairs, whose acknowledged leadership in thought and business makes them typical representatives of business elements that voluntarily work together for the general good." As defined by this organization, welfare work is something given to the employee by the employer for the welfare of both. It is not something the employee himself does to improve his own working conditions.

We are told that employees should assume the management of welfare work.

Should they install sanitary conveniences? Of course not.

Would they know the need of a wash room in a factory if they never had had one? No.

Should they manage lunch rooms? A few employers have attempted unsuccessfully to turn over the management of the lunch rooms to the employees, the result being that one self-sacrificing subofficial in each concern would find the burden entirely on his shoulders before working hours, during working hours, and after working hours. Employees cannot attend committee meetings during working hours, and they are unwilling to do so afterwards, for they generally have outside engagements. Furthermore, the employees know nothing about the restaurant business. If they did, they would probably be engaged in it instead of in their different trades. All experiments along this line of which we have heard have failed. The so-called "democratic idea," purely a fad, never has been successfully operated.

Many employers would introduce welfare work into their establishments were it not for the time and trouble needed for its organization. The employment of a welfare director removes this obstacle. Successful prosecution of welfare work requires concentration of responsibility. All of its branches must be under the supervision of one person, or efforts in different directions may conflict, or special and perhaps pressing needs may escape attention. Pressure of daily business routine usually relegates welfare work to the last consideration, but the average employer is interested in his men and is willing to improve their condition if only their needs are brought to his attention.

[223]

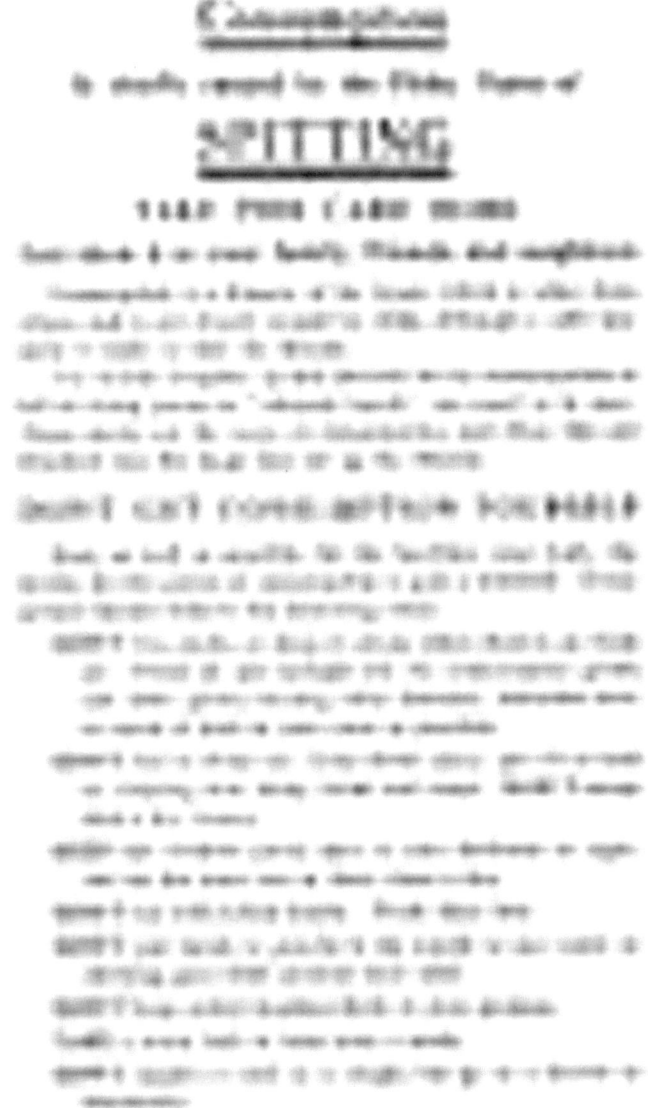

FIRST LESSONS IN INDUSTRIAL HYGIENE

HOW TO GET WELL IF YOU HAVE CONSUMPTION

If you or any one in your family have consumption, you must obey the following rules if you wish to get well:

DON'T waste your money on patent medicines or advertised cures for consumption, but go to a doctor or dispensary (see last page). If you go in time, you can be cured; if you wait, it may be too late.

DON'T drink whisky or other forms of liquor.

DON'T sleep in the same bed with any one else, and, if possible, not in the same room.

Good food, fresh air, and rest are the best cures. Keep out in the fresh air and in the sunlight as much as possible.

KEEP your windows open winter and summer, day and night.

IF properly wrapped up you will not catch cold.

GO to a sanatorium while you can and before it is too late.

The careful and clean consumptive is not dangerous to those with whom he lives and works.

Don't give consumption to others.

Many grown people and children have consumption without knowing it, and can give it to others. Therefore every person, even if healthy, should observe the following rules:

DON'T SPIT on the sidewalks, playgrounds, or on the floors or hallways of your home or school. It spreads disease, and is dangerous, indecent, and unlawful.

WHEN YOU MUST SPIT, spit in the gutters or into a spittoon half filled with water.

DON'T COUGH OR SNEEZE without holding a handkerchief or your hand over your mouth or nose

WELFARE WORK THAT COUNTS

[225]This method of promoting the welfare of the worker may have been a necessary step in the development of industrial hygiene. Undoubtedly it has succeeded, in many cases, in bringing to an employer's consciousness the needs of his workmen, in accustoming employees to higher sanitary standards, and in teaching them to demand health rights from their employers. In many cases, however, "welfare work" has miseducated both employer and employee. The fact that "the so-called democratic idea, purely a fad, has never been successfully operated," is due to the interpretation given to "democratic idea." The two alternatives in the paragraph above quoted are lunch rooms, wash rooms, as gifts from employers to employees, or lunch rooms and wash rooms to be furnished by employees at their own expense. The true democratic idea, however, is that factory conditions detrimental to health shall be prohibited by factory legislation, and this legislation enforced by efficient factory inspectors, regardless of what may be given to employees above the requirement of hygiene.

Until employees are more active as citizens and more sensitive to hygienic rights, it is desirable that welfare directors be employed in factories to arbitrate between employer and employee, to raise the moral standard of a factory settlement, to organize amusements.

Welfare work at its best is a method of dividing business profits among all who participate in making these profits. Too often welfare secretaries teach employees how to be happy in the director's way, rather than in their own way. This adventitious position increases suspicion on both sides, [226]disturbs the discipline of the foreman, weakens rather than strengthens the worker's efficiency, because it depends upon other things than work well done and the relation of health to efficiency. In a small factory town the owner of a large cotton mill has recognized the financial benefit of physically strong workers, and is trying the experiment of a welfare director. The man himself works "with his sleeves up." The social worker has an office in the factory. A clubhouse is fitted up for the mill hands to make merry in. A room in the factory is reserved for a lunch room, with plants, tables, and chairs for the comfort of the women. Parties are given by the employer to the employees, which he himself attends. He has thrown himself into whatever schemes his director has suggested. The director complained that the reason the new lunch room was not more popular was because a piano was needed. A second-hand one would not do, for that would cultivate bad taste in music. This showed the employer that soon everything would be expected from the "big house on the hill." An event which happened at the time when the pressure was greatest on him for the piano, convinced him that his employees could supply their real needs without any trouble or delay. The assistant manager was about to leave, and in less than a week five hundred dollars was raised among the workers for his farewell gift. Walking home that night late from his office the owner was attracted by the sound of jollity, and saw a little room jammed full of mill people enjoying the improvised music of a mouth organ played to the accompaniment of heels. He resolved henceforth to train his employees to do his work well and to earn more pay, — and to let them amuse themselves. From that time on he refused to be looked upon as the *deus ex machina* of the town. He decided that the best way to give English lessons to foreigners was to improve the school. His beneficence in supplying them with pure water at the mill did [227]not prevent a ravaging typhoid epidemic because the town water was not watched. He saw that the best way to improve health was to strengthen the health board and to make his co-workers realize that they were citizens responsible for their own privileges and rights.

Emergency hospitals and Y.M.C.A. buildings are sad substitutes for safety devices and automatic couplers. Christmas shopping in November is less kind than prevention of overwork in December. Night school and gymnastic classes are a poor penance for child labor and for work unsuited to the body. The left hand cannot dole favors enough to offset the evils of underpay, of unsanitary conditions, of inefficient enforcement of health laws tolerated by the right hand.

Just because a man is taking wages for work done, is no reason why he should forfeit his rights as a citizen, or allow his children, sisters, neighbors, to work in conditions which decrease their efficiency and earning power. What the employee can do for himself as a citizen, having equal health rights with employers, he has never been taught to see. Factory legislation is state direction of industries so far as relates to the safety, health, and moral condition of the people,—and which embraces to-day, more than in any other epoch, the opinion of the workers themselves. No government, however strong, can hope successfully to introduce social legislation largely affecting personal interests until public opinion has been educated to the belief that the remedies proposed are really necessary. Until schools insist upon a better ventilation than the worst factories, how can we expect to find children of working age sensitive to impure air? Where work benches are more comfortable than school desks, where drinking water is cleaner and towels more sanitary, however unsanitary they may be, than those found in the schoolhouse, the worker does not realize that they menace his right to earn a living wage as much as does a temporary shut-down.

[228]Employers are by no means solely to blame for unhealthy working conditions. A shortsighted employee is as anxious to work overtime for double pay as a shortsighted employer is to have him. Among those who are agitating for an eight-hour day are many who, from self-interest or interest in the cause, work regularly from ten to sixteen hours.

Would it help to punish employees for working in unhealthy places? The highest service that can be rendered industrial hygiene is to educate the industrial classes to recognize hygienic evils and to coöperate with other citizens in securing the enforcement of health rights.

[229]

THE LAST DAYS OF TUBERCULOSIS

If the historian Lecky was right in saying that the greatest triumphs of the nineteenth century were its sanitary achievements, the Lecky of the twenty-first century will probably honor our generation not for its electricity, its trusts, and its scientific research, but for its crusade against the white plague and for its recognition of health rights. Thanks to committees for the prevention of tuberculosis,—local, state, national, international,—we are fast approaching the time when every parent, teacher, employer, landlord, worker, will see in tuberculosis a personal enemy,—a menace to his fireside, his income, and his freedom. Just as this nation could not exist half slave, half free, we of one mind now affirm that equal opportunity cannot exist where one death in ten is from a single preventable disease.[13]

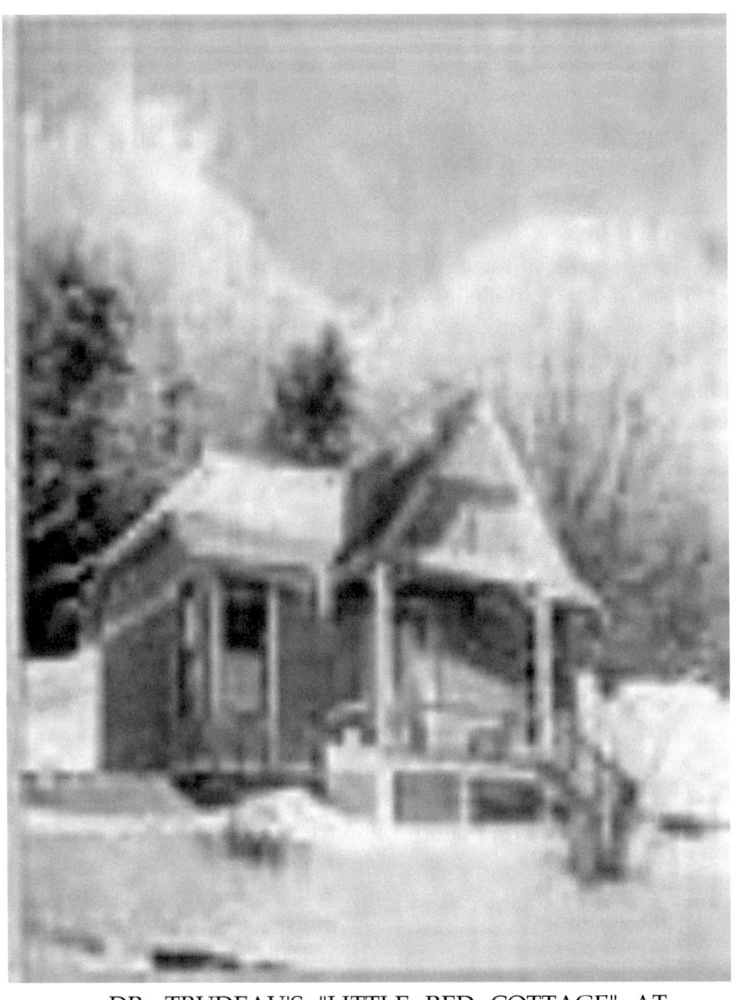

DR. TRUDEAU'S "LITTLE RED COTTAGE" AT
SARANAC—BIRTHPLACE OF OUT-OF-DOOR
TREATMENT IN AMERICA

Of no obstacle to efficient living is it more true than of tuberculosis, that the remedy depends upon enforcing rather than upon making law, upon practice rather than upon precept, upon health habits
rather than upon medical remedies, upon coöperation of lay citizens

rather than upon medical science or isolated individual effort. Without learning another fact about tuberculosis, we can stamp it out if we will but apply, and see that officers of health apply, lessons of cleanliness and natural living already known to us.

[230]Perhaps the most striking results yet obtained in combating tuberculosis are those of the Massachusetts General Hospital in Boston. To visit its tuberculosis classes reminds one more of the sociable than the clinic. In fact, one wonders whether the milk diet and the rest cure or the effervescing optimism and good cheer of the physicians and nurses should be credited with the marvelous cures. The first part of the hour is given to writing on the blackboard the number of hours that the class members spent out of doors the preceding week. So great was the rivalry for first place that the nurse protested that a certain boy in the front row gave himself indigestion by trying to eat his meals in ten or fifteen minutes. It was then suggested that twenty hours a day would be enough for any one to stay out of doors, and that plenty of time should be taken for meals with the family and for cold baths, keeping clean, etc. Interesting facts gathered by personal interviews of two physicians with individual patients are explained to the whole class. Next to the number of hours out of doors, the most interesting fact is the number of hours of exercise permitted. A man of forty, the head of a family, beamed like a school child when told that, after nearly a year of absolute rest, he might during the next week exercise ten minutes a day. A graduate drops in, the very picture of health, weighing two hundred pounds. An apparently hopeless case would brighten up and have confidence when told that this strong, handsome man has gained fifty pounds by rest, good cheer, fresh air, all on his own porch. One young man, just back from a California sanatorium where he progressively lost strength in spite of change of climate, is now returning to work and is back at normal weight.

[231]

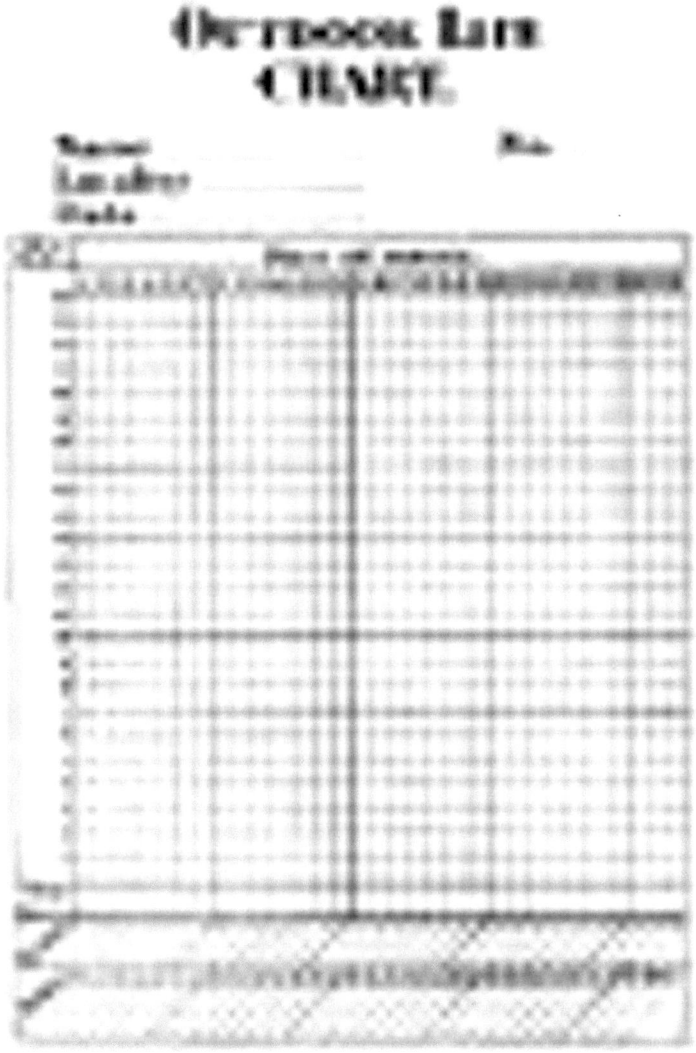

OUTDOOR LIFE CHART.

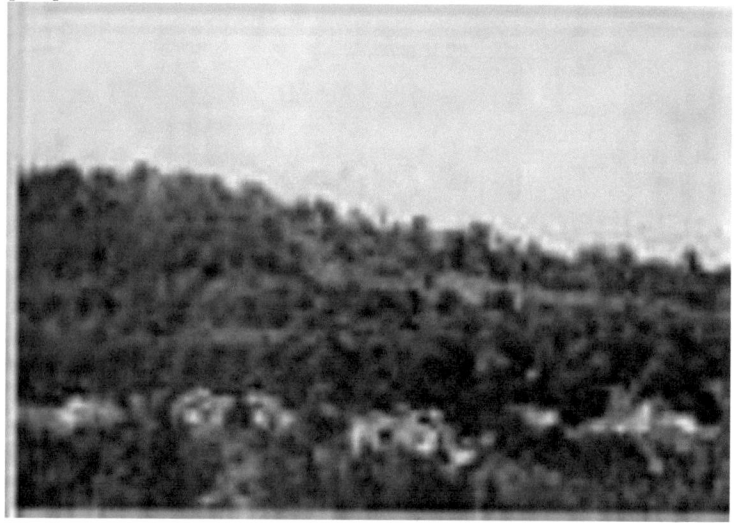

FIGHTING TUBERCULOSIS IN THE MOUNTAINS—SARANAC

Every patient keeps a daily record, called for by the following instructions:

Make notes of temperature and pulse at 8, 12, 4, and 8 o'clock, daily; movements of bowels; hours in open air; all food taken; total amount of milk; total amount of oil and butter; appetite; digestion; spirits; cough (amount, chief time); expectoration (amount in 24 hours, color, nature); exercise (if allowed), with temperature and pulse 15 minutes after exercise; sweats; visitors.

The following simple instructions can be followed in any home, even where open windows must take the place of porches:

Rest out of doors is the medicine that cures consumption. Absolute rest for mind and body brings speedy improvement. It [233]stops the cough and promotes the appetite. The lungs heal more quickly when the body is at rest. Lie with the chest low, so the blood flow in the lungs will aid to the uttermost the work of healing. The rest habit is soon acquired. Each day of rest makes the next day of rest easier, and shortens the time necessary to regain health.

The more time spent in bed out of doors the better. Do not dress if the temperature is above 99 degrees, or if there is blood in the sputum. It is life in the open air, not exercise, that brings health and strength. Just a few minutes daily exercise during the active stage of the disease may delay recovery weeks or months. Rest favors digestion, exercise frequently disturbs digestion. When possible have meals served in bed. Never think the rest treatment can be taken in a rocking-chair. If tired of the cot, shift to the reclining chair, but sit with head low and feet elevated. Do not write letters. Dictate to a friend. Do not read much and do not hold heavy books. While reading remain in the recumbent posture.

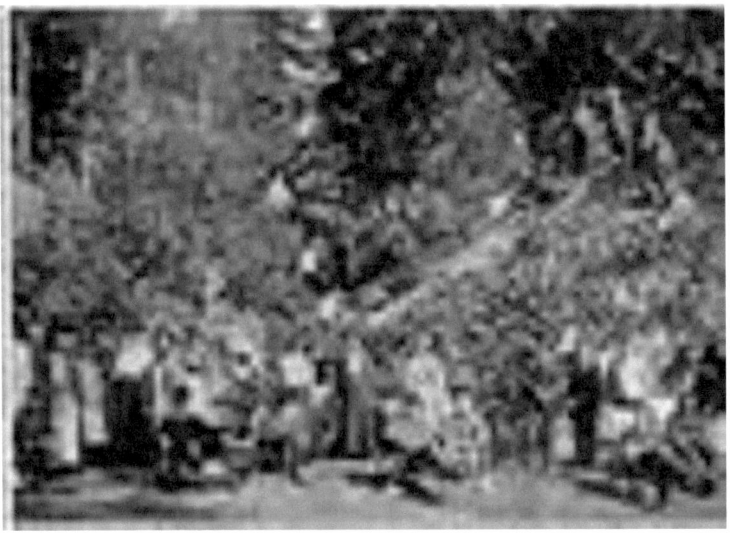

FIGHTING TUBERCULOSIS IN DAY CAMPS – BOSTON

Once having learned the simple facts that must be noted and the simple laws that must be followed, once [234]having placed oneself in a position to secure the rest, the fresh air, and the health diet, no better next steps can be taken than to observe the closing injunction in the rules for rest:

There are few medicines better than clouds, and you have not to swallow them or wear them as plasters, – only to watch them. Keeping your eyes aloft, your thoughts will shortly clamber after them, or, if they don't do that, the sun gets into them, and the bad ones go a-dozing like bats and owls.

THE BACK OF A STREET-CAR TRANSFER, SUNDAYS, NEW YORK CITY

Important as are sanatoriums in mountain and desert, day or night camps within and near cities, milk and egg clinics, home visiting, change of air and rest for those who are known to be tuberculous, their importance is infinitesimal compared with the protection that comes from clean, healthy environment and natural living for those not known to be tuberculous. This great fact has been recognized by the various bodies now engaged in popularizing the truth about tuberculosis by means of stationary and traveling exhibits, illustrated lectures, street-car transfers, advertisements, farmers' institutes, anti-spitting signs in public vehicles and public buildings, board of health instructions in many languages, magazine stories, and press reports of conferences. This brilliant campaign of education shows what can be done by national, state, and county superintendents of schools, if they will make the most of school hygiene and civics.

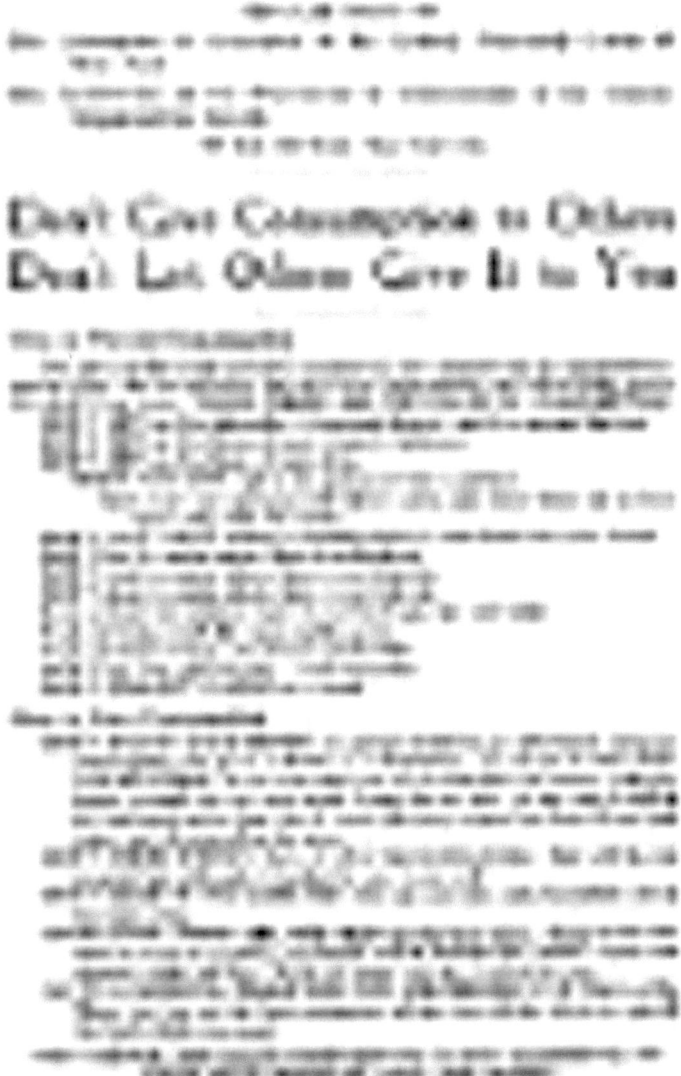

Don't Give Consumption to Others
Don't Let Others Give It to You

AN EXAMPLE IN COÖPERATION THAT ANTI-TUBERCULOSIS CRUSADERS SHOULD FOLLOW

[236]Is it not significant that America's national movement is due primarily to the organizing capacity of laymen in the New York Charity Organization Society rather than to schools or hospitals? Most of the local secretaries are men whose inspiration came from contact with the non-medical relief of the poor in city tenements. The secretary of the national association is a university professor of anthropology, who has also a medical degree. The child victim's plea — Little Jo's Smile — was nationalized by an association of laymen, aided by the advertising managers of forty magazines. The smaller cities of New York state are being aroused by a state voluntary association that for years has visited almshouses, insane asylums, and hospitals. These facts I emphasize, for they illustrate the opportunity and the duty of the lay educator, whether parent, teacher, labor leader, or trustee of hospital, orphanage, or relief society.

Three fundamental rules of action should be established as firmly as religious principles:

1. The public health authorities should be told of every known and every suspected case of tuberculosis.

2. For each case proved by examination of sputum to be tuberculous, the public-health officers should know that the germs are destroyed before being allowed to contaminate air or food.

3. Sick and not yet sick should practice habits of health that build up vitality to resist the tubercle bacilli and that abhor uncleanliness as nature abhors a vacuum.

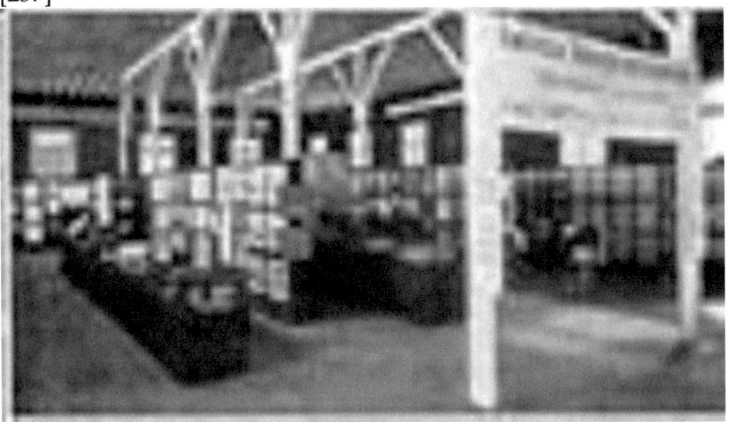

FIGHTING TUBERCULOSIS WITH A NATIONAL ORGANIZATION

All laws, customs, and environmental conditions opposed to the enforcement of these three principles must be modified or abolished. If the teachers of America will list for educational use in their own communities the local obstacles to these rules of action, they will see exactly where their local problem lies. The illustrations that are given in this book show in how many ways these rules of action are now being universalized. Three or four important steps deserve especial comment:

1. Compulsory notification of all tuberculous cases.

2. Compulsory removal to hospital of those not able at home to destroy the bacilli, or compulsory supervision of home care.

3. Examination of all members of a family where one member is discovered to be tuberculous.

4. Special provision for tuberculous teachers.

5. Protection of children about to enter industry but predisposed to tuberculosis.

6. Prohibition of dry cleaning of schools, offices, and streets.

7. Tax provision for educational and preventive work.

Compulsory notification was introduced first in New York City by Hermann M. Biggs, M.D., chief medical [238]officer: 1893, partially voluntary, partially compulsory; 1897, compulsory for all. Physicians who now hail Dr. Biggs as a statesman called him persecutor, autocrat, and violator of personal freedom fifteen years ago. Foreign sanitarians vied with American colleagues in upbraiding him for his exaggeration of the transmissibility of consumption and for his injustice to its victims. As late as 1899 one British expert particularly resented the rejection of tuberculous immigrants at Ellis Island, and said to me, "Perhaps if you should open a man's mouth and pour in tubercle bacilli he might get phthisis, but compulsory notification is preposterous." In 1906 the International Congress on Tuberculosis met in Paris and congratulated New York upon its leadership in securing at health headquarters a list of the known disease centers within its borders; in 1906 more than twenty thousand individual cases were reported, ten thousand of these being reported more than once. To know the nature and location of twenty thousand germ factories is a long step toward judging their strength and their probable product. To compulsory notification in New York City is largely due the educational movements of the last decade against the white plague, more particularly the growing ability among physicians to recognize and to treat conditions predisposing to the disease. As in New York City, the public should provide free of cost bacteriological analysis of sputum to learn positively whether tuberculosis is present. Simpler still is the tuberculin test of the eyes, with which experiments are now being made on a large scale in New York City, and which bids fair to become cheap enough to be generally used wherever physical examinations are made. This test is known as Calmette's Eye Test. Inside the eyelid is placed a drop of a solution—95 per cent alcohol and tuberculin. If conjunctivitis develops in twenty-four hours, the patient is proved to have tuberculosis. Some physicians still fear to use this test. Others question its proof. The "skin test" is also being thoroughly tried in several American cities and, if finally found trustworthy, will greatly simplify examination for tuberculosis. Dr. John W. Brannan, president of Bellevue and Allied Hospitals, New York City, is to report on skin and eye tuberculin tests for children at the International Congress on Tuberculosis, mentioned later.

Bring this Card with you.

Bringe diese Karte jedesmal mit.

Portate questa Carta con voi.

ברענג ריא קאר טע

Clinics for the Treatment
of Tuberculosis.

MANHATTAN.

NOTE.—Manhattan applicants for examination or treatment should apply at the dispensary in the district in which they live. Location of dispensaries is shown on the map.

DISPENSARIES.

Department of Health.
　　Weekdays 10 A. M. to 4 P. M.
　　Mon., Wed., Fri., 8 to 9 P. M.

Bellevue Hospital Dispensary.
　　Weekdays 1 to 4.30 P. M.

Gouverneur Hospital Dispensary.
　　Mon., Wed., Fri., 2 to 4 P. M.

Presbyterian Hospital Dispensary.
　　Mon., Wed. Fri., 1.30 to 3.30 P. M.

Harlem Hospital Dispensary.
　　Weekdays 3 to 4 P. M.

Vanderbilt Clinic.
　　Weekdays 2 to 3 P. M.
　　Tues., Thurs., Sat., 9 to 10.30 A. M.

New York Dispensary
　　Weekdays 11 A. M. to 12.30 P. M.

New York Hospital Dispensary.
　　Weekdays 2 to 4 P. M.

Health Department, BRONX.
　　3d Avenue and St. Paul's Place.
　　Weekdays 2 to 4 P. M.

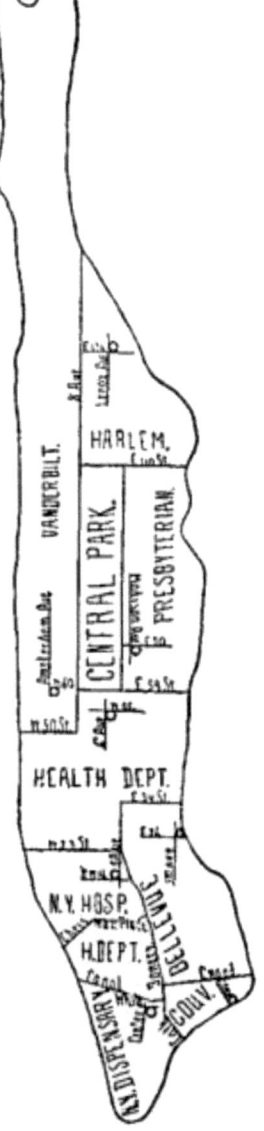

FIGHTING TUBERCULOSIS BY ORGANIZED COÖPERATIVE DISPENSARY WORK

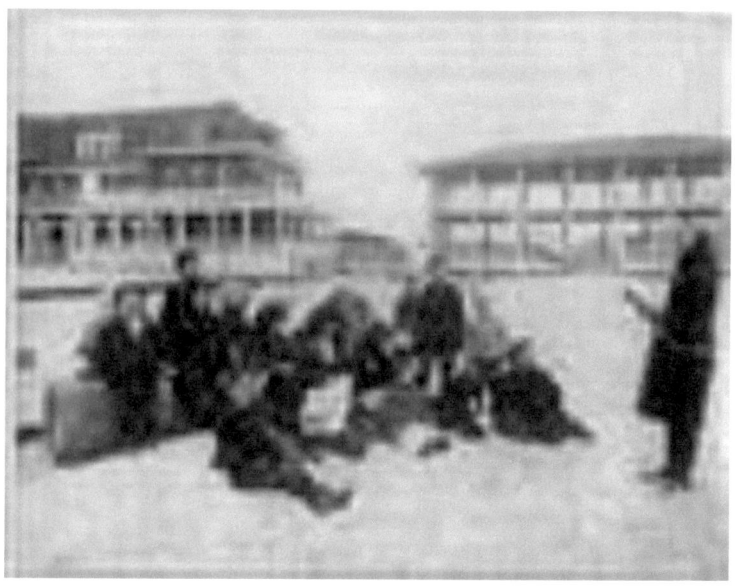

FIGHTING BONE TUBERCULOSIS AT SEA BREEZE, WHERE EYE AND SKIN TUBERCULIN TESTS ARE BEING MADE

[240]Compulsory removal of careless consumptives is yet rare. One obstacle is the lack of hospitals. In New York ten thousand die annually from tuberculosis and fifty thousand are known to have it, yet there are only about two thousand beds available. So long as the patients anxious for hospital care exceed the number of beds, it does not seem fair to give a bed to some one who does not want it. On the other hand, it should not be forgotten that patients are taken forcibly to smallpox and scarlet-fever hospitals, not for their own good, but for the protection of others. The last person who should be permitted to stay at home is the tuberculous person who is unable, unwilling, or too ignorant to take the necessary precautions for others' [241]protection. A rigid educational test should be applied as a condition of remaining at home without supervision.

The objections to compulsory removal are two: (1) it is desired to make sanatorium care so attractive that patients will go at the earliest stage of the disease; (2) an unwilling patient can defeat the sanitarian's effort to help him and others. The alternative for compulsory removal is gratuitous, and, if need be, compulsory, supervision of home care, such as is now given in New York City. In Brighton, England, Dr. Newsholme treats his municipal sanatorium as a vacation school, giving each patient one month only. Thus one bed helps twelve patients each year. Almost any worker can spare one month and in that time can be made into a missionary of healthy living.

Family examining parties were begun in New York by Dr. Linsly R. Williams, for the relief agency that started the seaside treatment of bone tuberculosis. Many of the crippled children at Sea Breeze were found to have consumptive fathers or mothers. In one instance the father had died before Charlie had "hip trouble." Long after we had known Charlie his mother began to fail. She too had consumption. Family parties were planned for 290 families. Weights were taken and careful examination made, the physician explaining that predisposition means defective lung capacity or deficient vitality. Of 379 members, supposedly free from tuberculosis, sixteen were found to have well-marked cases. (Of twenty Boston children whose parents were in a tuberculosis class, four had tuberculosis.) In one instance the father was astonished to learn not only that he was tuberculous, but that he had probably given the disease to the mother, for whom he was tenderly concerned. Of special benefit were the talks about teeth and nourishment, and about fresh air and water as germ killers. One examination of this kind will organize a family crusade against carelessness.

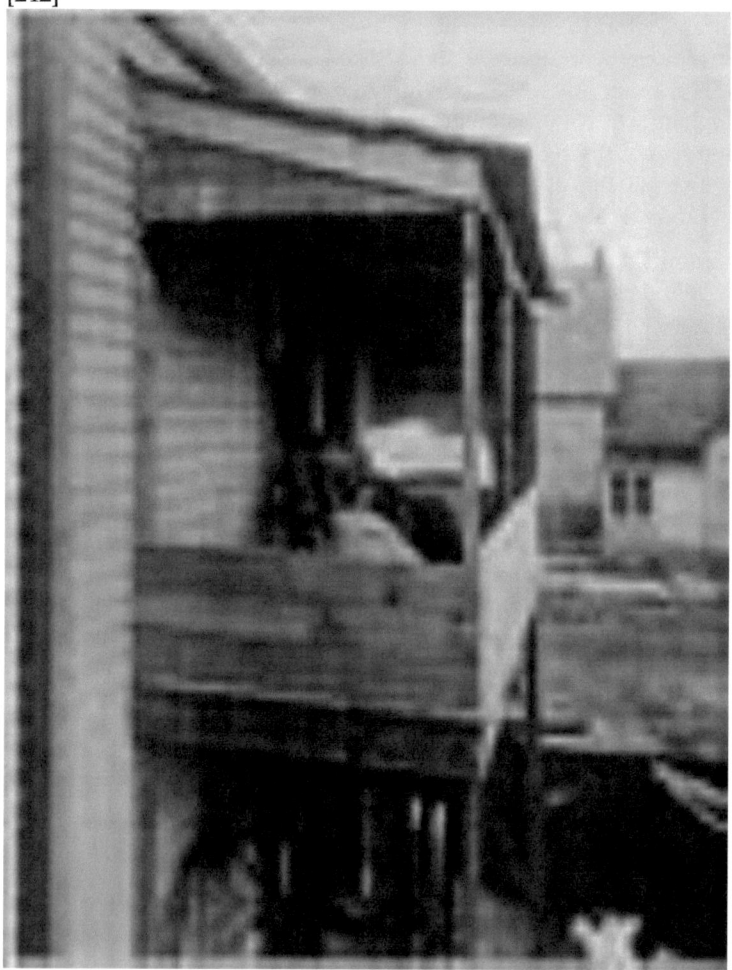

FIGHTING TUBERCULOSIS IN SMALL CITIES
New York State Charities Aid Association

Tuberculous teachers ought to be excluded from schoolrooms not merely because they may spread tuberculosis, but because they cannot do justice to school work without sacrifices that society ought not to accept. A tuberculous teacher ought to be generous enough to permit public hospitals to restore her strength or enterprising enough [243]to join tuberculosis classes. It is selfish to demand independence at the price which is paid by schools that employ tuberculous teachers.

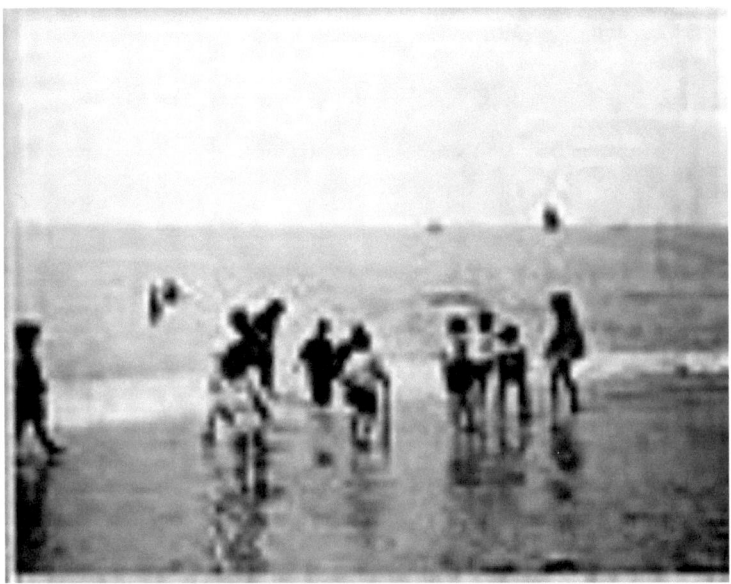

FIGHTING BONE TUBERCULOSIS WITH SALT WATER AND SALT AIR

Predisposition to tuberculosis should be understood by every child before he is accepted as an industrial soldier. Many trades now dangerous would be made safe if workers knew the risk they run, and if society forbade such trades needlessly to exhaust their employees. A perfectly sound man is predisposed to tuberculosis if he elects to work in stale, dust-laden air. Ill-ventilated rooms, cramped positions, lack of exercise in the open air, prepare lungs to give a cordial reception to tubercle bacilli. Rooms as well as persons become infected. Fortunately, opportunities to work are so varied in most localities that workers predisposed to tuberculosis may be sure of a livelihood in an occupation suited to their vitality. Destruction of germs in the air, in carpets, on walls, on streets, is quite as important as [244]destruction of germs in lungs. Why should not tenants and workers require health certificates stating that neither house nor working place is infected with tubercle bacilli? Some cities now compel the disinfection of premises occupied by tuberculous persons *after* their removal. Landlords, employers, tenants, and employees can easily be taught to see the advantage of disinfecting premises occupied by tuberculous cases *before* detection.

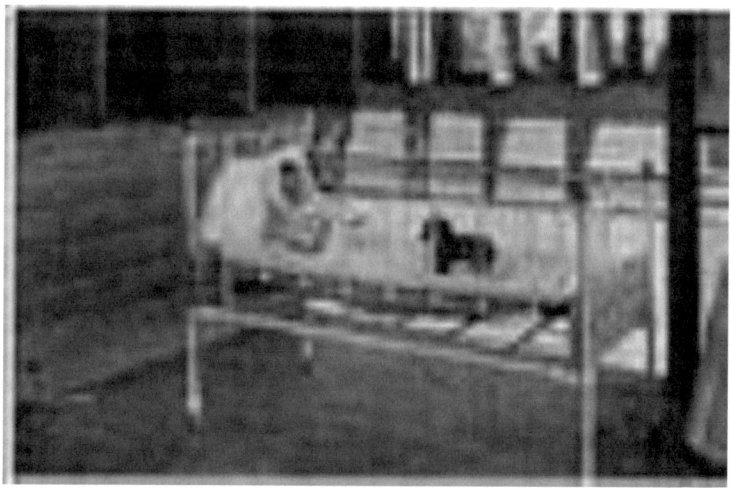

FIGHTING FEATHER DUSTERS IS ONE OBJECT OF SEA-AIR HOSPITALS FOR BONE TUBERCULOSIS

Dry cleaning, feather dusters, dust-laden air, will disappear from schoolrooms within twenty-four hours after school-teachers declare that they shall disappear. We have no right to expect street cleaners, tenement and shop janitors, or overworked mothers to be more careful than school-teachers. Last year I said to a janitress, "Don't you realize that you may get consumption if you use that feather duster?" Her reply caused us to realize our carelessness: "I don't want any more than I've got now." Shall we some day have compulsory examination and instruction of all cleaners, starting with school cleaners?

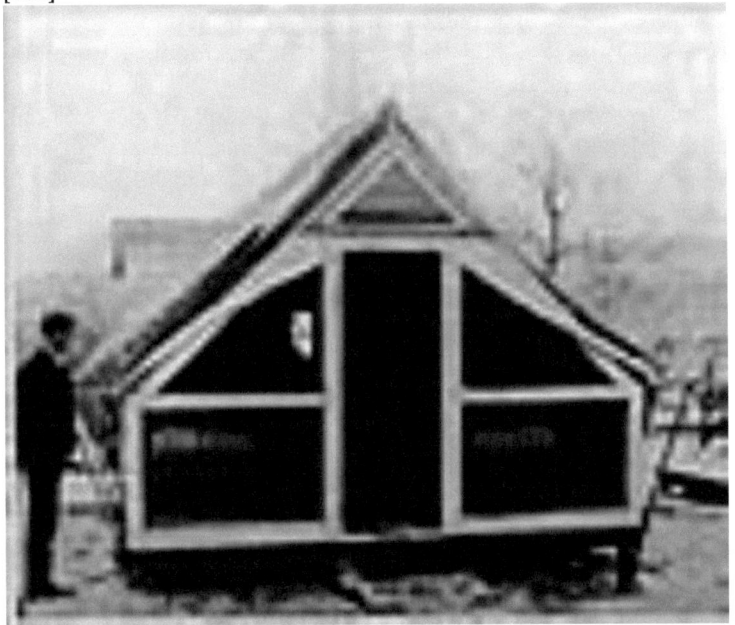

FIGHTING TUBERCULOSIS IN OPEN TENTS

Taxing is swift to follow teaching in matters of health. Teachers can easily compute what their community loses from tuberculosis. The totals will for some time prove a convincing argument for cleanliness of air, of body, and of building wherever the community is responsible for air, building, and body. The annual cost of tuberculosis to New York City is estimated at $23,000,000 and to the United States at $330,000,000. The cost of exterminating it will be but a drop in the bucket if school-teachers do their part this next generation with the twenty million children whose day environment they control for three fourths of the year, and whose habits they can determine.

The first meeting in America of the International Congress on Tuberculosis was held at Washington, D.C., September 21 to October 12, 1908. For many years the [246]proceedings of this congress will undoubtedly be the chief reference book on the conquest of tuberculosis.[14]

How many aspects there are to this problem, and how many kinds of people may be enlisted, may be seen from the seven section names: I. Pathology and Bacteriology; II. Sanatoriums, Hospitals, and Dispensaries; III. Surgery and Orthopedics; IV. Tuberculosis in Children — Etiology, Prevention, and Treatment; V. Hygienic, Social, Industrial, and Economic Aspects; VI. State and Municipal Control of Tuberculosis; VII. Tuberculosis in Animals and Its Relation to Man.

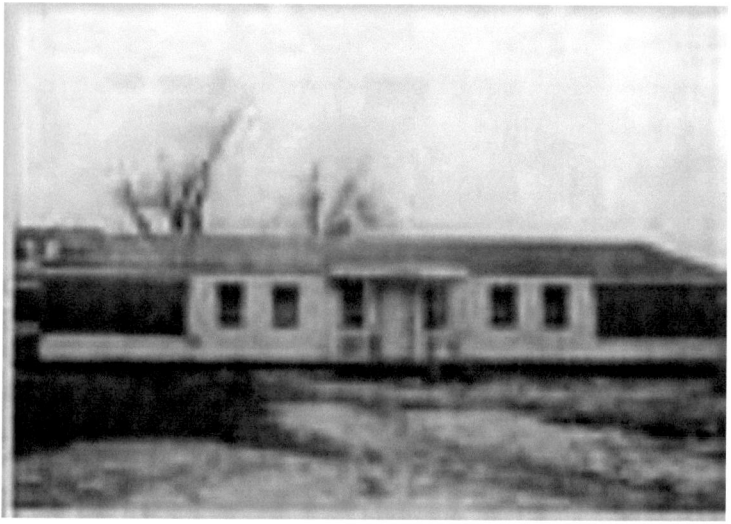

FIGHTING TUBERCULOSIS IN CHEAP SHACKS, $125 PER BED, OTISVILLE, NEW YORK

[247]How many-sided is the responsibility of each of us for stamping out tuberculosis is shown by the preliminary programme of the eight sessions of Section V. These topics suggest an interesting and instructive year's study for clubs of women, mothers, or teachers, or for advanced pupils.

I. Economic Aspects of Tuberculosis

1. The burdens entailed by tuberculosis:

a. On individuals and families.
b. On the medical profession.

c. On industry.
d. On relief agencies.
e. On the community.
f. On social progress.

2. The cost of securing effective control of tuberculosis:

a. In large cities.
b. In smaller towns.
c. In rural communities.

II. Adverse Industrial Conditions

1. Incidence of tuberculosis according to occupation.

2. Overwork and nervous strain as factors in tuberculosis.

3. Effect of improvements in factory conditions on the health of employees.

4. Legitimate exercise of police power in protecting the life and health of employees.

III. The Social Control of Tuberculosis

1. Outline of a comprehensive programme for:

a. National, state, and municipal governments.
b. Departments of health and departments of public relief.
c. Private endowments.
d. Voluntary associations for educational propaganda.
e. Institutions, such as schools and relief agencies, which exist primarily for other purposes.

[248]2. A symposium on the relative value of each of the features in an aggressive campaign against tuberculosis:

a. Compulsory registration.
b. Free sputum examination.
c. Compulsory removal of unteachable and dangerous cases.
d. Laboratory research.
e. Hospital.
f. Sanatorium.

g. Dispensary.

h. The tuberculosis class.

i. Day camp.

j. Private physician.

k. Visiting nurse.

l. After-care of arrested cases.

m. Relief fund.

n. Climate.

o. Hygienic instruction, — personal and in class.

p. Inspection of schools and factories.

q. Educational propaganda.

IV. Early Recognition and Prevention

1. Importance of discovering the persons who have tuberculosis before the disease has passed the incipient stage.

2. Examination of persons known to have been exposed or presumably predisposed.

3. Systematic examination of school children during their course and on leaving school to go to work.

4. Professional advice as to choice of occupation in cases where there is apparent predisposition to disease.

V. After-Care of Arrested Cases

1. Instruction in healthful trades in the sanatorium.

2. Training for professional nursing in institutions for the care of tuberculous patients.

3. Farm colonies.

4. Convalescent homes or cottages.

5. Aid in securing suitable employment on leaving the sanatorium.

6. How to deal with the danger of a return to unfavorable home conditions.

[249]VI. Educational Methods and Agencies

1. Special literature for general distribution.

2. Exhibits and lectures.

3. The press.

4. Educational work of the nurse.

5. Labor organizations.

6. Instruction in schools of all grades.

7. Presentation and discussion of leaflets awarded prizes by the congress.

VII. Promotion of Immunity

1. Development of the conception of physical well-being.

2. Measures for increasing resistance to disease:

a. Parks and playgrounds.
b. Outdoor sports.
c. Physical education.
d. Raising the standards of living: housing, diet, cleanliness.

3. Individual immunity and social conditions favorable to general immunity.

VIII. Responsibility of Society for Tuberculosis

1. A symposium of representative

a. Citizens.
b. Social workers.
c. Employers.
d. Employees.
e. Physicians.
f. Nurses.
g. Educators.
h. Others.

Cash prizes of one thousand dollars each are offered: (1) for the best evidence of effective work in the prevention or relief of tuberculosis by any voluntary association since 1905; (2) for the best exhibit of a sanatorium for working classes; (3) for the best exhibit of a furnished home for the poor, designed primarily to prevent, but also to permit the cure of tuberculosis.

[250]

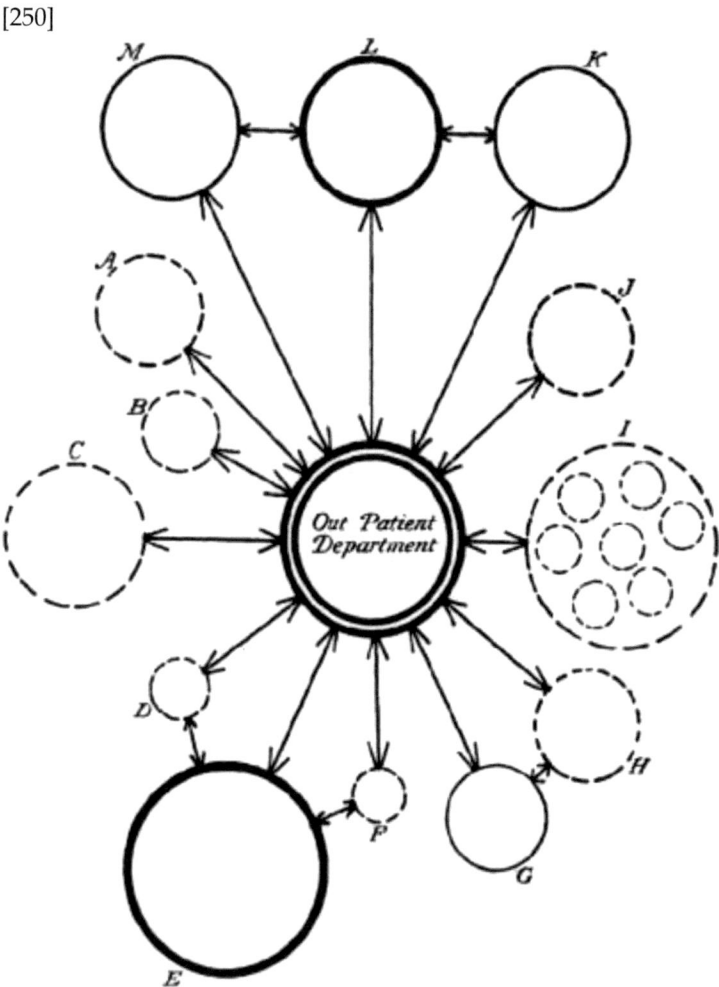

BOSTON FIGHTS TUBERCULOSIS WITH A COMPREHENSIVE PLAN
A-D, F, H-J, private hospitals and agencies reporting cases to the official center; *E*, home care; *K, L, M*, day camp and hospitals for incipient and advanced cases

A white-plague scrapbook containing news items, articles, and photographs will prove an interesting aid to self-education or to instruction of children, working girls' clubs, or mothers' meetings. Everybody ought to enlist in this war, for the fight against tuberculosis is a fight for cleanliness [251]and for vitality, for a fair chance against environmental conditions prejudicial to efficient citizenship.

So sure is the result and so immediate the duty of every citizen that Dr. Biggs wrote in 1907: *In no other direction can such large results be achieved so certainly and at such relatively small cost. The time is not far distant when those states and municipalities which have not adopted a comprehensive plan for dealing with tuberculosis will be regarded as almost criminally negligent in their administration of sanitary affairs and inexcusably blind to their own best economic interests.*

FOOTNOTES:

[13] The best literature on tuberculosis is in current magazines and reports of anti-tuberculosis crusaders. For a scientific, comprehensive treatment, libraries and students should have *The Prevention of Tuberculosis* (1908) by Arthur Newsholme, M.D. A popular book is *The Crusade against Tuberculosis*, by Lawrence F. Flick, of the Henry Phipps Institute for the Study, Treatment, and Prevention of Tuberculosis.

[14] Those desiring copies this year or hereafter will do well to write to The National Association for the Study and Prevention of Tuberculosis, 105 East 22d St., New York City. The congress is under the control of the National Association and is managed by a special committee appointed by it. Even after a national board of health is established, the National Association for the Study and Prevention of Tuberculosis will continue to be a center for private interest in public protection against tuberculosis. One of its chief functions is the preparation and distribution of literature to those who desire it.

[252]

THE FIGHT FOR CLEAN MILK

"With the approval of the President and with the coöperation of the Department of Agriculture,[15] the [national quarantine] service has undertaken to prepare a complete report upon the milk industry from farm to the consumer in its relation to the public health." This promise of the United States Treasury insures national attention to the evils of unclean milk and to the sanitary standards of farmer and consumer. Nothing less than a national campaign can make the vivid impression necessary to wean dairymen of uncleanly habits and mothers of the ignorant superstition that babies die in summer just because they are babies. When two national bureaus study, learn, and report, newspapers will print their stories on the first page, magazines will herald the conclusions, physicians will open their minds to new truths, state health secretaries will carry on the propaganda, demagogues and quacks will become less certain of their short-cut remedies, and *everybody will be made to think.*

The evolution of this newly awakened national interest in clean milk follows the seven stages and illustrates the seven health motives presented in Chapter II. I give the story of Robert M. Hartley because he began and prosecuted his pure-milk crusade in a way that can be duplicated in any country town or small city.

Robert M. Hartley was a strong-bodied, strong-minded, country-bred man, who started church work in New York City almost as soon as he arrived. He distributed religious [253]tracts among the alleys and hovels that characterized lower New York in 1825. Meeting drunken men and women one after another, he first wondered whether they were helped by tracts, and then decided that the mind befogged with alcohol was unfit to receive the gospel message. Then for fifteen years he threw himself into a total-abstinence crusade, distributing thousands of pamphlets, calling in one year at over four thousand homes to teach the industrial and moral reasons for total abstinence. Finally, he began to wonder whether back of alcoholism there was not still a dark closet that must be explored before men could receive the message of religion and self-control. So in 1843 he organized the New York Association for Improving the Condition of the Poor, which ever since has remembered how Hartley found alcoholism back of irreligion, and how back of alcoholism and poverty and ignorant indifference [254]he found indecent housing, unsanitary streets, unwholesome working conditions, and impure food.

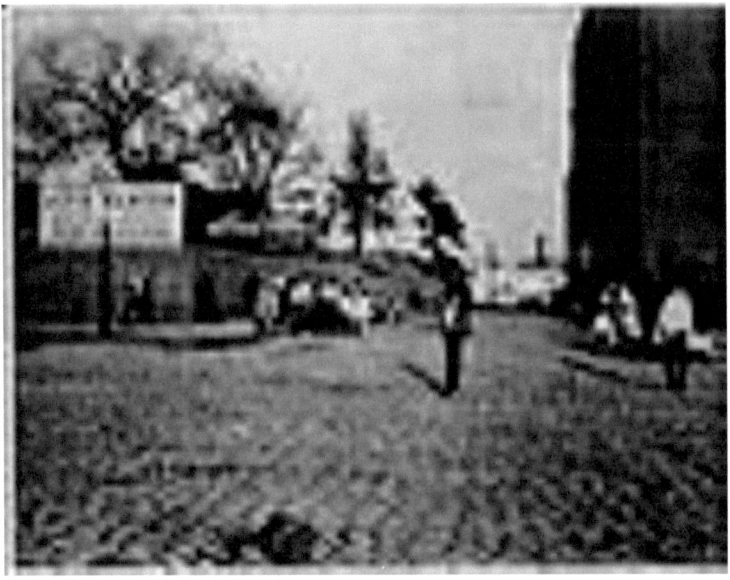

FIGHTING INFANT MORTALITY BY A SCHOOL FOR MOTHERS IN THE HEART OF NEW YORK CITY,—JUNIOR SEA BREEZE

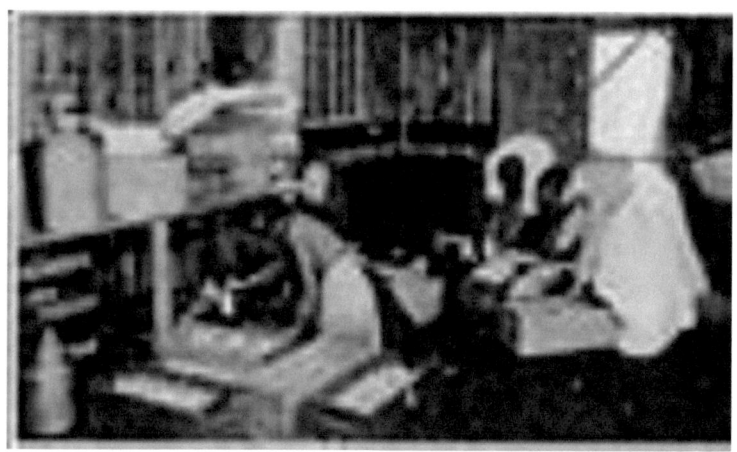

PROVIDING AGAINST GERM GROWTH AND ADAPTING MILK TO THE INDIVIDUAL BABY'S NEED,—ROCHESTER'S MODEL DAIRY

Hartley's instinct started the first great pure-milk agitation in this country. While visiting a distillery for the purpose of trying to persuade the owner to invest his money in another business, he noticed that "slops smoking hot from the stills" were being carried to cow stables. He followed and was nauseated by the sights and odors. Several hundred uncleaned cows in low, suffocating, filthy stables were being fed on "this disgusting, unnatural food." Similar disgust has in many other American cities caused the first effort to better dairy conditions. Hartley could never again enjoy milk from distillery cows. Furthermore, his story of 1841 made it impossible for any readers of newspapers in New York to enjoy milk until assured that it was not produced by distillery slops. The instinctive loathing and the discomfort of buyers awakened the commerce motives of milk dealers, who covered their wagons with signs declaring that they "no longer" or "never" fed cows on distillery refuse. But Hartley could not stop when the anti-nuisance stage was reached. He did not let up on his fight against impure or adulterated milk until the state legislature declared in 1864 that *every baby, city born or country born, no matter how humble its home, has the right to pure milk.*

Clean Milk for New York City

CONFERENCE

ROOM 44, N. Y. ACADEMY OF MEDICINE
NO. 17 WEST 43D STREET

November 20th, 1906, Tuesday 3 p.m. and 8 p.m.

ESSENTIAL FACTS AS TO NEW YORK CITY

Manhattan's Infant Mortality
(UNDER 5 YRS.)

June to September, 1904, 4428
June to September, 1905, 4687
June to September, 1906, 4428

Daily Consumption of Milk

1,000,000 qts.
½ in quart bottles
⅔ in 40-quart cans
" Certified," 10,000 quarts
" Inspected," 3,000 quarts
24 to 48 hours old on arrival

Comes from

30,000 dairies, 40 to 400 miles distant
600 creameries — 105 proprietors
10 city railroad depots

Sold in

12,000 places, mostly from cans
Sale of skim milk prohibited

Milk Law Violations, 1905

Destroyed, 39,618 quarts
Arrests, 806
Fines, $16,435

New York City Inspectors

14 in country since July; might make rounds not oftener than
once a year
(For 3 yrs. before, only 2; previously none)
16 in city, might make rounds in 30 to 40 days
(Before July, 14)

POINTS OF AGREEMENT

Cleanliness is the supreme requisite, from cow to consumer

Cows must be healthy, persons free from contagious diseases, premises clean, water pure, utensils clean, cans and bottles sterile, shops sanitary

Temperature is second essential

50° F. or lower at dairy
45° F. at creamery
45° F. or less during transportation
Not above 50° when sold to the consumer

As to Pasteurization

Not necessary for absolutely clean milk
Destroys benign as well as harmful germs
Disease germs develop more rapidly than in pure raw milk
True, 155° for 30 minutes to 167° for 20 minutes
Cost per quart, estimated, $\frac{1}{4}$ to $\frac{1}{2}$ ct.
Commercial, 165° for 15 seconds
Cost per quart, negligible

As to Inspection

Some inspection needed within the city
Some inspection needed of dairy and creamery

WHAT NEXT STEPS SHOULD NEW YORK TAKE?

Skim Milk

Should its sale be permitted?
Under what conditions?
How would this affect price of whole milk?

Pasteurization

Should pasteurization be made compulsory?
For what portion of the supply?
At whose expense?
Would it increase price of milk?
Does it render inspection unnecessary?
Does it reduce need for inspection?
Should sale of repasteurized milk or cream be permitted?
Should bottles show whether true or commercial pasteurization is used?

Infants' Milk Depots

Should they use pasteurized or clean milk?
Are municipal depots desirable?
Should private philanthropy support depots?
How many depots would be required in New York City?
Is Rochester experience applicable to New York City?
What educational work is possible in connection with milk depots?

Model Milk Shops

What may safely be sold in connection with milk?
Should law discourage other than model shops?
Are present sanitary laws rigid enough?
Should private capital be encouraged to establish shops?
Is it practicable to prohibit use of cans?
What provision can be demanded for proper refrigeration?
What for receiving milk before business hours when delivered
from stations?
What for sterilization of utensils and bottles?
What for attendants' dress and care of person?
Would such restrictions increase price?

Inspection

Is it practicable by inspection alone to secure a clean milk
supply?
Will it protect against more dangerous forms of infection?
How many inspectors does New York City need?
Within the city?
Among country dairies and creameries?
How many inspectors should the state employ?

Legislation

What needed as to diseased cattle?
What as to diseases of persons producing or handling milk?
Is present sanitary code sufficient?
Shall law require sterilization of all milk cans and bottles by
milk company or creamery before returned to farms or
refilled?
Shall sealing cans at creameries be required?
Shall transferring from one can to another or from can to
bottle in open street be made a misdemeanor?
Shall pollution of milk cans and bottles be made a misde-
meanor?
Shall bacterial standard be established?
Is state supervision now adequate?
What further legislation is needed?
Does present law prescribe adequate penalties?

Education

Should state system of lectures before agricultural institutes
be extended?
Should Maryland plan of traveling school be adopted as means
of reaching producer?
What can be done to assist Teachers College in its plan for
milk exhibit?
What can be done to teach mothers to detect unclean milk and
to care properly for milk purchased?
How can tenement mothers keep milk at proper temperature?
Can nothing be done to increase the supply and cheapen the
price of ice?
Is it desirable that a local committee be formed to coöperate
with the Department of Health and County Medical Society?

[258]Unfortunately Hartley and his contemporaries had never heard of disease germs that are carried by unclean milk into the human stomach. Science had not yet proved that many forms of barnyard filth could do quite as much harm as distillery refuse. Commerce had not invented milk bottles of glass or paper. The law of 1864 failed in two particulars: (1) it did not demand cleanliness from cow to consumer; (2) it did not provide means for its own enforcement, for learning whether everything and everybody that had to do with milk was clean. Not knowing of germs and their love for a warm climate and warm food, they naturally did not prohibit a temperature above fifty degrees from the time of milking to the time of sale. How much has been left for our generation to do to secure pure milk is illustrated by the opening sentence of this chapter, and more specifically by the programme of a milk conference held in New York in November, 1906, the board of health joining in the call. The four-page folder is reproduced in facsimile (excepting the names on the fourth page), because it states the universal problem, and also because it suggests an effective way to stimulate relevant discussion and to discourage the long speeches that spoil many conferences.

This conference led to the formation of a milk committee under the auspices of the association founded by Hartley. Business men, children's specialists, journalists, clergymen, consented to serve because they realized the need for a continuing public interest and a persisting watchfulness. Such committees are needed in other cities and in states, either as independent committees or as subcommittees of general organizations, such as women's clubs, sanitary leagues, county and state medical societies. Teachers' associations might well [259]be added, especially for rural and suburban districts where they are more apt than any other organized body to see the evils that result from unclean milk. The New York Milk Committee set a good example in paying a secretary to give his entire time to its educational programme,—a paid secretary can keep more volunteers and consultants busy than could a dozen volunteers giving "what time they can spare." Thanks chiefly to the conference and the Milk Committee's work, several important results have been effected. The general public has realized as never before that two indispensable adjectives belong to safe milk,—*clean* and *cool*. Additional inspectors have been sent to country dairies; refrigeration, cans, and milk have been inspected upon arrival at night; score cards have been introduced, thanks to the convincing explanations of their effectiveness by the [260]representatives of the Bureau of Animal Industry of the national Department of Agriculture; 8640 milch cows were inspected by veterinary practitioners (1905-1907), to learn the prevalence of bovine tuberculosis (of these thirty-six per cent reacted to the tuberculin test); state societies and state departments have been aroused to demand an efficient live-stock sanitary board; magistrates have fined and imprisoned offenders against the milk laws, where formerly they "warned"; popular illustrated milk lectures were added to the public school courses; illustrated cards were distributed by the thousand, telling how to keep the baby well; finally, private educational and relief societies, dispensaries, settlements, have been increasingly active in teaching mothers at home how to prepare baby's milk. In 1908 a Conference on Summer Care of Babies was organized representing the departments of health and education, and fifty private agencies for the care of sick babies and the instruction of mothers. The superintendent of schools instructed teachers to begin the campaign by talks to children and by giving out illustrated cards. Similar instructions were sent to parochial schools by the archbishop.

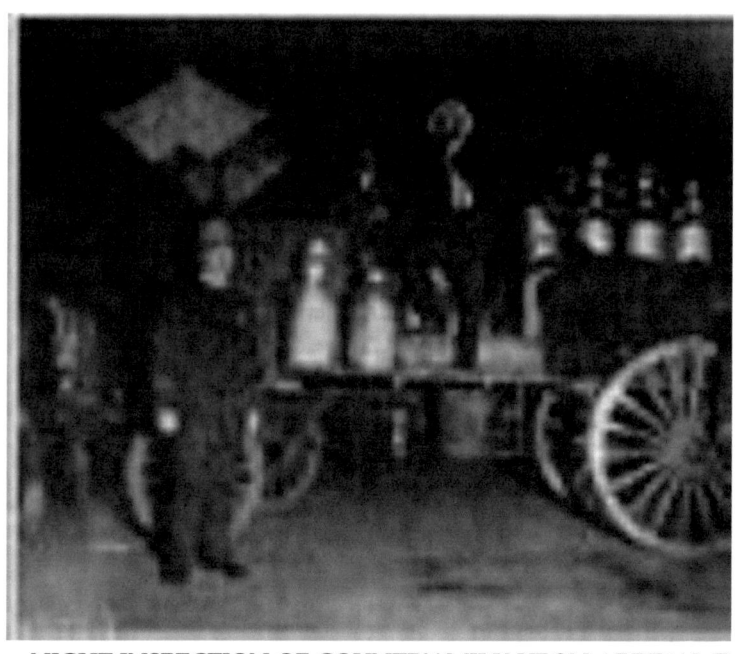

NIGHT INSPECTION OF COUNTRY MILK UPON ARRIVAL IN
NEW YORK CITY

As elsewhere, there are two schools of pure-milk crusaders: (1)
those who want cities to *do things*, to pasteurize all milk, start milk
farms, milk shops, or pure-milk dispensaries; and (2) those who
want cities and states to *get things done*. So far the New York Milk
Committee has led the second school and has opposed efforts to
municipalize the milk business. The leader of the other school is the
noted philanthropist, Nathan Strauss, who has established pasteurization plants in several American and European cities. The discussion of the two schools, similar in aim but different in method, is
made more difficult, because to question philanthropy's method
always seems to philanthropy itself and to most bystanders an un-
gracious, ungrateful act. As the issue, however, is clean milk, not
personal motive, it is important [261]that educators and parents in
all communities benefit from the effective propaganda of both
schools, using what is agreed upon as the basis for local pure-milk
crusades, reserving that which is controversial for final settlement

by research over large fields that involve hundreds of thousands of tests.

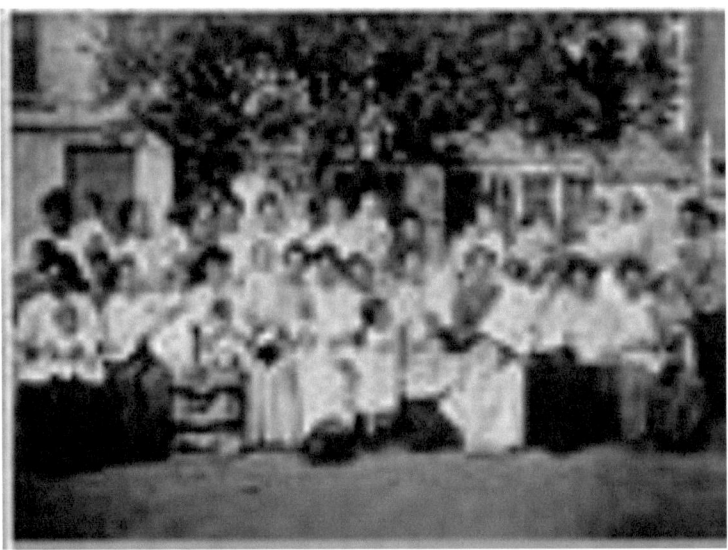

A NEW YORK MILK COMMITTEE'S INFANT DEPOT AND SCHOOL FOR MOTHERS

Pasteurization, municipal dairies, municipal milk shops, municipal infant-milk depots, are the four chief remedies of the *doing things* school. European experience is cited in support of each. We are told that cow's milk, intended by nature for an infant cow with four stomachs, is not suited, even when absolutely pure, to the human infant's single stomach. Cow's milk should be modified, weakened, diluted, to fit the digestive powers of the individual infant; hence the municipal depot or milk dispensary that provides exactly the right milk for each baby, prescribed by municipal physicians and nurses who know. That the well-to-do and the just-past-infancy may have milk as safe as babies receive [262]at the depot, municipalization of farm and milk shop is advocated. Some want the city to run only enough farms and milk shops to set a standard for private farmers, as has been done in Rochester. This is city ownership and operation for educational purposes only. Finally, because raw milk even from clean dairies may contain germs of typhoid, scarlet fever, or tuberculosis, pasteurization is demanded to kill every germ. There are advocates of pasteurization that deprecate the practice and deny that raw milk is necessarily dangerous; they favor it for the time being until farms and shops have acquired habits of cleanliness. Likewise many would prefer private pasteurization or laws compelling pasteurization of all milk offered for sale; but they despair of obtaining safe milk unless city officials are held [263]responsible for safety. Why wait to discuss political theories about the proper sphere for government, when, by acting, hundreds of thousands of lives can be saved annually? These methods of *doing things* will not add to the price of milk; it is, in fact, probable that the reduction in the cost of caring for the sick and for inspecting farms and shops will offset the net cost of depots, farms, and dairies.

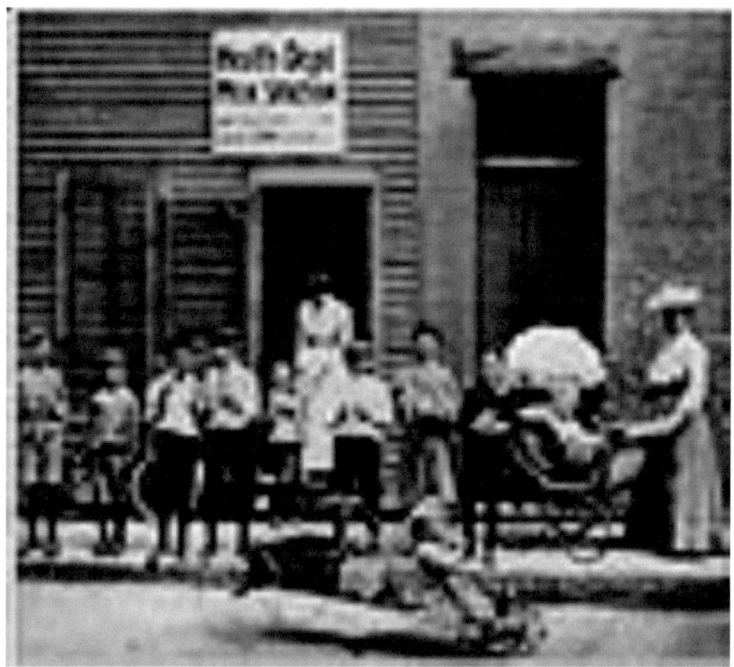

ONE OF ROCHESTER'S SCHOOLS IN CLEANLINESS

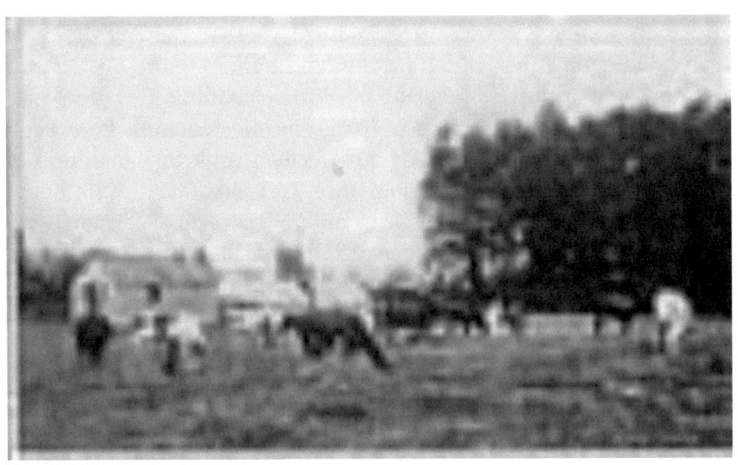

ROCHESTER'S MODEL DAIRY FARM

As to pasteurization, its cost is negligible, while the cost of cleanliness is two, four, or ten cents a quart. Whether ideally clean milk is safe or not, raw milk that is not clean is unfit for human consumption. All cities should compel evidence of pasteurization as a condition of sale. Large cities should have their own pasteurizing plants, just as many cities now have their own vaccine farms and antitoxin laboratories. Parents in small towns and in the country should be taught to pasteurize all milk.

The *getting things done* school admits the need for modified milk of strength suited to the infant's stomach; affirms the danger of milk that contains harmful germs; demands educational work by city, state, and nation; confesses that [264]talk about cleanliness will not make milk safe. On the other hand, it denies that raw milk is necessarily dangerous; that properly modified, clean, raw milk is any safer when pasteurized; that talking about germ-proof milk insures germ extinction. It maintains that pasteurization kills benign germs essential to the life of milk, and that after benign germs are killed, pasteurized milk, if exposed to infection, is more dangerous than raw milk, for the rapid growth of harmful germs is no longer contested by benign germs fighting for supremacy. While it is admitted that raw milk produced under ideal conditions may become infected by some person ignorant of his condition, and before detection may cause typhoid, scarlet fever, or consumption, it has not been proved that such instances are frequent or that the aggregate of harm done equals that which pasteurized milk may do. Pasteurization does not remove chemical impurities; boiling dirt does not render it harmless. The remedy for germ-infected milk is to keep germs out of milk. The remedy for unclean milk is cleanliness of cow, cow barn, cowyard, milker, milk can, creamery, milk shop, bottle, nipple. If the sale of unclean milk is prevented, farmers will, as a matter of course, supply clean milk. By teaching farmers and milk retailers the economic advantages of cleanliness they will cultivate habits that guarantee a clean milk supply. By punishing railroads and milk companies that transport milk at a temperature which encourages germ growth, and by dumping in the gutter milk that is offered for sale above 50 degrees, the refrigerating of milk will be made the rule. Purging magistrates' courts of their leniency toward dealers in impure, dangerous milk is better than purging milk of germs. Boiling milk receptacles will save more babies than boiling milk. Teaching mothers about the care of babies will bring better results than giving them a false sense of safety, because only one of many dangers has been removed by pasteurization. Educating consumers to demand [265]clean milk and to support aggressive work by health departments leaves fewer evils unchecked than covering up uncleanliness by pasteurization.

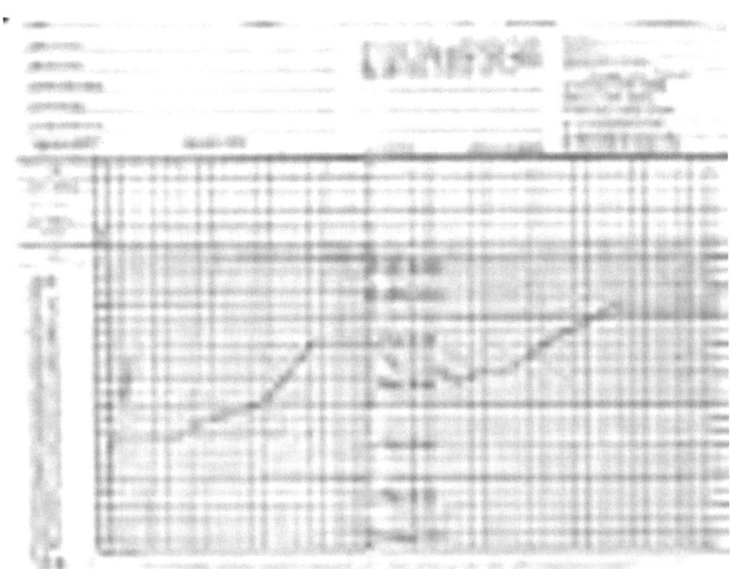

NEW YORK MILK COMMITTEE'S GRAPHIC METHOD OF SHOWING BABIES' PROGRESS

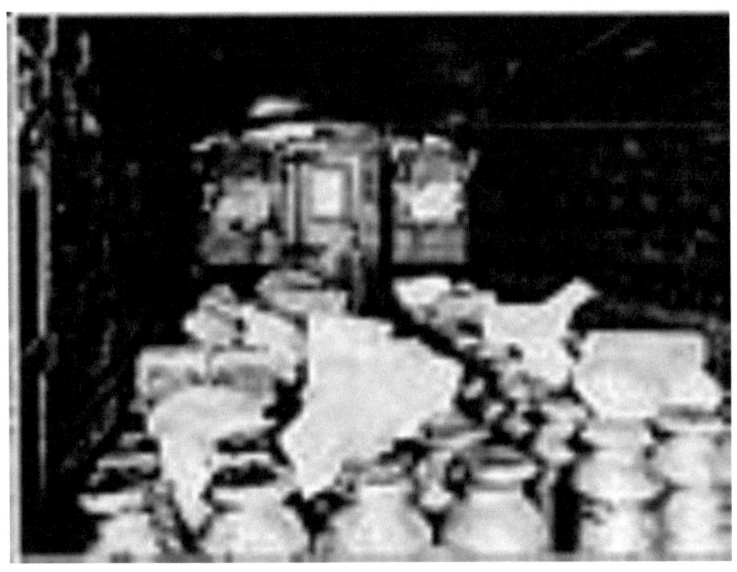

PRODUCING WINTER CONDITIONS IN MIDSUMMER BY PROPER REFRIGERATION FOR MILK IN FREIGHT CARS

When doctors disagree what are we laymen to do? We can take an intelligent interest in the inquiries that are now being made by city, state, and national governments. Because everybody believes that clean milk is safer than unclean milk, that milk at 50 degrees will not breed harmful germs, we can demand milk inspection that will tell our health officers and ourselves which dealers sell only clean milk at 50 degrees and never more than 60 degrees, that never shows over 100,000 colonies to the cubic centimeter. We can get our health departments to publish the results of their scoring of dairies and milk shops in the papers, as has been done in Montclair. We can tell our health officers that the best results in fighting infant mortality are at Rochester, which city, winter and summer, [266]by inspection, correspondence, and punishment, educates farmers and dealers in cleanliness, not only censuring when dirty or careless, but explaining how to make more money by being clean. Finally, mothers can be taught at home how to cleanse the bottles, the nipples, all milk receptacles, and all things in rooms where milk is kept. Absolutely clean milk of proper temperature *at the shop* may not safely be given to a baby in a dirty bottle. Infant milk depots, pasteurization, the best medical and hospital care, breast feeding itself, cannot prevent high baby mortality if mothers are not clean. The most effective volunteer effort for pure milk is that which first makes the health machinery do its part and then teaches, teaches, teaches mothers and all who have to do with babies.

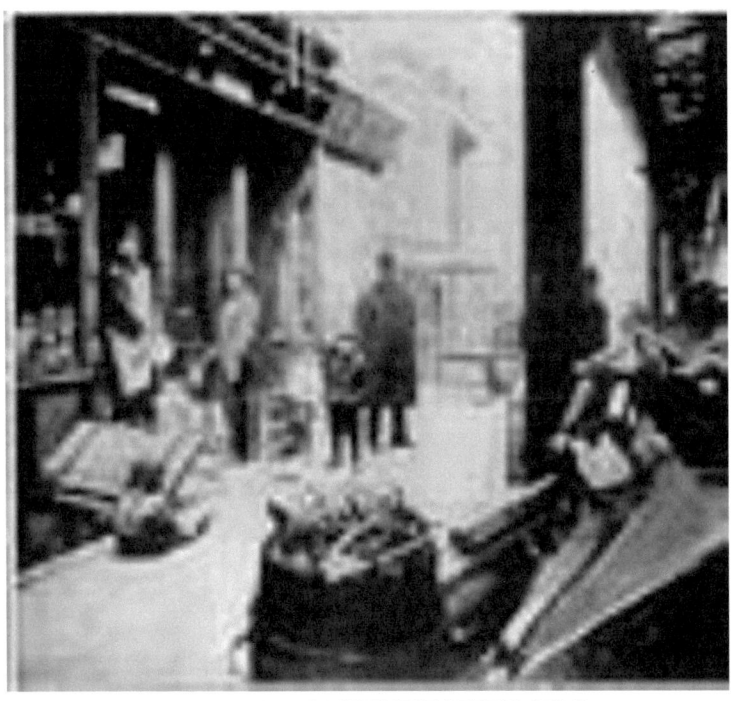

NEITHER PASTEURIZATION NOR
INSPECTION CAN MAKE IT SAFE TO
SELL "DIP MILK" UNDER SUCH UN-
CLEAN CONDITIONS

[267]"Clean air, clean babies, clean milk," has been the slogan of Junior Sea Breeze,—a school for mothers right in the heart of New York's upper East Side. In the summer of 1907 twenty nurses went from house to house telling 102,000 mothers how to keep the baby well. This was the only district that had fewer baby deaths than for 1906. Had other parts of the city shown the same gain, there would have been a saving of 1100 babies. The following winter a similar work was conducted by nurses from the recently founded Caroline Rest, which has an educational fund for instruction of mothers in the care of babies, especially babies not yet born and just born. Heretofore the baby has been expected to cry and to have summer complaint before anybody worried about the treatment it received.

If the baby lived through its second summer, it was considered great good fortune. Junior Sea Breeze and Caroline Rest start their educational work before the baby is sick, in fact, before it is born. Their results have been so notable that several well-to-do mothers declare that they wish they too might have a school. Dispensaries and diet kitchens and more particularly maternity wards of hospitals, family physicians, nurses, and midwives, should be required to know how to teach mothers to feed babies regularly, the right quantities, under conditions that insure cleanliness whether the breast or the bottle is used. Perhaps some day no girl will be given a graduating certificate, or a license for work, teaching, or marriage, until she has demonstrated her ability to give some mother's baby "clean air, clean body, clean milk."

FOOTNOTES:

[15] Libraries should obtain all reports on milk, Bureau of Animal Industry, Washington, D.C.

[268]

CHAPTER XXVIToC

PREVENTIVE "HUMANIZED" MEDICINE: PHYSICIAN AND TEACHER

No profession, excepting possibly the ministry, is regarded with greater deference than the medical profession. Our ancestors listened with awe and obedience to the warnings and behests of the medicine man, bloodletter, bonesetter, family doctor. In modern times doctors have disagreed with each other often enough to warrant laymen in questioning the infallibility of any individual healer or any sect, whether homeopath, allopath, eclectic, osteopath, or scientist. Yet to this day most of us surround the medical profession or the healing art with an atmosphere of necromancy. Even after we have given up faith in drugs or after belief is denied in the reality of disease and pain, we revere the calling that concerns itself, whether gratuitously or for pay, with conquering bodily ills.

Self-laudation continues this hold of the medical profession upon the lay imagination. One physician may challenge another's faults, ridicule his remedies, call his antitoxin dangerous poison, but their common profession he proudly styles "the most exalted form of altruism." Young men and women beginning the study or the practice of medicine are exhorted to continue its traditions of self-denial, and in their very souls to place human welfare before personal or pecuniary advancement. Newspapers repeat exhortation and laudation. We laymen pass on the story that we know is not universally true, — physicians know, physicians apply what they know without consciousness of error, physicians must be implicitly trusted.

[269]For a physician to give poison when he means to give food is worse, not better, than for a layman to make the same mistake. Neither the moral code nor the law of self-preservation enjoins a tuberculous mother to take alcohol or to sleep in an unventilated room, even if an uninformed physician prescribes it. Instruction in physiology and hygiene would be futile if those who are educated as to

the elementary facts of hygiene and physiology must blindly follow blind physicians. A family doctor who gives cod-liver oil for anæmia due to adenoids may do a child as much harm as a nurse who drugs the baby to make it sleep. The physician who refuses to tell the board of health when smallpox or typhoid fever first breaks out takes human life just as truly as if he tore up the tracks in front of an express train. This is another way of saying that parents and teachers must fit themselves to know whether the family physician and their community's physicians are efficient practitioners and teachers. Every one can learn enough about the preventable causes of sickness and depleted vitality to insist upon the ounce of education and prevention that is better than a pound of cure.

For its sins of omission, as for its sins of commission, the medical profession shares responsibility with laymen. For years leading educators, business men, hospital directors, public officials, have known that communicable diseases could be stamped out. The methods have been demonstrated. There is absolutely no excuse to-day for epidemics of typhoid in Trenton, Pittsburg, or Scranton, for epidemics of scarlet fever in the small towns of Minnesota, for uninterrupted epidemics of tuberculosis everywhere. Had either laymen, physicians, or school-teachers made proper use of the knowledge that has been in text-books for a generation, this country would be saving thousands of lives and millions of dollars every year. Our *doing* and *getting done* have lagged behind our *knowing*.

[270]The failure of physicians to "socialize" or "humanize" their knowledge is due to two causes: (1) no one has been applying *result tests* to the profession as a whole and to the state in its capacity as doctor, testing carefully the sickness rate, the death rate, and the expense rate of preventable diseases; (2) physicians themselves have not needed to know, either at college or in practice, the tax levied upon their communities by preventable sickness. Public schools can do much to secure result tests for individual physicians, for the profession as a whole, and for boards of health. Schooling in preventive medicine, or, better named, schooling in preventive hygiene, will fit physicians to do their part in eradicating preventable disease.

Preventive hygiene is not an essential part of the training of American physicians or nurses to-day. Not only are there no colleges of preventive hygiene, but medical schools have not provided individual courses. It is possible for a man to graduate with honors from our leading medical colleges without knowing what "vital statistics" means. Even boards of health, their duties and their educational opportunities, are not understood by graduates; it is an accident if the "social and economic aspects of medical practice," "statistical fallacies," "hospital administration," "infant mortality," are familiar terms. It is for this reason, rather than because physicians are selfish, that indispensable and beneficent legislation is so generally opposed by them when the prerogatives of their profession seem in danger. Practically every important sanitary advance of the past century has been fought at the outset by those whose life work should have made them see the need. Physicians bitterly attacked compulsory vaccination, medical inspection of schools, compulsory notification of communicable diseases. What is perhaps more significant of the physician's indifference to preventive hygiene is the fact that most of the sanitary movements that have [271]revolutionized hygienic conditions in America owe their inception and their success to laymen, for example, tenement-house reform, anti-child labor and anti-tuberculosis crusades, welfare work in factories, campaigns for safety appliances, movement for a national board of health, prison, almshouse, and insane-asylum reform, schools for mothers, and milk committees. The first hospital for infectious diseases, the first board of health, the first out-of-door sea-air treatment of bone tuberculosis in the United States, were the result of lay initiative.

Dr. Hermann M. Biggs says that in America the greatest need of the medical profession and of health administration is training that will enable physicians and lay inspectors to use their knowledge of preventive hygiene for the removal of living and working conditions that cause preventable sickness. A physician without knowledge of preventive hygiene is simply doing a "general repair" business.

For a few months in 1907 New York City had a highly efficient commissioner of street cleaning, who, in spite of the unanimous protests and appeals of the press, refused to give up the practice of medicine. Hitherto the board of health of that city has been unable to obtain the full time of its physicians because professional standards give greater credit to the retail application of remedies than to the wholesale application of preventives.

Statesmanship as well as professional ability is expected of physicians in the leading European cities, more particularly of those connected with health departments. There it is not felt that a medical degree is of itself a qualification for sanitary or health work. After the professional course, physicians must take courses in preventive hygiene and in health administration. Medical courses include such subjects as vital statistics, duties of medical officers of health, sanitary legislation, state medicine.

[272]The needless cost for one year of "catching" diseases in New York City would endow in perpetuity all the schools and lectureships and journals necessary to teach preventive hygiene in every section of this great country. That city alone sacrifices twenty-eight thousand lives annually to diseases that are officially called preventable. The yearly burial cost of these victims of professional and community neglect is more than a million dollars. When to the doctor bills, wages lost, burial cost of those who die are added the total doctor bills, wages lost, and other expenses of the sick who do not die, we find that one city loses in dollars and cents more every year from communicable diseases than is spent by the whole United States for hospitals and boards of health.

Many diseases and much sickness are preventable that are not communicable. Indigestion due to bad teeth is not itself communicable, but it can be prevented. One's vitality may be sapped by irregular eating or too little sleep; others will not catch the trouble, although too often they imitate the harmful habits. Adenoids and defective vision are preventable, but not contagious. Spinal curvature and flat foot are unnecessary, but others cannot catch them. Preventive hygiene, however, should teach the physician's duty to educate his patient and his community regarding all controllable conditions that injure or promote the health.

In the absence of special attention to preventive medicine new truth is forced to fight its way, sometimes for generations, before it is accepted by the medical profession. So strong are the traditions of that profession and so difficult is it for the unconventional or heterodox individual to retain the confidence of conservative patients, that the forces of honorable medical practice tend to discourage research and invention. The man who discovers a surgical appliance is forced by the ethics of his profession either [273]to commercialize it and lose his professional standing, or to abide the convenience of his colleagues and their learned organizations in testing it. Rather than be branded a quack, charlatan, or crank, the physician keeps silent as to convictions which do not conform to the text-books. Many a life-saving, health-promoting discovery which ought to be taken up and incorporated into general practice from one end of the country to the other, and which should be made a part of the minimum standard of medical practice and medical agreement, must wait twenty-five or fifty years for recognition.

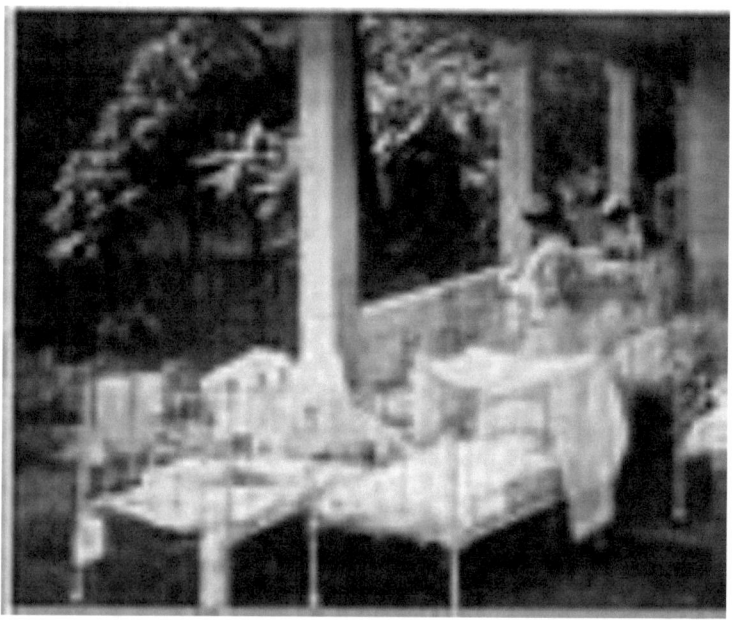

THE DISCIPLE OF FRESH AIR AND HOME INSTRUCTION IS STILL AN OUTCAST IN SCORES OF HOSPITALS

For want of a school of preventive medicine to emphasize universally every new truth, the medical colleges are permitted to remain twenty-five or fifty years behind absolutely demonstrated facts as to medical truth and medical [274]practice. In 1761 a German physician, Avenbruger, after discovering that different sounds revealed diseased tissue, used "chest tapping" in the diagnosis of lung trouble. In 1815 Lëannec discovered that sound from the chest was more distinct through a paper horn. On that principle the modern stethoscope is built. He made an accurate diagnosis of tuberculosis, and while suffering from that disease treated himself as a living clinical study. In 1857 Pasteur proved the presence of germs "without which no putrefaction, no fermentation, no decay of tissue takes place." In 1884 Trudeau started the first out-of-door care of pulmonary tuberculosis in America. In 1892 Biggs secured the compulsory notification of pulmonary tuberculosis. In 1904 began our first out-of-door sea-air treatment for bone tuberculosis. Yet there are thousands of physicians to-day who sincerely believe that they are earning their fees, who, from houses shut up like ovens, give advice to patients for treatment of tuberculosis, who prescribe alcohol and drugs, who diagnose the disease as malaria for fear patients will be scared, who oppose compulsory registration, and who never look for the tuberculous origin of crippled children. Just think of its being possible, in 1908, for a tuberculous young man of thirty to pay five dollars a day to a sanatorium whose chief reliance is six doses of drugs a day!

In 1766 America's first dentist came to the United States. By 1785 itinerant dentists had built up a lucrative practice. In 1825 a course of lectures on dentistry was delivered before the medical class at the University of Maryland. As early as 1742 treatises were written "Upon Dentition and the Breeding of Teeth in Children." In 1803 the possibility of correcting irregularities was pointed out, as was the pernicious effect of tartar on the teeth in 1827. In 1838 attempts were made to abolish, "in all common cases, the pernicious habit of tooth drawing." In 1841 treatises were written on the importance of regulating [275]the teeth of children before the fourteenth year and on the importance of preserving the first teeth. Yet in 1908 it is necessary to write the chapter on Dental Sanitation. Few physicians, whether in private practice or hospitals or just out of medical college, consider it necessary to know the conditions of the mouth before prescribing drugs for physical illness.

Osteopathy furnishes an up-to-date illustration. Discredited by the medical profession, by medical journals and medical schools, it has in fifteen years built up a practice of eight thousand men, having from one to three years' training, including over one hundred physicians with full medical training plus a course in osteopathy. There were means of learning fifteen years ago what was truth and what was quackery about the practice of osteopathy. By refusing to look for its truth and by concentrating attention upon its quackery the medical profession has lost fifteen years. Whereas the truth of osteopathy should have been adopted by the medical colleges and a knowledge of its possibilities and limitations required of every practicing physician, a position has been reached where alleged quackery seems in several important points to be discrediting the sincerity, the intelligence, and the efficiency of orthodox medicine. No appeal to the natural can be stronger, no justification of schools of preventive medicine more complete, than the following paragraph from an osteopathic physician who is among the small number who, having both the medical and osteopathic degrees, see both the possibilities and limitations of manual surgery and demand the inclusion of this new science in the medical curriculum.

The physical method of treating disease presents a tremendous and significant departure from the empiricism of medicine and the experimentation of dietetics, the restricted fields of electricity, suggestion, water cures, and massage. The patient as an individual is not treated; the disease as a disease is not treated; the [276]symptoms are not treated; but the entire physical organism, with its many parts and diverse functions, is exhaustively examined until each and every abnormal condition, whether of structure or of function, causing disease and maintaining symptoms, is found and administered to with the skill of a definite art, based upon the data of an exact science.

Likewise the truths underlying Christian Science have been disdained by medical schools and medical experts, just as its spiritual truth has been disdained by religious leaders, until it has grown to such strength that laymen are almost forced to question the sincerity and the efficacy of the conventional in religion as well as medicine. In May, 1907, the Emmanuel Church in Boston organized a clinic for the purpose of utilizing for neurasthenics particularly both the spiritual and the physical truths underlying religion and the various branches of medical science. Daily papers and magazines are giving a great deal of space to this experiment in "psychotherapy," which is discussed in the chapter on Mental Hygiene. Schools and chairs in preventive hygiene would soon give to the medical profession a point of view that would welcome every new truth, such as the alliance of religion and medicine, and estimate its full worth promptly. Truth seeking would be not only encouraged but made a condition of professional standing.

Just what attitude any particular physician takes can be learned by the teacher or parents whose children he treats. If he pooh-poohs or resents board of health regulations as to isolation of scarlet-fever patients, he is a dangerous man, no matter how noble his personal character. If he says cross-eyes will straighten, weak eyes will strengthen, or nose-stopping adenoids "absorb," he is bound to do harm. If he says tuberculosis is incurable, noncommunicable, hereditary, or curable by drugs, or if he tries to cure cancer by osteopathy, he can do more injury than an insane criminal. If he fails to teach a mother how to bathe, feed, [277]and clothe the baby, how to ventilate a room for the sick or the well, he is an expensive luxury for family or for school, and belongs to an age that knew neither school nor preventive hygiene. If he takes no interest in health administration; if he overlooks unclean milk or unclean streets, open sewers, and unsanitary school buildings, street cars, churches, and theaters; if he does not help the health board, the public hospitals, the schools, the factory, and tenement departments enforce sanitary laws, he is derelict as a citizen and as a member of an "exalted profession." [278]If he sees only the patients he himself treats or one particular malady, he is derelict as a teacher, no matter how charming his personality or how skilled in his specialty. If a school physician is slovenly in his work, if he spends fifteen minutes when he is paid for an hour, should the efficient school-teacher conceal the fact from her superiors because he is a physician? If private hospitals misrepresent facts or compromise with political evils for the sake of a gift of public money, their offense is more heinous because of their exalted purpose. The test of a physician's worth to his patients and to his community is not what he is or what he has learned, and not what his profession might be, but what happens to patient and to community. Human welfare demands that the medical profession be judged by what it does, not by what it might do if it made the best possible use of its knowledge or its opportunity.

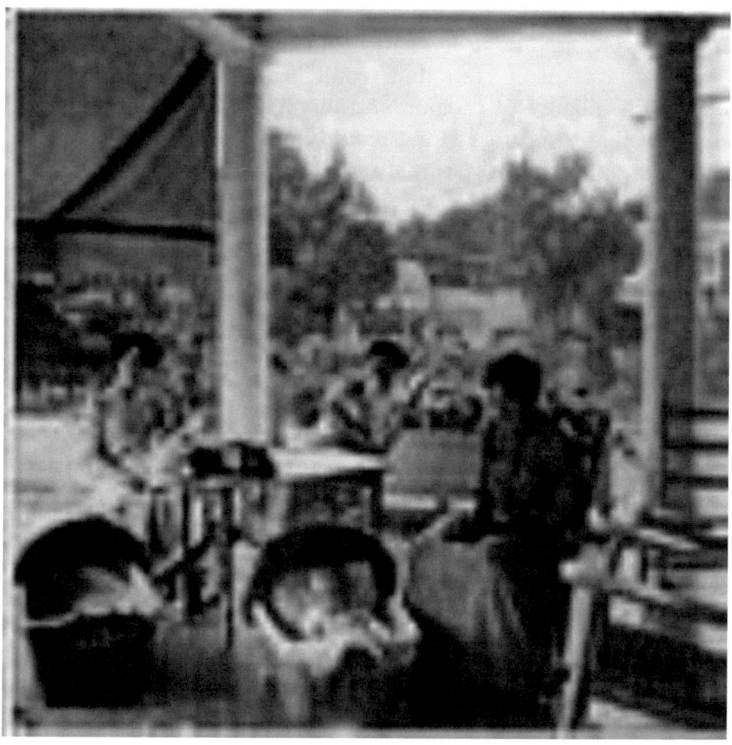

TOO MANY PHYSICIANS AND EVEN MATERNITY HOSPITALS FAIL TO TEACH MOTHERS, EITHER BEFORE OR AFTER BABIES ARE BORN
Caroline Rest Educational Fund was given to show the value of such teaching

A dispensary that treats more patients than it can care for properly is no better than a street-car company that chronically provides too few seats and too many straps. Unless physicians test themselves and their profession by results, we shall be compelled to "municipalize the medical man." Preventable sickness costs too much, causes too much wretchedness, and hampers too many modern educational and industrial activities to be neglected. If the medical profession does not fit itself to serve general interests, then cities, counties, and states will take to themselves the cure as well as the prevention of communicable and other preventable sickness. Human life and public health are more precious than the medical profession, more important even than theories and traditions against public interference in private matters. The unreasoning opposition of medical men to government protection of health, their concentration on cure, and their tardy emphasis on prevention have forced many communities to stumble into the evil practices mentioned in Chapter XVI. Incidentally, [279]the best physicians have learned that the prosperity of their profession increases with every increase in the general standard of living. It is the man in the ten-room house not the man in one room who supports physicians in luxury. It is the healthy man and the healthy community that value efficient medical service.

Many American cities maintain dispensaries and hospitals for the poor. Whether they will go to the logical conclusion of engaging physicians to give free treatment to all regardless of income depends largely upon what the next generation of private physicians do. The state already says when a physician's training fits him to practice. It will soon expect him to pass rigid examinations in the social and economic aspects of his profession, — its educational opportunity, vital statistics, sick and death rates. Will it need to municipalize him in order to protect itself?

Obviously the teacher or parent should not begin cooperation with physicians by lecturing them or by assuming that they are selfish and unwilling to teach. The best first step is to ask questions that they should be able to answer:

What causes cholera morbus or summer complaint? When does milk harm the baby? How can unclean milk be made safe? Whose fault is it that the milk is sold unclean and too warm? What agencies help sick babies? What is the health board doing to teach mothers?

Or, if a school physician, the teacher can ask:

Why not remove these adenoids? What causes them? When will they disappear by absorption? What harm can they do in the meantime? How long would an operation take? Would it hurt very much? What would be the immediate effects? Why not act at once? What provisions are there in town for such operations? Why have the physicians paid so little attention to breathing troubles? What could your state do to interest physicians in school hygiene? Will the school physician talk to a [280]mothers' meeting? What agencies will give outings to sick children? What dispensaries are accessible? Who is the proper person to organize a public health league?

Physicians love to teach. If teachers and parents will love to learn and will ask the right questions, all physicians can be converted into hygiene missionaries, heralds of a statesmanship that guarantees health rights to all.

Licensing the Practitioner

Three parties are interested in setting a high standard for physicians, dentists, druggists, nurses, and veterinary surgeons—the profession itself, the schools that educate, and the general public on whom the arts are practiced. The schools and the practitioners are, for the most part, primarily interested in protecting a monopoly of skill. Their interest in restrictive legislation is analogous to that of the labor union which limits the number of apprentices. This trade unionism among professional colleges and professional graduates of these colleges has gradually developed a higher and higher standard that results in greater protection to the public. The first step is generally to demand that all persons entering a profession after a given date shall prove to the state their ability to "practice" without injury to clients. It is almost impossible to get such laws through unless the original law exempts all persons by whatever name, who are practicing the art in question at the time the law is passed. Whether we are speaking of medicine, law, dentistry, accountancy, osteopathy, or barbering, this has been the history of compulsory restriction and of state examinations.

As with regard to most other legislation, the enforcement of the law lags behind its definition. Moreover nothing is done after a man has passed a certain examination to see that he remains fit and safe to treat the public. Because no supervision is provided except on the day of [281]examination, it is possible for men and women to fill their brains for a week or two weeks with the information necessary to pass what coaches and tutors have learned will, in all probability, be asked. Forever after, the public is left to protect itself. Out of this condition have arisen the evil, unethical, and unprofessional practices represented particularly by painless dentists, by ignorant or dishonest physicians, and by osteopaths and careless nurses.

The machinery for preventing these evils is discussed in Chapter XXIX. Suffice it here to present to parents and teachers the need for examination in advance of certification that will show whether or not those who make a livelihood by caring for others' health are equipped to mitigate rather than aggravate evils, and for further tests by which the public can learn from time to time which, among those professional men who are protected by the public against competition, continue to be safe. Finally, if, as will be clearly seen, it is desirable that what we call professional ethics persist and that self-advertisement be discouraged, society must, for its own protection, adopt some other means than epithets to correct the evils of self-advertisement and quackery. Even though we admit the responsibility of each citizen when he goes to the house of a private practitioner who has made no other effort to lure him thither than to place a card in the window, it must be seen that we cannot hold responsible for their choice men and women who receive through newspapers, magazines, or circulars convincing notices that Dr. So-and-So or the Integrity Company or the Peerless Dental Parlor will place at their disposal, at prices within their reach, skill and devotion absolutely beyond their reach at the office of an efficient private practitioner. Some way must be found by which departments of health will currently impose tests of methods and results upon physicians, opticians, pharmacists, manufacturers of medicine, and dentists.

[282]As laymen become more intelligent regarding their own bodies and healthy living, it grows harder and harder for quacks and incompetents to mislead and exploit them. Better than any possible outside safeguard is hygienic living. Fortunately, we can all learn the simple tests of environment and of living necessary to the selection of physicians, dentists, and opticians, or other "architects of health" whose efficiency and integrity are beyond question.

[283]

PART IV. OFFICIAL MACHINERY FOR ENFORCING HEALTH RIGHTS

CHAPTER XXVIIToC

DEPARTMENTS OF SCHOOL HYGIENE

The term "school hygiene" generally suggests no other school than the public school. State laws say nothing about compulsory hygiene in military academies, ladies' seminaries, or other preparatory and finishing schools. Yet when one thinks of it, one must conclude that the right to health and to healthful school environment cannot equitably be confined to the children whose tuition is given at public expense. There is a better way to check "swollen" fortunes than by ruining the health of "fortune's children." The waste and danger of slow-minded, noticeably inefficient children are no less when parents are rich than when parents are poor. There is no justification for neglecting the health of children in parochial schools, in private schools for the well-to-do or rich, or in commercial schools for the ambitious youth of lower income strata. Nor has the commercial, parochial, private school, or college, any clearer right than the public school to injure or to fail to promote pupils' health. So far as school hygiene is advisable, so far as it is right to make hygiene compulsory, its personal and social benefits should be shared by children of school age without regard to income, and its laws should be enforced by all teachers, principals, and officers that have [284]to do with school. In presenting a programme for school hygiene this chapter refers to the hygiene taught, the hygiene practiced, the hygiene not taught, and the hygiene not practiced in buildings and on grounds where children and youth are at school, whether these children are in kindergarten or high school, in reformatory or military academy, in charitable school, or in finishing and preparing center for society's juniors.

The question of the local, state, and national machinery by which proper standards of school hygiene shall be made effective will be taken up after we have considered individual steps in a comprehensive programme for school hygiene.

1. *Thorough physical examination of all candidates for teachers' positions and periodic reëxamination of accepted teachers.*

Teachers would be grateful to be told in time their own physical needs and the relations of their vitality to the vitality of their pupils. Are your teachers examined? Do they know the laws of health and the signs of child health? Are they permitted to continue in schoolrooms after tuberculosis is discovered? Are normal graduates given physical tests before being permitted to teach and before being permitted to give four years to preparation for teaching?

2. *Thorough physical examination of every single child in every single school upon entering and periodically during school life.*

We believe a vast number of things that "ain't so" about the health of country children as compared with city children, of private-school children as compared with public-school children. Where do we find more degenerate men, physically and morally, than in so-called "American settlements," where, for generations, children have had all outdoors to play in, except when in homes and schoolhouses that are seldom cleansed and seldom ventilated? Open [285]mouths and closed minds clog the "little red schoolhouse"; there headaches do not suggest eye strain; there deafness and running ears are frankly attributed to scarlet fever which everybody must have with all the other "catching" diseases, the earlier the better; there colds begin in December and run until March, to the serious injury of attendance and promotion records; there bone tuberculosis is called "knee trouble" or "spine trouble in the family"; there boys like my little friend Fred count the bottles of cod-liver oil they take to cure adenoids that could be removed in two minutes.

The index to community life and community living conditions should be read in the country, not only for the country's sake, but also for the sake of the city whose milk and water, poisoned in the country, cause thousands of deaths annually, besides annual sick bills exceeding many times over the Russell Sage and Carnegie Foundations, which we rightly call munificent. Reading the index of private schools and colleges is important for their children and youth, but still more important for the community upon which unbridled passion, inability to work or to spend properly, inconsequential thinking, mediæval ideals of caste, etc., can inflict greater injuries than can typhoid fever or cholera.

The physical record of each child should be kept from date of entrance to date of leaving school, showing condition at successive examinations, absence because of illness, etc.

3. *Thorough physical examination of children when leaving school, or when passing compulsory school age, as a condition to "working papers" and to "coming out."*

To give working papers to children seriously handicapped by physical defects is to buy future industrial trouble, hospital and poorhouse bills. A boy with adenoids, a girl with eye trouble, should not be permitted to begin the fight for self-support without at least being clearly shown that the [286]correction of these defects will increase their earning power. At present a schoolgirl with incipient tuberculosis, or predisposed to that disease, can get working papers, go to a hammock or tobacco factory, work long hours, breathe bushels of dust, deplete her vitality, spread tuberculosis among her co-workers and home associates, infect a tenement,— and all this without any help or advice or any protection from society until she is too sick to work and her physician notifies the health department that she is a danger center. We may disagree about society's right to control a child's act after the defects are discovered, but who will question society's duty to tell that child and her parents the truth about her physical needs before it accepts her labor or permits her to "enter society"?

4. *Supervision by physicians of hygiene practiced in schoolrooms and on playgrounds.*

Superintendent Maxwell, of New York City, and other educational leaders urge teachers to do their utmost to learn the physical conditions and home environment of the individual child, and to fit school treatment to the individual possibilities and handicaps. But experience proves conclusively that try as they will, teachers and principals have neither the special knowledge nor the time to acquire the special knowledge requisite to use the facts disclosed by the physical examination of school children. Physicians and nurses are needed, not so much for treating children, as for teaching children, parents, teachers, family and dispensary physicians.

Private schools have visiting physicians who may be consulted; they need physicians to supervise, with power to examine or to require certificates of examination. The Committee on the Physical Welfare of School Children found that when a visitor was detailed for that purpose it was easy to secure the coöperation of parents, teachers, family physicians, dispensaries, school boards, and [287]charitable societies. The Hawthorne Club's school secretary has been similarly successful in Boston, as have those of Hartley House, Greenwich House, and the Public Education Association in New York.

5. *Restriction of study hours at school and at home to limits compatible with health.*

Whether the hours of study at school and at home are excessive cannot be learned from treatises on pedagogics or physiology. Because children differ in vitality as in ability to learn, the maximum limit for study hours should be determined by the individual child's physical condition. When the Japanese went to war with Russia the highest authority in the field was the army surgeon. To this fact was largely due the astonishingly small amount of sickness and the high fighting capacity and endurance of the Japanese, working under unfavorable conditions. No board of school superintendents or board of directors, no state superintendent of schools or college professor, has the right to compel or to allow study hours beyond the maximum compatible with the individual student's physical condition and endurance. The physician responsible for school hygiene should have an absolute veto upon any educational policy, method, or environment demonstrably detrimental to children's vitality.

6. *Establishment of a "follow-up" plan to insure action by parents to correct physical defects and to attend to physical needs.*

The advantages of *getting things done* over *doing things* have been repeatedly emphasized. In smaller cities and in rural districts it is particularly important for schools to get things done better by existing local agencies, such as churches, health and street-cleaning departments, hospitals, clinics, medical and sanitary societies, trade unions, young people's societies, and women's clubs. Where parents who have been followed up and taught, obstinately or [288]ignorantly refuse to attend to their children's needs, the segregation of the physically defective or needy will encourage the coöperation of children themselves in persuading parents to act intelligently for the child's sake. No child wants to remain "queer" or "dopey" or behind his peers. The city superintendent of schools for New York City has asked for laws compelling parents to permit operations and punishing them for neglecting to take steps, within their power, to remove physical defects discovered at school.

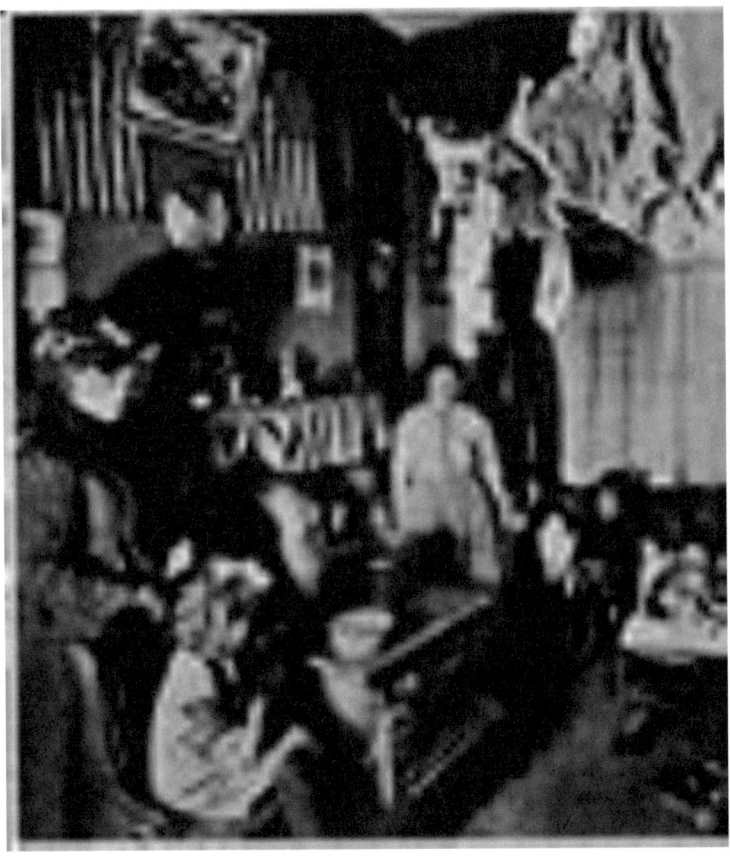

TEACHING A MOTHER TO CARE FOR ONE CHILD INSURES BETTER CARE FOR ALL HER CHILDREN

[289]7. *Physiological age should influence school classification and school curriculum.* On this subject the studies of Dr. C. Ward Crampton, referred to in the chapter on Vitality Tests, are invaluable and as convincing as they are revolutionary. Scientists accept his proof that our present high school curriculum is ill adapted to a large proportion of children; the "physiologically too young" drop out; only the physiologically mature succeed. The two physiological ages should be given different work. Children whose bodies yearn for pictures, muscular and sense expression, should be given a chance in school for normal development. Analysis should wait for action. Organized play and physical training antedated physical examination in our schools. Like the curriculum they often disregard physiological age, doing harm instead of good. Facts as to physical condition and physiological development would enable us to utilize the momentum of these two to broaden school hygiene and to insure proper physical supervision. Only good would result from adopting Leipsic's plan of having school children examined without clothing, in the presence of parents if parents desire. Expensive? Not so expensive as high school "mortality" due to maladjusted curriculums that force the great majority of boys and girls to drop out before graduation and ruin the health of a large fraction of those who remain.

8. *Construction of school building and of curriculum so that, when properly conducted, they shall neither produce nor aggravate physical defects.*

When the state for its own protection compels a child to go to school, it pledges itself not to injure itself by injuring the child. Thousands of children are now being subjected to conditions in school far more injurious than the factory and shop conditions against which the national and state child labor committees have aroused universal indignation. Two illuminating studies of school buildings in New [290]York City were made last year by the Committee on the Physical Welfare of School Children, and later by the Board of Education. Similar studies should be made of every schoolroom. Whereas our discussions of buildings and curriculum have hitherto proceeded largely from abstract principles of light, ventilation, heating, and pedagogics, these two reports deal with rooms, equipment, courses of study, and school habits as they are, with obvious detrimental effects on child victims. Numerous questions that it is practicable to answer are given in Chapter XIV.

What and when to build can be better determined after we have learned the what and the where of present equipment.

In passing it is worth while to note that in large cities teachers are frequently forced to choose between bad ventilation and street noises. From Boston comes the suggestion that we avoid noises and evils of congestion by building schoolhouses for city children on the outskirts in the midst of fields, transporting, and, if necessary, feeding children at public expense. While it is true that the public funds now spent in attempting to cure physical and moral ills would purchase ample country reservations, the practical next step seems to be to provide ample play space and breathing space within the city for every school building already erected, and without fail for all buildings to be erected hereafter.

9. *Hygiene should be so taught that children will cultivate habits of health and see clearly the relation of health and vitality to present happiness and future efficiency.* Social rather than personal, public rather than private, health needs emphasis. Children can be shown how their health affects their neighbor; why money spent for health boards is a better investment than money given to corrupt politicians; that the cost of accepting Thanksgiving turkey or a park picnic from a political leader who encourages inefficient government is sickness, misery, deficient schooling, lifelong [291]handicap; that children and adults have health rights in school and factory, on street and playground, which the law will protect if only they know when these rights are infringed.

10. *Central supervision of school hygiene.* In private and public, boarding and day, country and city, reformatory and military, commercial and high schools, the index — physical welfare of school children — should be read and interpreted. Headquarters should learn whether or not physical examinations are made and whether harmful conditions are corrected. So far as public schools are concerned, "headquarters" means for cities the fact center that informs city superintendent or school board; for rural schools, it means the

county superintendent's office. Whether city or county headquarters have the facts and act accordingly should be known by state superintendents. Whether state superintendents are demanding the facts and educating the county and city headquarters of their states should be known to the national commissioner of education and by him published for all the world. Some people think the state health board should be responsible, others the state educational authority. The important thing is to make some one officer responsible. Methods can be easily worked out if the need is conceded. Legislatures will gladly confer the powers necessary to reading the index of all public schools.

As for parochial and private schools, they may resent for a time public supervision of their hygiene teaching and practice. However, the case could be so presented that they would ask for it, because it would help not only their pupils and society but the schools themselves. No religious belief or private investment can afford to admit that it disregards child health; state supervision would require nothing more than evidence of adequate school hygiene.

11. *Information gained at school regarding conditions prejudicial to community health should be published and [292]made the basis of an aggressive campaign for the enforcement of sanitary laws.* Ten thousand uses can be made of the information gained at school, ten thousand forces can be made to do educational work, but only a few kinds of work can be done effectively at school. Franklin Ford has said: "You can relate school to all life, but you cannot bring all life under the school roof." As Chapters XVI-XVIII make clear, to socialize the point of view of dispensaries and hospitals is more effective than to put clinics in school buildings. To *do for* or *give to* people who can help themselves is to *give up* and *do up* power of self-help.

Machinery that must some day exist for the execution of this programme will be approximately the following:

I. National Machinery

1. Clearing house for facts regarding school hygiene as taught and practiced in all schools under the Stars and Stripes; this to be a part of the National Bureau of Education.

2. Scientific research to be conducted by the National Bureau of Education or by the future National Board of Health.

II. State Machinery

1. Clearing house for facts regarding school hygiene taught and practiced in all schools within state limits; this to be maintained by the state educational authorities.

2. Agents to make special inquiries as to practice and teaching of school hygiene.

3. Agents to inspect and to instruct county superintendents, county physicians, teachers, normal schools, etc.

4. A bureau of experts — architect, sanitarian, teacher — whose approval must be obtained before any school building can be erected. (A plan which brought excellent results when applied by state boards to charitable institutions, hospitals for the insane, etc.)

5. Standard making by normal schools, state universities, hospitals, or other educational and correctional institutes under direct state management.

[293]III. County Machinery

1. Clearing house for facts regarding school hygiene taught and practiced in all schools within county limits; this to be maintained by the county superintendent of schools.

2. Physician and nurse to organize inspection and instruction for rural schools, to give lessons and make demonstrations at county institutes, to show teachers how to interest physicians, dentists, health officers, and parents in the physical welfare of school children.

IV. Town and Township Machinery

1. Teachers intelligent as to physical needs, as to sanitation of buildings, etc.

2. An examining physician, to be salaried where the population justifies; elsewhere to work as a volunteer in coöperation with teacher and with county physician.

3. Physical history of each child from date of entrance to date of leaving school, to be kept up to date by teacher.

V. City Machinery

1. A division to be known as the Department of School Hygiene, headed by an officer who gives his entire time to that department.

2. A subcommittee of the Board of Education.

3. Clearing house for facts regarding school hygiene taught and practiced in all schools within city limits.

4. Specialists to examine applicants for teaching positions, and to reëxamine teachers to determine fitness for continuance, for promotion, and for special assignments.

5. A bureau for inspection and control of all hygiene of school buildings, old and new, with power to compel repairs or to reject plans that do not make adequate sanitary provision.

6. Similar supervision of curriculum and of study hours prescribed.

7. A bureau for the inspection and control of curriculum, required home study, exercise, physical training, etc., so far as relates to the health of pupils, and to the physical ability of children to be in certain grades or to be promoted. This will decide [294]the duration of lessons, frequency of intermissions, sequence of subjects, time and method of recess throughout the various grades.

8. Supervision of indoor and outdoor playgrounds, roof gardens, indoor and outdoor gymnasiums, swimming pools, etc.

9. Supervision of instruction in school hygiene.

10. A staff of inspectors for communicable diseases of pupils and teachers, to be subject to the board of education or the board of health.

11. A staff of examiners adequate to examine all children and teachers at least once a year for defects of eye, ear, teeth, nose, throat, lungs, spine, bones, glands, etc., and for weight and height to be under the control of the board of education or the board of health. The expense would not be as great as the penalty paid for omitting such examination.

12. A staff of nurses to assist medical examiners to give children practical demonstrations in cleanliness, to teach mothers the care of children both at their homes and in mothers' meetings, to enlist the coöperation of family physician and neighborhood facilities, such as hospitals, dispensaries and relief agencies, magistrates' courts and probation officers, — all to be under the control of the board of education or the board of health.

Whether inspectors, examiners, and nurses shall be directed by the board of education or the board of health is a question that it is impossible to decide without knowledge of local conditions. So far as state and county organizations are concerned, it is clear that whatever the boards of health may do, it will be necessary for state and county superintendents of education to equip themselves with the machinery above recommended. In cities it is quite clear that a board of education should be responsible for all of the machinery suggested, excepting the three divisions that have to do with work hitherto considered as protection against transmissible diseases, namely, inspection, examination, district visiting. In Cleveland these are school duties. In New York they are duties of the health department. Boston has school nurses and health [295]department physicians. The state law of Massachusetts provides that where health boards do not examine school children, school boards may spend money for the purpose.

As to inspection for transmissible diseases, it seems quite clear that health boards should not delegate their authority or responsibility to any other body, for they alone are accountable to their communities for protection against contagion. It is clear, too, that in the interest of community health, departments of health are justified in pointing out in advance of contagion those children most likely to become a menace. Similar grounds of public interest justify the health boards in sending nurses and physicians to the home as a means of getting things done.

Dr. Biggs feels that responsibility for the physical welfare of school children will strengthen health work in all cities, and, given proper interest on the part of school officials, should make possible universal coöperation in a constructive programme. On the other hand, he believes that division of responsibility between school and health boards will weaken both in their appeals for funds and for support of a constructive programme. I have heard principals and superintendents maintain also that the moral effect of a visit to the school by a representative of the health board vested with powers of that board was much greater than a visit by a representative of the school board. They further allege that a physician coming from the outside is more apt to see things that need correction and less apt to accept excuses than an inspector who feels that he belongs to the same working group as the school-teacher. Because the follow-up work in the homes incident to successful use of knowledge gained at school involves so many sanitary remedies, it is theoretically better organization to hold the health authority responsible.

[296]

PRESENT ORGANIZATION OF SCHOOL HYGIENE IN NEW YORK CITY

Many of the elements of the machinery outlined in the preceding chapter already exist in New York City. All of them brought together, either by amalgamation or by proper coördination, would present a very strong front. Unfortunately, however, there is not only unsatisfactory team work, but the efficiency of individual parts is seriously questioned by the heads of the health and school departments.

The inspection for contagious diseases, the examination for physical defects, the follow-up work by nurses and physicians, are in charge of the department of health. Physical training and athletics for elementary and high schools, winter recreation centers, and vacation playgrounds are under directors and assistants employed by the board of education. Heretofore inadequate powers and inadequate assistance for training or for research have been given to the physical director.

The city superintendent of schools, in his report for the year 1907, presented to the board of education in January, 1908, declares that the "present arrangements have been inadequate.... In only 248 schools — less than half the total number — were any examinations for possible diseases made. In these 248 schools not more than one third of the pupils were examined. It is only a few months since any examinations for physical defects were made outside of the boroughs of Manhattan and The Bronx, and then only on account of the New York Committee on the Physical Welfare of School Children."

[297]As is so often the case, it is difficult to decide the merits of a method that has not been efficiently executed. The department of health has not hitherto done its best in its school relations. The commissioner of health, in a public interview, expresses resentment

at the strictures by the school authorities. Yet in 1907 he permitted to accumulate an unexpended balance of $33,000 specifically voted for school inspectors, and repeatedly tried to have this amount transferred to other purposes. The interest of the Bureau of Municipal Research in municipal budgets that tell for what purposes money is voted and then prevent transfers without full publicity, preserved this particular fund. Moreover, the discussion that prevented its diversion from physical examinations strengthened the health department's interest in this important responsibility. Neither physicians nor nurses have been adequately supervised. Instead of seeing that defects were removed, the department of health sent out postal cards like the following:

"This Notice Does NOT Exclude This Child From School"

DEPARTMENT OF HEALTH
THE CITY OF NEW YORK

To prevent

Oct. 2, _____ 190 6

The parent or guardian of _____
of _____ attending P. S. 51 _____
is hereby informed that a physical examination of this child seems to show an abnormal condition of the _Eyes, Nose, Throat and teeth_

Remarks _No Anaemia_

Take this child to your family physician for treatment and advice.
Take this card with you to the family physician.

THOMAS DARLINGTON, M. D.,
HERMANN M. BIGGS, M. D.,   **Commissioner of Health.**
General Medical Officer

From 118,000 such notices sent out only 9600 replies were received, of which only one in twenty stated that attention had actually been given the needy child. The [298]department had been satisfied with evidence that family physicians had advised parents properly, as in the case of the child above reported:

TAKE THIS CARD TO YOUR PHYSICIAN

The Physician in charge is requested to fill out and forward this postal after he has examined this child.

I have this day examined_____
of P. S.___57___and find the following condition:

As reported. Also enlarged cervical glands,

and advised as follows: *Operation for adenoids and tonsils,
Dental treatment at Cornell. Fresh air
outing at Sea Breeze. Eyes wait.*

Respectfully yours, *C. L. O.*

Date __Oct. 9, 1906__

For a candid, complete criticism of the medical examination work up to June, 1908, consult the report of the Bureau of Municipal Research, presented to the Washington Congress of Public Education Associations in October, 1908, by Commissioner of Health, Dr. Darlington. The bureau's study is entitled *A Bureau of Child Hygiene*, and, in addition to the story of medical examination in New York City schools, gives the blank forms adopted for use in September, 1908. Important as are the facts given in this study, its greatest value, its authors declare, is in its account of "the method of intelligent self-criticism and experiment which alone enables a public department to keep its service abreast of public needs."

The Bureau of Municipal Research made its study for the purpose of learning whether the disappointing results emphasized by the school authorities were due to "dual responsibility in the school — that of the board of education and that of the department of health" — and to "lack of power or inclination to compel parents to remedy defects," [299]or to *deficient administration* of power and inclination by health officials. Coöperating with school physicians and nurses in three schools, 1442 children were examined, of whom 1345, or 93.2 per cent, had 3458 defects that needed treatment. The postal-card notice was followed by an interview with the parent either at school or at home. Only 4.2 per cent of the total number of parents refused to act, 81 per cent secured or permitted treatment for one or more defects, while 15 per cent promised to take the proper steps at the earliest possible date. Three fourths of the parents acted after one personal interview. "The net average result of a day's work by a nurse was the actual treatment of over five children, three of them completely, and two of them for one or more defects," — sixty cents per child!

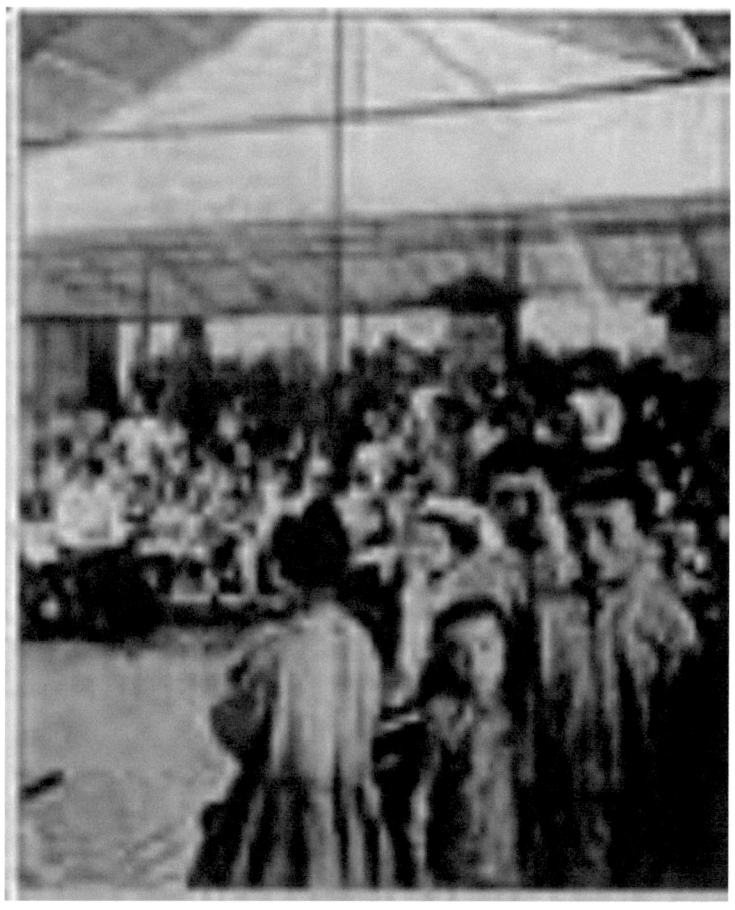

A PHOTOGRAPH OF MOUTH BREATHING MAY MAKE COMPULSION UNNECESSARY

Having established the willingness—even eagerness—of parents to do all in their power to remove defects that handicapped their children, it was obviously the duty of the health department so to organize its work that it could insure the education of parents. The new Bureau of Child Hygiene gives foremost place to instruction of parents in care of babies, in needs of school children, and in the importance of physical examination when enlisting in the industrial army. Whether this work is well done is learned by result tests applied at headquarters, where work done [300]and results are reported daily and summarized weekly. No longer will it be possible, without detection, for one physician to find only eye trouble and to neglect all other defects; for two inspectors examining different children in the same school to report results differing by 100 per cent; for physicians in different schools to find one 18 per cent, another 100 per cent with defects; for two inspectors examining identical children to agree on 51 out of 101 cases of vision, on 49 out of 96 cases of adenoids, or 3 out of 10 cases of skin disease.

So conclusive were the results of follow-up work efficiently supervised by the department of health, that school officials are, for the present, inclined to waive the demand for the transfer of physicians and nurses to the board of education, and to substitute education for compulsion with parents who obstinately refuse to take proper remedial measures for their children when reported defective.

This present plan requires the entire working time of inspectors and nurses for school work. Thus New York has for the present definitely abandoned the plan of having the district inspection for contagious diseases done by school physicians. The purpose of the change is not to reduce danger of infection, which was negligible, but to increase the probability of scientific attention to school children.

Before a final settlement is made for New York City there should be tests showing what the school authorities would do if physicians and nurses were subordinate to them. It is conceivable that one physician working from nine to five would accomplish more than six physicians working the alleged three hours a day. So imperative are the demands of school hygiene that it seems probable that in

New York and in other large cities school physicians, whether paid by the board of health or the board of education, must be expected to be at the service of school children, subject to the call of school officers, during as many [301]hours of the day as teachers themselves must give. It is even conceivable that effective use of the knowledge gained by physical examinations of school children, and by those responsible for school hygiene, will require evening office hours or evening visits to homes, and regular Saturday office hours and Saturday visits by school physicians and nurses. Finally, it must be expected that the programme for school hygiene will need the special attention of physicians and nurses during the summer months, and other vacation periods when children and parents alike have time to receive and to carry out their instructions.

One danger in New York City is that the board of education, like the board of health, when compelled to choose between so-called standard, necessary, traditional duty and school hygiene, will sacrifice the latter. The school authorities, without any more funds and without physicians and nurses, could already have made, had they desired, eye tests and breathing tests sufficiently accurate to detect the majority of children needing attention. The outcome of the discussion as to the jurisdiction of the two boards will undoubtedly be to interest both in their joint responsibility for children's welfare, and to increase the attention given by both to the physical condition of the child when he presents himself for registration as a wage earner.

[302]

OFFICIAL MACHINERY FOR ENFORCING HEALTH RIGHTS

The argument for *getting things done* presumes adequate active machinery, official and private, for *doing things* that schools are being urged to do. The chapter on Departments of School Hygiene suggests local, county, state, and national machinery necessary (1) to protect the child from injuries due to school environment, school methods, and school curriculum; (2) to getting those things done for the child at home and on the street, need for which is disclosed by physical and vitality tests at school. It is unreasonable to confine the school to the activities above outlined unless health machinery, adequate to the demands placed upon it by school and other community needs, is devised and kept in order.

Generally speaking, adequate health machinery is already provided for by city charters and by the state laws under which villages, townships, and counties are organized. Quite as generally, however, machinery and methods of adequate administration are undeveloped. How much machinery has already been set to work by New York City is shown by the accompanying chart. A useful exercise for individuals or school classes wishing to study health administration would be to chart in this way the machinery actually at work in their locality, county, and state. Even for New York it should be remembered that this chart does not include national quarantine, the state protection of the port, the state dairy and health commissions, or the state and national food inspection. [303]To get an idea of the vast amount of attention given to health in New York City there should be added to this chart the work of many departments other than the department of health. The building bureau, tenement-house department, board of water supply, sewage commission, street cleaning, public baths and comfort stations, the department of water, gas, and electricity, and finally the department of hygiene and physical training in the public schools.

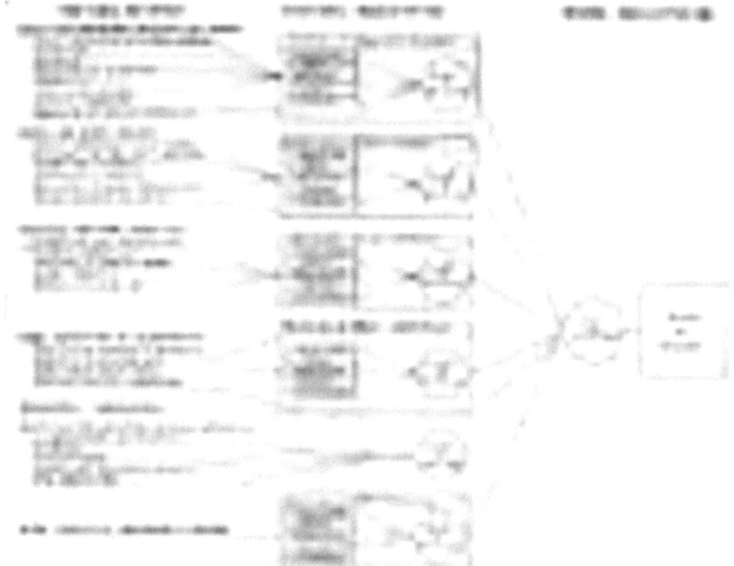

CHART SHOWING HOW NEW YORK CITY'S DEPARTMENT OF
HEALTH EXERCISES IT'S AUTHORITY
Courtesy of Bureau of Municipal Research

Five elements of adequate machinery are generally lost sight of:

1. The voter.

2. The nonvoter, subject to health laws and often apt to violate them.

3. The mayor, governor, or president who appoints health officers.

4. The council, board of aldermen, legislature, or congress that enacts health laws.

5. The police courts and the judiciary—police, circuit and supreme—that decide whether society has suffered from violation of law and what penalties should be inflicted for such violation.

Legislative bodies have hitherto slighted their responsibilities toward public health. The chairman of a committee on public health of a state legislature was heard to remark, "I asked for that committee because there isn't a blooming thing to do." If voters, nonvoters, and health officials will follow the suggestion of this book to secure school and health reports that will disclose community and health needs, it will be increasingly difficult for legislators to refuse funds necessary to efficient health administration.

To the courts tradition has required such deference that one hesitates to find out in how far they have been responsible in the past for the nonenforcement of health laws. Yet nothing is more obstructive of sanitary progress than the failure of magistrates to enforce adequate [304]penalties for truancy, adulteration of milk, maintaining a public nuisance, defiling the air with black smoke, offering putrid meats for sale, running an unclean lodging house, defying tenement-house or factory regulations, working children under age and overtime, spitting in public places, or failing to register transmissible diseases.[16]

The appointing officer cannot, of course, be held responsible unless voters and nonvoters know in how far his appointees are inefficient, and in how far he himself has failed to do his utmost to secure funds necessary to efficiency. Too frequently appointments to health positions have been made on political grounds, and catastrophes have been met by blundering incapacity. The political appointee has been made the scapegoat, and the appointing officer, whether mayor, governor, or president, has regained public confidence by replacing an old with a new incompetent.

In order to have health machinery work properly, the appointing officer should not be allowed to shift responsibility for failure to his subordinates. For example, it was recently found in New York City that while the tenement-house commissioner was being condemned for failing to enforce the law, he had turned over to the corporation counsel, also appointed by the mayor, for prosecution ten thousand "violations" to which no attention whatever had been paid!

The voter, nonvoter, appointing officer, legislative officer, and judicial officer determine the character and purpose of machinery and are analogous to the surveyors, stock-holders, directors, and constructors who provide railroads with tracks and with running stock. The actual running force of health department or railroad is what is meant by its official machinery. What this machinery should be depends, of course, upon the amount of business to be [305]done, and differs with the size of the district and the character of population to be served.

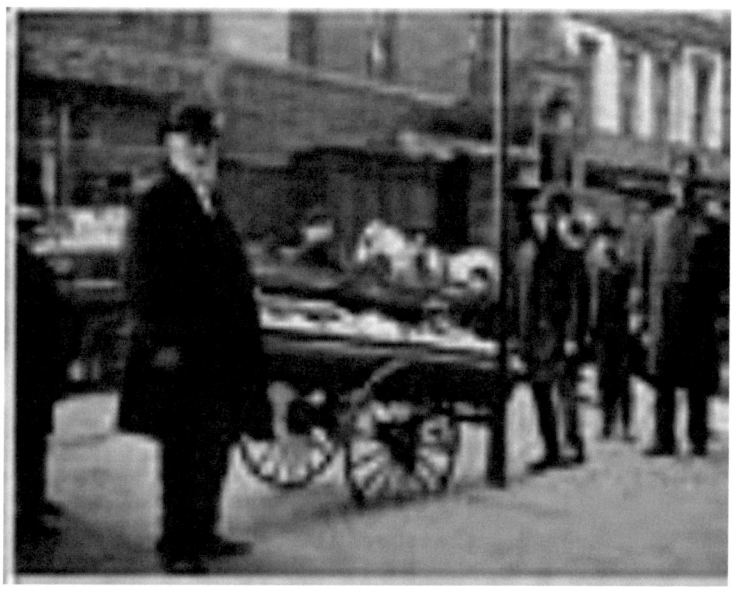

FOR PUSH-CART FOOD, INSPECTION IS PARTICULARLY NEEDFUL

Local health machinery should guarantee protection against the evils mentioned in preceding chapters. In general, one man is better than three to execute, although three may be better than one to legislate. Where small communities do not wish to have the entire state sanitary code rigidly administered, they can adopt New York's method of a legislative board of three members, headed by an executive, whose business it is to act, not talk; to watch subordinates, and to enforce rigidly and continuously ordinances passed by the board. The National Bureau of Census places under the general heading Health and Sanitation the following activities: health administration, street cleaning and refuse disposal, sewers and sewage disposal. Sanitarians generally emphasize also the health significance of efficient water service.

[306]A community's health programme should be clearly outlined in the annual budget. Where health work is given funds without specification of the kinds of work to be done, serious evils may be overlooked and lesser evils permitted to monopolize the energies of health officers. Again, after money has been voted to prevent an evil, records should be made of work done when done, and of money spent when spent, so that any diversion will be promptly made known. The best present guides to budget making, to educational health reports, and to records that show efficiency or inefficiency of health administrators are the budget and report of the department of health for New York City, and the story of their evolution told in *Making a Municipal Budget*, by the Bureau of Municipal Research.

To find out whether local machinery is adequate, the reader must enumerate the things that need to be done in his community, remembering that in all parts of the United States to-day there are sanitary laws offering protection against dangers to health, excepting some dangers not understood until recently, such as child labor, dangerous trades, lack of safety devices. Adequate local protection, however, will not become permanent until adequate state machinery is secured.

State health machinery should be of two kinds,—fact-gathering and executive supervision through inspection. The greatest service of state boards of health is to educate localities as to their own needs, using the experience of all communities to teach each community in how far its health administration menaces itself and its neighbors. In addition to registration of contagious diseases, facts as to deaths and births should be registered. State health boards should "score" communities as dairies and milk shops are now being scored by the National Bureau of Animal Industries and several boards of health. When communities persist in maintaining a public nuisance and [307]in failing to enforce health laws, state health machinery should be made to accomplish by force what it has failed to accomplish by education.

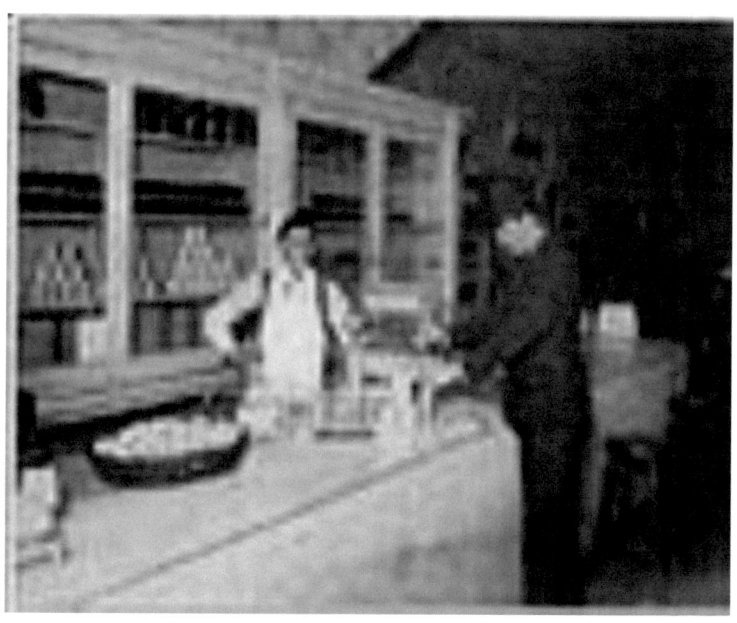

NATIONAL MACHINERY HAS STIMULATED LOCAL MILK
INSPECTION AND STATE DAIRY INSPECTION

States alone can cope adequately with dangers to milk and water sources and to food. The economic motive of farmers has developed strong veterinary boards for the protection of cattle. Similar executive precaution must soon be taken by cities for the protection of babies and adults of the human species. It is far more economical to insure clean dairies, clean water sources, and wholesome manufactured foods by state inspectors than by local inspectors. At present the task of obtaining clean milk and clean water falls upon the few cities enlightened enough and rich enough to finance the inspection of community foods. Once tested, it would be very easy to prove that [308]properly supported state health authorities will save many times the cost of their health work in addition to thousands of lives.

County or district machinery is little known in America. For that reason rural sanitary administration is neglected and rural hospitals are lacking. In the British Isles rural districts are given almost as careful inspection as are cities. Houses may not be built below a certain standard of lighting, ventilation, and conveniences. Outbuildings must be a safe distance from wells. Dairies must be kept clean. Patients suffering from transmissible diseases may be removed by force to hospitals. What is more to the point, rural hospitals have proved that patients cared for by them are far more apt to recover than patients cared for much more expensively and less satisfactorily at home, while less likely to pollute water and milk sources or otherwise to endanger health.

With national machinery the chapter on Vital Statistics has already dealt. We shall undoubtedly soon have a national board of health. Like the state boards, its first function should be educative. In addition, however, there are certain administrative functions where inefficiency may result in serious losses to nation, state, and locality. National quarantine, national inspection of meats, foods, and drugs are administrative functions of vital consequence to every citizen. Authorities are acquainted at the present time with the fact that the sanitary administration of the army and navy is unnecessarily and without excuse wasteful of human energy and human life. In the Spanish American War 14 soldiers died of disease for 1 killed in battle; in the Civil War 2 died of disease to 1 killed in battle; during the wars of the last 200 years 4 have died of disease for 1 killed in battle. Yet Japan in her war with Russia, by using means known to the United States Army in 1860, gave health precedence over [309]everything else and lost but 1 man to disease for 4 killed in battle. Diseases are still permitted to make havoc with American commerce because the national government does not apply to its own limits the standards which it has successfully applied to Cuba and Panama.

"The Japanese invented nothing and had no peculiar knowledge or skill; they merely took occidental science and used it. The remarkable thing is not what they did, but that they were allowed to do it. It is a terrible thing that Congress should choose to make one of its rare displays of economy in a matter where a few thousand dollars saved means, in case our army should have anything to do, not only the utterly needless and useless loss of thousands of lives, but an enormous decrease of military efficiency, and might, conceivably, make all the difference between victory and defeat."

FOOTNOTES:

[16] The technic and principles of municipal engineering have been treated in detail in *Principles of Sanitary Science and the Public Health,* by William T. Sedgwick, and in *Municipal Sanitation in the United States*, by Charles N. Chapin, M.D.

[310]

SCHOOL AND HEALTH REPORTS

For every school-teacher or school physician responsible for the welfare of children at school, there are fifty or more parents responsible for the physical welfare of children at home. Therefore it is all important for parents to know how to read the index for their own children, for their children's associates, and for their community. School reports and health reports should tell clearly and completely the story of the school child's physical needs.

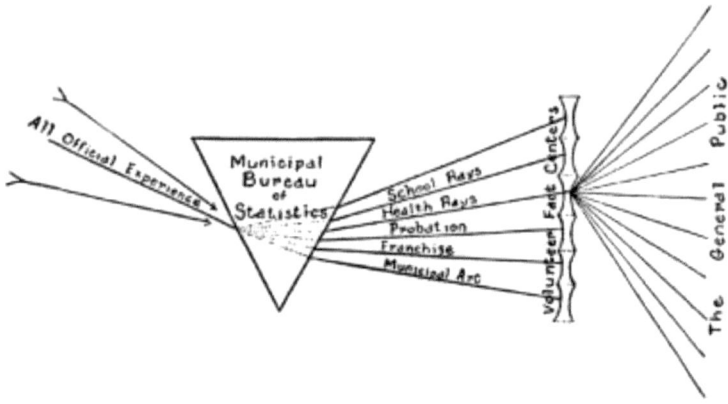

NECESSARY TO EFFICIENT DEMOCRACY

It is impracticable at the present time to expect a large number of men and women to be interested in the reports published by school and health boards, for, with few exceptions, little effort is made to write these reports so that they will interest the parent. Fortunately, a small number of persons wishing to be intelligent can compel public officials to ascertain the necessary facts and to give them to the public. So backward is the reporting of public business [311]that at the present time there is probably no service that a citizen can render his community which would prove of greater importance than to secure proper publicity from health and school boards.

Generally speaking, these published reports fail to interest the citizen, not because officials wish to conceal, but because officials do not believe that the public is interested. A mayor of Philadelphia once furnished a notable exception. He called at the department of health and complained against publishing the number of cases of typhoid and smallpox lest stories in the newspapers "frighten the city and injure business." A sanitary inspector who was in the room asked if Philadelphia's business was more important than the health of Philadelphia's citizens. As a result of her "impertinence" the inspector was removed. That same year an epidemic of smallpox spread through all the rural districts and cities of Pennsylvania, because physicians thought it would be kinder to the patients not to make known to their neighbors the presence of so disagreeable a disease. Almost all health and school authorities, however, can be made to see the advantage of taking the public into their confidence, because public confidence means both public recognition and greater success in obtaining funds. With more funds comes the power to do more work.

Other details with regard to health reports will be found in the chapter on Vital Statistics. As to school reports, little thought has been given in the past to their educational possibilities. A book was recently published—*School Reports and School Efficiency*—by the Committee on the Physical Welfare of School Children, which tells the origins of school reports; contains samples of reports from one hundred cities; gives lists of questions frequently answered, occasionally answered, and never answered; and shows how to study a particular report so as to learn whether or not important questions are answered. The United States commissioner [312]of education has organized among state and city superintendents special committees on uniform and adequate reporting. His aggressive leadership is welcomed by school men generally, and promises vast benefits.

Just because the physical welfare of the school child is an index to health needs, the school report can put into one statement for a city or a state the story told by the index. The accompanying card tells facts that the individual teacher and individual parent want to know about a child, what a superintendent wants to know about all children, and what a community wants to know about all children. A modification of this card will soon be adopted in New York City. It is both a card index and a card biography of the individual boy or girl. It is expected to follow the child from class to class, each teacher telling the story of his physical welfare and his progress. When the boy goes to a new school or new grade, his new teacher can see at a glance not only what subjects have given him trouble, but what diseases or physical defects have kept him out of school or otherwise retarded his progress. With this card it is easy to take a hundred children of the same age and the same grade, to put down in one column those who have eye defects, and in another those who have no eye defects, for every school, every district, and for the schools as a whole. Schools that use these record cards are enabled, by thus classifying the total, to learn where the defects of children are, how serious the problem is, how many days children lose from school because of preventable defects, and in what section of the city the defects are most prevalent.

The mere reporting of facts will stimulate teachers, principals, and parents to give attention. For example, assume a table:

Field of Inspection

Total number of public schools	7
Public schools under inspection	3
Public schools not under inspection	4

The reader wonders why four schools are neglected and which particular schools they are. Let the next table read:

Examination

Total registration in all schools	1500
Number of children examined	500
Number of children not examined	1000

Parents begin to wonder whether or not their children were examined, and why the taxes spent for school examination of all children go to one third of the children. The next table arrests attention:

Treatment

Number needing treatment	200
Number known to have been treated	50
Number not known to have been treated	150

We ask, at once, if examination is worth while, and if treatment really corrects the defects, saves the pupil's time and teacher's time, discovers many defects; and we want to find out whether the one hundred and fifty reported not treated have since been attended to.

[313]

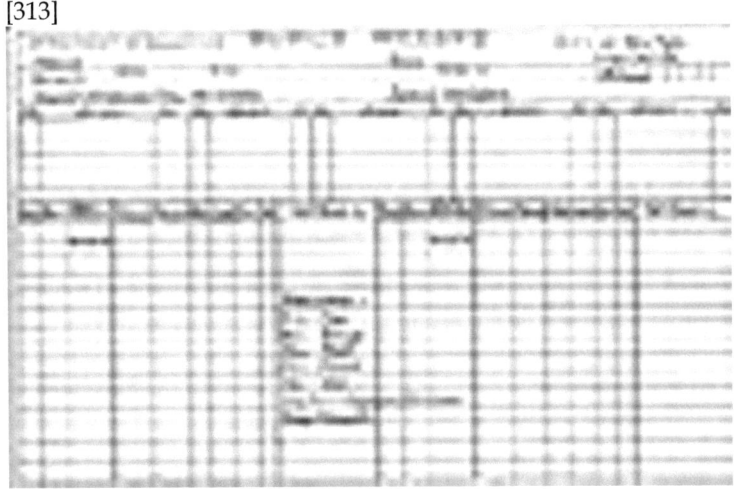

[315]Again, if three out of five of those examined need treatment, people will wonder whether among the thousand not examined there is the same proportion—three out of five, or six hundred—who have some trouble that needs attention. Having begun to wonder, they will ask questions, and will expect the board of health or the school physicians to see that the questions are answered. As has been proved in New York, taxpayers and the press will go farther and will demand that the annual budget provide for making general next year the benefits found to result last year from a test of health policies.

The story of the prevalence of contagious diseases in school children could be told by a table such as is now in use by New York's department of health:

Table XII[316]

Prevalence of Contagious Diseases in School Children

(Case rate schools)

School	General Communicable Diseases 1		Communicable Diseases of Eye and Skin2	
	Number	Number	Number	Number

	Found by Inspectors		Reported by Attending Physician	Total	per 1000 Registered in Schools Inspected	found by Inspectors and Nurses	per 1000 Registered in Schools Inspected
	In School	Among Absentee					
A							
B							
C							

1 Smallpox, diphtheria, scarlet fever, measles, chicken pox, mumps, and whooping cough; excluded when found.

2 Trachoma and other contagious eye diseases, ringworm, impetigo, scabies, favus, and pediculosis; excluded only for persistent nontreatment.

Another table shows the following facts for each disease:

Table XIII

Contagious Diseases Found in Schools by Inspectors and Nurses

(Number and disposition of cases)

General Communicable Diseases

Diphtheria	Scarlet fever	Measles	Smallpox	Chicken pox	Whooping cough	Mumps	T

in

ed

rea-

n-
d in

ol or
ence of
ment
ished
nber of
ments
nber of
uctions

Communicable Diseases of Eye and Skin							
Eye		Skin					
Trachoma	Other	Ringworm	Impetigo	Scabies	Favus	Pediculosis	Mi

n

ed

rea-

n-
d in
or
e of
nt
ed
r of
nts
r of
ions

[317]The story of noncontagious physical defects found and treated is set forth in the following table:

Table XIV

Medical Examination of School Children: Noncontagious Physical
Defects Found and Treated, 1906

| fects | School A | | | | School B | | | | School C | | | |
| | Found | | Reported Treated | | Found | | Reported Treated | | Found | | Reported Treated | |
	No.	% of Total Defects Found	No.	% of Total Defects Found	No.	% of Total Defects Found	No.	% of Total Defects Found	No.	% of Total Defects Found	No.	% of Total Defects Found
enoids												
sal athing												
per-phied sils												
fective ate												
fective aring												
fective ion												
fective th												
d nutri-n												
eased erior vical nds												
eased sterior vical												

357

| glands |
| Heart disease |
| Chorea |
| Pulmonary disease |
| Skin disease |
| Deformity of spine |
| Deformity of chest |
| Deformity of extremities |
| Defective mentality |
| Total |

The effect of a report telling what schools have enough seats, proper ventilation, adequate medical inspection, safe drinking water, ample play space, and what schools are without these necessities is to cause the reader to rank the [318]particular school that he happens to know; i.e. he says, "School A is better equipped than School B; or, School C is neglected." County and state superintendents in many states have acquired the habit of ranking schools according to the number of children who pass in arithmetic, algebra, etc. It would greatly further the cause of public health and, at the same time, advance the interest of education if state superintendents would rank individual schools, and if county superintendents would rank individual schools, *according to the number of children found to have physical defects, the number afflicted with contagious diseases, and the number properly treated.*

It is difficult to compare one school with another, because it is necessary to make subtractions and divisions and to reduce to percentages. It would not be so serious for a school of a thousand pupils as for a school of two hundred, to report 100 for adenoids. To make it possible to compare school with school without judging either unfairly, the state superintendent of schools for Connecticut has made tables in which cities are ranked according to the number of pupils, average attendance, per capita cost, etc. As to each of these headings, cities are grouped in a manner corresponding to the line up of a battalion, "according to height." A general table is then shown, which gives the ranking of each city with respect to each important item. Applied to schools, this would work out as follows:

Table XV

Table of Ranking-Schools Arranged Alphabetically

| School | Rank in | | | | |
	Register	Defects Found	Children Needing Treatment	Children Treated	Children not Treated
A	10	11	11	12	6
B	20	22	22	24	12
C	30	33	30	36	18

[319]Such a table fails to convey its significance unless the reader is reminded that rank 18 in children not treated is as good a record for a school that ranks 30 in register as is rank 6 for a school that ranks 10 in register.

The Connecticut report makes a serious mistake in failing to arrange schools according to population. If this were done, schools of a size would be side by side and comparison would be fair. When, as in the above table, schools are arranged alphabetically, a school with four thousand pupils may follow or precede a school with four hundred pupils, and comparison will be unfair and futile.

Where, on the other hand, schools are arranged in order of register, a table will show whether schools confronted with practically the same problems, the same number of defects, the same number of children needing treatment, are equally successful, or perhaps equally inactive, in correcting these defects. The following table brings out clearly marked unequal achievement in the face of relatively equal need.

Table XVI

Table of Ranking-Schools Arranged according to Register, not Alphabetically

| School | Rank in | | | | |
	Register	Defects Found	Children Needing Treatment	Children Treated	Children not Treated
A	9	9	9	9	9
X	10	10	10	14	6
H	11	11	11	17	3

If the number of schools in a state is so large that it is unlikely that people will read the table of ranking because of the difficulty of finding their own school, an alphabetical table might be given that would show where to look in the general ranking table for the school or schools in which the reader is interested.

[320]Experience will demonstrate to public school superintendents the strategic advantage of putting together all the things they need and of telling the community over and over again just what needs there are, what penalties are paid for want of them, and what benefits would result from obtaining them. If health needs of school children were placed side by side with mental results, the relation would come out so clearly that parents, school boards, and taxpayers would realize how inextricably they are bound together and would see that health needs are satisfied. To this end superintendents should require teachers to keep daily reports of school conditions.

Table XVII

Weekly Class-Room Schedule

| | Temperature | | | Cleaning | | | Exercise | |
	10.30	12.00	2.00	Dry	Wet	Disinfecting	In Room	Out of Room
Monday								
Tuesday								
Wednesday								
Thursday								
Friday								

The teacher's daily report of the temperature of a schoolroom, taken three times a day, tells the parent exactly what is the efficiency of the ventilating and heating apparatus in the particular school in which he is interested; whereas the report of the department of buildings gives only the number of schools which have an approved system of ventilation and steam heat. School authorities may or may not know that this system of ventilation is out of order, that the thermometer in the indoor playground of School A stood at forty degrees for many days in winter. But they must know it when the principal of School A sends in a daily record; the school board, the parents, or the press [321]will then see that the condition is remedied. If the condition is due to lack of funds, funds will never be forthcoming so long as the condition is concealed.

Similar results will follow publicity of overcrowding, too little play space, dry cleaning of school buildings, etc. The intent of such reporting is not to "keep tabs" on the school-teacher, the school child, the janitor, the principal, superintendent, or board, but to insure favorable conditions and to correct bad conditions. This is done best by giving everybody the facts. The objective test of the efficiency of a method throws emphasis on the method, not on the motive of those operating it. The blackboard method of publishing facts concentrates attention upon the importance of those facts and enlists aid in the attainment of the end sought.

[322]

CHAPTER XXXIToC

THE PRESS

The president of Princeton University declares that for several decades we have given education that does not instruct and instruction that does not educate. Others tell us that because we read daily papers and magazines our minds become superficial, that our power to concentrate or memorize is weakened, — that we read so much of everything that we learn little of anything. As the habit of reading magazines and newspapers is constantly increasing, I think we must assume that it has come to stay. If we cannot check it, we can at least turn it to good advantage, systematize it, and discipline ourselves.

Among the subjects continually described in newspapers and magazines, and even on billboards and in street-car advertising, is the subject of hygiene. No greater service can be rendered the community than for those who are conducting discussions of health to teach people how to read correctly this mass of information regarding health, to separate misinformation from information, and to apply the lessons learned to personal and public hygiene. There is no better way of doing this than to teach a class or a child to clip out of magazines and newspapers all important references to health, and then to classify these under the subject-matter treated. A teacher, parent, or club leader might practice by using the classification of subjects outlined in the Contents of this book. It is surprising how rapidly one builds up a valuable collection serviceable for talks or papers, but more particularly for giving one a vital and intelligent interest in practical health topics.

[323]Interested in comparing the emphasis placed on health topics in a three-cent paper having a small circulation with a penny paper having twenty times the circulation, I made during one week thirty-eight clippings from the three-cent paper and ninety-five from the penny paper. The high-priced paper had no editorial

comment within the field of health, whereas the penny paper had three columns, in which were discussed among other things: *The Economics of Bad Teeth*; *Need for Individual Efficiency*; *"Good Fellows" Lower Standard of Living by Neglecting their Families*. The penny paper advertised fifty-two foods, garments, whiskies, patent medicines, or beautifiers urged upon health grounds. In the three-cent paper twenty-six out of thirty-eight items advertised food, clothing, patent medicine, or whisky. One issue of a monthly magazine devoted to woman's interests contained twenty-eight articles and editorials and fifty-five advertisements that concern health, — thirty-seven per cent of total reading matter and thirty-seven per cent of total advertisement.

Excellent discipline is afforded by this clipping work. It is astonishing how few men and women, even from our better colleges, know how to organize notes, clippings, or other data, so that they can be used a few weeks later. There is a satisfaction in seeing one's material grow, as is remembered by all of us, in making picture scrapbooks or collections of picture postal cards and stamps. "Collections" have generally failed for want of classification, — putting things of a kind together. Chronological arrangement is uninteresting because unprofitable. One never knows where to find a picture, or a stamp, or a health clipping. Clippings, like libraries, will be little used if not properly catalogued so that use is easy. If a health-clipping collection is attempted, there are four essentials: (1) arrangement by topic; (2) inclusion of advertisements; (3) inclusion of items from magazines; (4) cross references.

[324]For classification, envelopes can be used or manila cards 10×12 inches. The teacher, parent, or advanced student will probably think the envelope most useful because most easily carried and filed, — most likely to be used. But clippings should be bound together in orderly appearance, or else it will be disagreeable working with them. Children, however, will like the pasting on sheets, which show clearly the growth of each topic. Envelopes or cards should not have clippings that deal with only one health topic. Unless a test is made to see how many health references there are in a given period, it should be made a rule not to clip any item that does not contain something new, — some addition to the knowledge already collected.

Advertisements will prove interesting and educative. When newspapers and magazines announce some new truth, the commercial motive of manufacturer or dealer sees profit in telling over and over again how certain goods will meet the new need. Children will soon notice that the worst advertisements appear in the papers that talk most of "popular rights," "justice," and "morality." They will be shocked to see that the popular papers accept money to tell falsehoods about fake cures. They will be pleased that the best monthly magazines contain no such advertisements. They will challenge paper or magazine, and thus will be enlisted while young in the fight against health advertisements that injure health.

To clip articles from magazines will seem almost irreverent at first. But the reverence for magazines and books is less valuable to education than the knowledge concealed in them. Except where families preserve all magazines, clippings will add greatly to their serviceability.

The art of cross-referencing is invaluable to the organized mind. The purpose of classifying one's information is not to show how much there is, but to answer questions quickly and to guide constructive thinking. A clipping that deals [325]with *alcoholism, patent medicine*, and *tuberculosis* must be posted in three places, or cross-referenced; otherwise it will be used to answer but one question when it might answer three. If magazines may not be cut, it will be easy to record the fact of a useful article by writing the title, page, and date on the appropriate index card, or inclosing a slip so marked in the proper envelope.

While it is true that the most important bibliography one can have in his private library is a classification of the material of which he himself has become a part while reading it, there are a number of health journals that one can profitably subscribe for. In fact, it is often true that the significant discoveries in scientific fields, or the latest public improvements, such as parks, bridges, model tenements, will not be appreciated until one has read in health journals how these improvements affect the sickness rate and the enjoyment rate of those least able to control their living conditions. The physician and nurse in their educational work for hospitals are distributors of health propaganda.

Wherever there is a local journal devoted to health, parents, teachers, educators, and club leaders would do well to subscribe and to hold this journal up to a high standard by quoting, thanking, criticising it. In New Jersey, for example, is a monthly called the *New Jersey Review of Charities and Corrections* that deals with every manner of subject having to do with public health as well as with private and public morality and education.

A similar journal, intended for national instruction, is *The Survey*, whose topical index for last year enumerates two hundred and thirty-two articles dealing with subjects directly connected with public hygiene, e.g.:

Schools, 6; school inspection, 3; eyes,—school children, 1; sex instruction in the schools, 2; psychiatric clinic, special children, 2; industrial education, 5; child labor, 18; playgrounds, 26; alley, crap, playing in streets, 3; labor conditions, 18; [326]industrial accidents, 10; wage-earner's insurance, 4; factory inspection, 1; consumer's league, 3; women's work, 6; tuberculosis, 23; hospitals, dispensaries (social), 5; tenement reform, 10; living conditions, 2; baths, 1; public comfort stations, 2; lodging houses, 1; clean streets, 6; clean milk, 6; smoke, 1; noises, 1; parks, 1; patent medicines, 2; sanitary code, 1; mortality statistics, 2; social settlements and public health, 1; midwives, 1; children's bureau, 1; juvenile and adult delinquent, 25; dependent, defective, and insane, 7; blind, 5; cripples, 1; homes for aged, 1; inebriates, 3; Traveler's Aid Committee, 1; infant mortality, 2; social diseases, 2.

The National Hospital Record, the *Dietetic and Hygienic Gazette*, the *Journal of Nursing*, are three other magazines primarily intended for nurses and physicians, but full of suggestive material for unprofessional readers. National magazines concerned with health, but seeking popular circulation, are *Good Health* and *Physical Culture*. In England there is a special magazine called *Children's Diseases*, which could be of great help to a school library for special reference. The same can be said of the *Psychological Clinic*, *Pediatrics*, and other technical journals published in this country. For many persons, to make the best use of any one copy of these magazines, clipping is of course impossible, but noting on a card or envelope is practicable.

Of late many of the national popular magazines have several columns devoted to health. We have not appreciated the educational possibilities of these columns. In most large cities there are monthly book reviews which may be profitably consulted in learning the new thought in the health field. If teachers would either write their experience or ask questions, if children knew that in a certain magazine or newspaper questions as to ventilation, bathing, exercise, would be answered, they would take a keen interest in the progress of discussions. The large daily papers make a great feature of their health hints. It is not [327]their fault if questioners care more about cosmetics and hair bleaches than about the fresh-air cure of headaches. They will coöperate with teachers and parents in securing more general discussion of other problems than beauty doctoring.

Finally, persons wanting not only to have intelligence as to matters promoting health, but actually to exert a helpful influence in their community, ought to want the published reports of the mayor, health department, the public schools, and other institutions, noting carefully all that is said about conditions relating to health and about efforts made to correct all unfavorable conditions. The best literature of our day, with regard to social needs, appears in the reports of our public and private institutions and societies. Of increasing value are the publications of the national government printing office. Because it is no one's business to find out what valuable material is contained in such reports, and because no educational museum is comparing report with report, those who live nearest to our health problems and who see most clearly the health remedies, are not stimulated to give to the public their special knowledge in an interesting, convincing way.

Teaching children how to find health lessons in public documents will advance the cause of public ethics as well as of public health. At the New York State Conference of Charities, of 1907, one official complained that the physicians made no educational use of their valuable experience for public education. He stated that a study of medical journals and health articles in popular magazines revealed the fact that the number of papers prepared by physicians in state hospitals averaged one to a doctor for every five or six years of service. This state of affairs is even more exaggerated in strictly educational institutions. Columbia University has recently instituted a series of lectures to be given by its professors to its professors, so that they may have a general knowledge of the work being done in other [328]fields besides their own at their own university. This is equally important for teachers and heads of departments in elementary schools. It is now admitted by most educators that elementary schools and young children present more pedagogical difficulties and pressing biological problems than higher schools. If teachers and parents would realize that their method of solving the health problems that arise daily in the schoolroom and in the home would interest other mothers and teachers, their spirit of coöperation would soon be reflected in school journals, popular magazines, and daily newspapers.

[329]

CHAPTER XXXIIToC

DO-NOTHING AILMENTS

"Men have died, from time to time, and worms have eaten them, but not for love" — *nor for work*. Work of itself never killed anybody nor made anybody sick. Work has caused worry, mental strain, and physical breakdown, only when men while working have been deprived of air, sun, light, exercise, sleep, proper food at the proper time, opportunity to live and work hygienically. Fortunately for human progress, doing nothing brings ailments of its own and has none of the compensations of work. As the stomach deprived of substantial food craves unnatural food, — sweets, stimulants, — so the mind deprived of substantial, regular diet of wholesome work turns to unwholesome, petty, fantastic, suspicious, unhappy thoughts. This state of mind, combined with the lack of bodily exercise that generally accompanies it, reacts unfavorably on physical health. An editor has aptly termed the do-nothing condition as a self-inflicted confinement:

A great deal of the misery and wretchedness among young men that inherit great fortunes is caused by the fact that they are practically in jail. They have nothing to do but eat, drink, and enjoy themselves, and they cannot understand why their lives are dull.

We have had the owner of a great railroad system pathetically telling the public that he is unhappy. That is undoubtedly true, [330]because with all his race horses, and his yachts, and all the things that he imagines to be pleasures, he is not really doing anything.

If he were running one little railroad station up the road, handling the freight, fussing about dispatches, living above the railroad station in two rooms, and buying shoes in a neighboring village for fifteen children he would be busy and happy.

But he cannot be happy because he is in prison,—in a prison of money, a prison that is honorable because it gives him everything that he wants, and he wants nothing.

A New York newspaper that circulates among the working classes where young men and women are inclined to associate health and happiness with doing nothing recently gave two columns to "Dandy Jim," the richest dog in the world. Dandy Jim's mistress left him a ten-thousand-dollar legacy. During his lifetime he wore diamonds. Every day he ate candy that cost eighty cents a pound. The coachman took him driving in the park sunny afternoons. He had no cares and nothing to work for. His food came without effort. He had fatty degeneration of the vital organs. He was pampered, coddled, and killed thereby. Thousands of men and women drag out lives of unhappiness for themselves and others because, like Dandy Jim, they have nothing to work for, are pampered, coddled victims of fatty degeneration. When President Butler of Columbia University finds it necessary to censure "the folly and indifference of the fathers, vanity and thoughtless pride of the mothers" who encourage do-nothing ailments; and when the editor of the *Psychological Clinic* protests that the fashionable private schools and the private tutor share with rich fathers and mothers responsibility for life failures,—it is time that educators teach children themselves the physical and moral ailments and disillusions that come from doing nothing.

Ten years ago a stenographer inherited two hundred and fifty thousand dollars. Her dream of nothing to do [331]was realized. She gave up her strenuous business life. Possessions formerly coveted soon clogged her powers of enjoyment. She imagined herself suffering from various diseases, shut herself up in her house, and refused to see any one. She grew morbid and was sure that every person who approached her had some sneaking, personal, hostile motive. Though always busy, she accomplished little. Desultory work, procrastination, and self-indulgence destroyed her power of concentration. She could not think long enough on one subject to think it out straight, therefore she was constantly deceived in her friends and interests. She first trusted everybody, then mistrusted everybody. Infatuation with every new acquaintance was quickly followed by suspicion. For years she was a very sick woman, a victim of do-nothing ailments.

Doing nothing has of late been seriously recommended to American business men. They are advised to retire from active work as soon as their savings produce reasonable income. It is true, this suggestion has been made as an antidote to greed rather than for the happiness of the business man. What retiring from business is apt to mean, is indicated by a gentleman who at the age of sixty decided to sell his seat on the New York Stock Exchange and to enjoy life. He became restless and very miserable. He threw himself violently into one thing after another; in less than a year he became an ill, broken old man, after trying vainly to buy back his business.

Both mind and body were made to work. The function of the brain is to think to a purpose, just as the function of the heart is to pump blood. The habit of doing nothing is very easily formed. The "out-of-work" soon become "the work-shy." Having too little to do is worse for the body and mind than having too little to eat. Social reformers emphasize the bad effect on society of vagrancy. Evils of indiscriminate relief to the poor are vividly described year [332]after year. The philanthropist is condemned, who, by his gifts, encourages an employee's family to spend what they do not earn, and to shun work. Yet the idleness of the tramp, street loafer, and professional mendicant is a negligible evil compared with the hindrance to human progress caused by the idleness of the well-to-do, the rich, the educated, the refined, the "best" people. It is as much a wrong to bring up children in an atmosphere of do-nothingism, as to refuse to have their teeth attended to or to have glasses fitted to weak eyes.

From the point of view of community welfare it is far more serious for the rich child to be brought up in idleness or without a purpose than for the poor child to become a public charge. Not only has society a right to expect more from rich children in return for the greater benefits they enjoy, but so long as rich children control the expenditure of money, they control also the health and happiness of other human beings. Unless taught the value and joy of wholesome work they cannot themselves think straight, nor are they likely to want to understand how they can use their wealth for the benefit of mankind. To quote President Butler again:

The rich boy who receives a good education and is trained to be a self-respecting member of the body politic might in time share on equal terms the chance of the poor boy to become a man of genuine influence and importance on his own account, just as now by the neglect, or worse, of his parents the very rich boy is apt to be relegated to the limbo of curiosities, and too often of decadence.

Nervous invalids make life miserable for themselves and for others, when often their sole malady is lack of the right kind of work to do.

Suiting work to interest and interest to work is an economy that should not be overlooked. The energy [333]spent in forcing oneself to do a distasteful task can be turned to productive channels when work is made pleasurable. The fact is frequently deplored that whereas formerly a man became a full-fledged craftsman, able to perform any branch of his trade, he is now confined to doing special acts because neither his interest nor his mind is called into play. Work seems to react unfavorably on his health. He has not the pride of the artisan in the finished product, for he seldom sees it. He does a task. His employer is a taskmaster. He decides that work is not good for him as easily as when a school-boy he grasped the meaning of escape from his lessons. By failing to fit studies to a student's interest, or by failing to insure a student's interest in his studies, schools and colleges miseducate young men and young women to look upon all work as tasks, as discipline, necessary but irksome, and to be avoided if possible. Just as there is a way of turning all the energy of the play instinct into school work, so there is a way of interesting the factory and office worker in his job. However mechanical work may be, there is always the interest in becoming the most efficient worker in a room or a trade. Routine—accurate and detailed work—does not mean the stultification of the imagination. It takes more imagination to see the interesting things in statistical or record work than to write a novel. Therefore employers should make it a point to help their employees to realize the significance of the perfection of each detail and the importance of each man's part. The other day a father said to me, "I want my boys to be as ashamed to do work in which they are not interested as to accept graft." When interest in work and efficiency in work are regarded as of more importance than the immediate returns for work, when it is as natural for boys and girls to demand enjoyment and complete living in work as it is to thrill at the sight of [334]the Stars and Stripes, do-nothing ailments will be less frequent and less costly.

Work—that one enjoys—is an invaluable unpatented medicine. It can make the sick well and keep the well from getting sick. It is the chief reliance of mental hygiene. "I should have the grippe if I had time," said a business woman to me the other day; but she did not have time, hence she did not have the grippe.

> If you're sick with something chronic,
> And you think you need a tonic,
> Do something.
> There is life and health in doing,
> There is pleasure in pursuing;
> Doing, then, is health accruing—
> Do something.
> And if you're seeking pleasure,
> Or enjoyment in full measure,
> Do something.
> Idleness, there's nothing in it;
> 'Twill not pay you for a minute—
> Do something.

[335]

HEREDITY BUGABOOS AND HEREDITY TRUTHS

One of the red-letter days of my life was that on which I learned that I could not have inherited tuberculosis from two uncles who died of consumption. For years I had known that I was a marked victim. Silently I carried my tragedy, suspecting each cold and headache to be the telltale messenger that should let others into my secret. He was a veritable emancipator who informed me that heredity did not work from uncle to nephew; that not more than a predisposition to consumption could pass even from parent to child; that a predisposition to consumption would come to nothing without the germ of the disease and the environmental conditions which favor its development; and that if those so predisposed avoid gross infection, lead a healthy life, and breathe fresh air they are as safe as though no tuberculous lungs had ever existed in the world. Some years later I learned to understand the other side of the case; I realized how I had been in real danger of contracting consumption in the darkened, ill-ventilated sick room of the uncle who taught me my letters and gave me my ideal of God's purpose in sending uncles to small boys.

There are two distinct things which make each individual life: the living stuff, the physical basis of life, handed down from parent to child; and the environmental conditions which surround it and play upon it and rouse its reactions and its latent possibilities. It is like the seed and the cultivation. You cannot grow corn from wheat, but you can grow the best wheat, or you may let your crop fail through careless handling.

[336]It is well that we should think seriously about the part played by heredity, for the living stuff of the future depends upon our sense of responsibility in this regard. The intelligent citizen would do well to read such a book as J. Arthur Thompson's *Heredity*

(1908), in which the latest conclusions of science are clearly and soundly set forth.

The main problem of to-day, however, is to use well the talents that we have. Here two things should always be kept in mind: First, the inhcrited elements which make up our minds and bodies are complex and diverse. Health and strength are inherited as well as disease and weakness; they have indeed a better chance of survival. In the most unpromising ancestry there are latent potentialities which may be made fruitful by effort. No limit whatever can be set to the possibilities of improvement in any individual.

In the second place, if science has shown anything more clearly than the importance of heredity, it is the importance of environment. This influence upon human lives is within our control, and it is a grave error to neglect what lies clearly within our power and to bemoan what does not. Science has wrought no benefits greater than those which result from drawing a clear line between heredity bugaboos and heredity truths. An overemphasis on the hereditary factor in development at the expense of the environmental factor, I call a heredity bugaboo; and it is a tendency which cannot be too strongly condemned. To fight against the sins and penalties of one's grandfather is a forlorn task that quickly discourages. To overcome diseases of environment, of shop and street, of house and school, seems, on the contrary, an easy task. Heredity bugaboos dishearten, enervate, encourage excesses and neglect. Heredity truths stimulate remedial and preventive measures.

We may well watch with interest the progress of eugenics, that new science which biologists and sociologists hope will some day remake the very living stuff of the human [337]race. But meanwhile let us take up with hope and courage and enthusiasm the great hemisphere of human fate which lies within our grasp. Good food and fresh air, well-built cities, enlightened schools and well-ordered industries, stable and free and expert government,—given these things, we can transform the world with the means now at our disposal. We can reap, if we will, splendid possibilities now going to waste, and by intelligent biological and sociological engineering we can hand on to the next generation an environmental inheritance which will make their task far easier than ours.

"Physical deterioration" is a bugaboo that is discovered by some in heredity and by others in modern industrial evils. The British director general called attention a few years ago to the fact that from forty to sixty per cent of the men who were being examined for military service were physically unfit. A Commission on Physical Deterioration was appointed to investigate the cause, and to learn whether the low physical standard of the would-be Tommy Atkins was due to inherited defects. The results of this study were published in a large volume called *Report on Physical Deterioration, 1904*, in which is set forth a positive programme for obtaining periodically facts as to the physique of the nation. In the course of the commission's exhaustive investigation there was found no evidence that any progressive deterioration was going on in any function of the body except the teeth. "There are happily no grounds for associating dental degeneracy with progressive physical deterioration." The increase in optical defects is attributed not to the deterioration of the eye, but to greater knowledge, more treatment, and better understanding of the connection between optical defects and headache.

[338]

Testing Environment—House Score Card

RATES OF INSPECTION

ROOMS*	I	II	III	IV	V	VI	VII	VIII	PERFECT SCORE							
*Light 10, gloomy 5, dark 0									10							
*Well ven. 15, poorly 7, badly 0									15							
*Repair good 5, fair 3, poor 1, bad 0									5							
Clean 10, soiled 5, dirty 2, filthy 0									10							
One person to room 10, 2 to room 8, 3 to room 4, 4 or more 0									10							
SINKS																
Construction: good 5, fair 2, bad 1									5							
WATER-CLOSET																
Construction: good 3, fair 2, poor 1, bad 0									3							
Condition: clean 3, dirty 1, filthy 0									3							
1 compartment for 1 family 3, for 2 families 1, for more than 2 families 0									3							
CLEANLINESS																
1 bath tub for 1 apartment 3, for more than 1 apartment 1, no bath 0									3							
Personal cleanliness: immaculate 7, fairly clean 5, dirty 2, filthy 0									7							
WASHING																
Stationary tubs 3, removable 2, no tubs 0									3							
Cleanliness of clothing: immaculate 7, fairly clean 5, dirty 2, filthy 0									7							
MEALS																
Regular 4, irregular 2, uncertain 0									4							
Amount and kind of food: good 4, fair 2, poor 2, bad 0									4							
Cooking: immaculate 4, clean 3, dirty 1, filthy 0									4							
Refrigeration: good 4, fair 2, poor 1, none 0									4							
									100							

*In estimating the light, ventilation, and repair of an apartment, divide the sum of the scores of each individual room by the number of rooms; this equals the perfect score for the apartment. — *New York Milk Committee.*

DEFINITIONS OF TERMS USED IN HOUSE SCORE CARD

LIGHT — Light enough to read easily in every part.

GLOOMY — Not light enough to read easily in every part, but enough readily to see one's way about when doors are closed.

DARK — Too dark to see one's way about easily when doors are closed.

WELL VENTILATED — With window on street or fair-sized yard (not less than 12 ft. deep for a five-story tenement house not on a corner), or on a "large," "well-ventilated" court open to the sky at the top: "large" being for a court entirely open on one side to the street or yard in a five-story basement, not less than 6 ft. wide from the wall of the building to the lot line; for a court inclosed on three sides and the other on the lot line in a five-story tenement, not less than 12x24 ft., "well ventilated" meaning either entirely open on one side to the street or yard, or else having a tunnel at the bottom connecting with the street or yard.

FAIRLY VENTILATED — With window opening on a shallow yard or on a narrow court, open to the sky at the top, or else with 3x3 inside window (15 ft. square) opening on a well-ventilated room in same apartment.

BADLY VENTILATED — With no window on the street, or on a yard, or on a court open to the sky, and with no window, or a very small window, opening on an adjoining room.

IN GOOD REPAIR — No torn wall paper, broken plaster, broken woodwork or flooring, nor badly shrunk or warped floor boards or wainscoting, leaving large cracks.

IN FAIR REPAIR — Slightly torn or loose wall paper, slightly broken plaster, warped floor boards and wainscoting.

IN BAD REPAIR — Very badly torn wall paper or broken plaster over a considerable area, or badly broken woodwork or flooring. (Rooms not exactly coinciding with any of the three classes are to be included in the one the description of which comes nearest to the condition.)

SINKS: GOOD — Iron, or iron supports with iron back sheet to prevent splashing of water on wall surface, in light location, used for one family. Water direct from city water mains or from a CLEAN roof tank.

BAD — Surrounded by wood rims with or without metal flushings, space beneath inclosed with wood risers; dark location, used by more than one family; water from dirty roof tank.

FAIR — Midway between above two extremes. (Sinks not exactly coinciding with any of the three classes are to be included in the one the description of which comes nearest to the condition.)

WATER-CLOSET: GOOD — Indoor closet. In well lighted and ventilated location, closet fixture entirely open underneath, abundant water flush.

FAIR — Indoor closet, poor condition — badly lighted and ventilated location, fixture inclosed with wood risers, or poor flush.

POOR — Yard closet — separate water-closet in individual compartment in the yard.

BAD — School sink — sewer-connected privy, having one continuous vault beneath the row of individual toilet compartments.

[340]The commission hoped "that the facts and opinions they have collected will have some effect in allaying the apprehensions of those who, as it appears, on insufficient grounds, have made up their minds that progressive deterioration is to be found among people generally." In regard to the facts which started the fear, the report says: (1) the evidence adduced in the director general's memorandum was inadequate to prove that physical deterioration had affected the classes referred to; (2) no sufficient material (statistical or other) is at present available to warrant any definite conclusions on the question of the physique of the people by comparison with data obtained in past times.

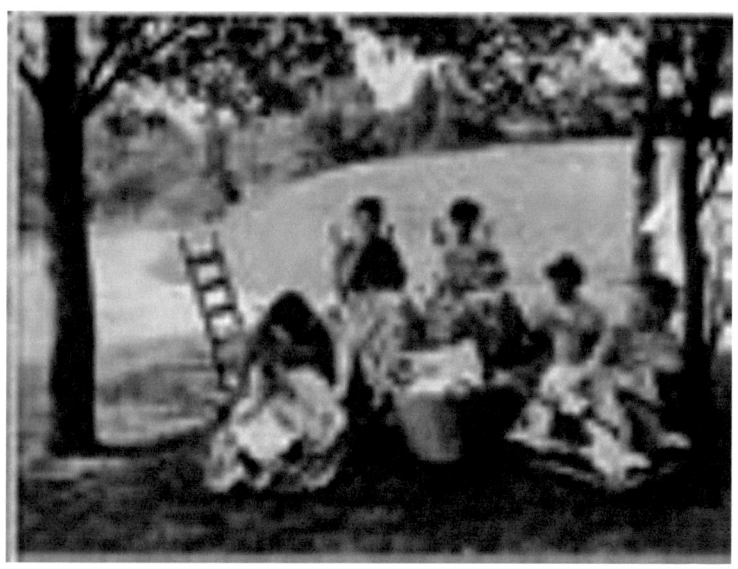

THE BEST INHERITANCE IS A MOTHER WHO KNOWS HOW
TO KEEP HER BABY WELL

The topics dealt with in the report refer to only a partial list of
conditions that need to be carefully studied before we can know
what environment heredity we are preparing for those who follow
us:

I. As to Babies

Training of mothers, provident societies and maternity funds,
feeding of infants, milk supply, milk depots, sterilization and
[341]refrigeration of milk, effect of mother's employment upon infant mortality, still births, cookery, hygiene and domestic economy,
public nurseries, crèches.

II. As to Children

Anthropometric measurements, sickness and open spaces, medical examination of school children, teeth, eyes, and ears, games and
exercises for school children, open spaces and gymnastic apparatus,
physical exercise for growing girls and growing boys, clubs and
cadet corps, feeding of elementary school children, partial exemp-

tion from school, special schools for "retarded" children, special magistrate for juvenile cases, juvenile smoking, organization of existing agencies for the welfare of lads and girls, education, school attendance in rural districts, defective children.

III. As to Living and Working Conditions

Register of sickness, medical certificates as to causes of death, overcrowding, building and open spaces, register of owners of buildings, unsanitary and overcrowded house property, rural housing, workshops, coal mines, etc., medical inspection of factories, employment of women in factories, labor colonies, overfatigue, food and cooking, cooking grates, adulteration, smoke pollution, alcohol, syphilis, insanity.

IV. As to Health Machinery

Medical officers of health, local, district, and national boards, health associations.

Scientists of the next generation will continue to differ as to heredity truths and heredity bugaboos unless records are kept now, showing the physical condition of school children and of applicants for work certificates and for civil service and army positions. The British investigators declared that "anthropometric records are the only accredited tests available, and, if collected on a sufficient scale, they would constitute the supreme criterion of physical deterioration, or the reverse.... The school population and [342]the classes coming under the administration of the Factory Acts offer ready material for the immediate application of such tests." In addition to the physical tests proposed in other chapters, there is great educational opportunity in the records of private and public hospitals. Every nation, every state, and every city should enlist all its educational and scientific forces to ascertain in what respects social efficiency is endangered by physical deficiencies that can be avoided only by restricting parenthood, and the environmental deficiencies that can be avoided by efficient health machinery.

The greatest of all heredity truths are these: (1) the deficiencies of infants are infinitesimal compared with the deficiencies of the world with which we surround them; (2) each of us can have a part in begetting for posterity an environment of health and of opportunity.

[343]

INEFFECTIVE AND EFFECTIVE WAYS OF COMBATING ALCOHOLISM

Wherever the Stars and Stripes fly over school buildings it is made compulsory to teach the evils of alcoholism. For nearly a generation the great majority of school children of the United States have been taught that alcohol, in however small quantities, is a poison and a menace to personal and national health and prosperity. Yet during this very period the per capita consumption of every kind of alcoholic beverage has increased. Whereas 16.49 gallons of spirituous liquors were consumed per capita of population in 1896, 22.27 gallons were used in 1906. Obviously the results of methods hitherto in vogue for combating alcoholism are disappointing.

Why this paradoxical relation of precept to practice? Why is this, the most hygiene-instructed country in the world, the Elysium of the patent-medicine and cocaine traffic? If we have only the expected divergence of achievement from ideal, then there is nothing for us to do but to congratulate ourselves and posterity upon the part played by compulsory legislation in committing all states and territories to hygiene instruction in all public schools. If, on the other hand, our disappointment is due to ineffective method, then the next step is to change our method.

The chief purpose of school hygiene has hitherto been not to promote personal and community health, but to lessen the use of alcohol and tobacco. Arguments were required against whisky, beer, cigars, and cigarettes. As the strongest arguments would probably make the most lasting impression upon the school child and the best profits for [344]author and bookseller, writers vied with one another in the rhetoric and hyperbole of platform agitation. What effect would it have upon you if you were exhorted frequently during the next eight years to avoid tobacco because a mother once killed a child by washing its head in tobacco water?

What is the effect on the mind of a boy or a girl who sees that the family doctor, the minister, the teacher, the judge, the governor, the President, and the philanthropist use tobacco and alcoholic beverages, when taught that "boys who use tobacco and alcoholic beverages will find closed in their faces the doors to strength, good health, skill in athletics, good scholarship, long life, best companions, many business positions, highest success"? It is probably true that "a boy once drank some whisky from a flask and died within a few hours." But that story is about as typical of boys and of whisky as that a boy once drank whisky from a flask and did not die for ninety years afterwards, or that George Washington drank whisky and became the Father of his Country.

How special pleading has dominated the teaching of school hygiene is illustrated by a recent book which, for the most part, successfully breaks away from the narrow point of view and the crude methods hitherto prevailing. It presents the following facts concerning New York City:

Saloons	10,821
Arrests	133,749
Expense of police department	$10,199,206
Police courts, jails, workhouses, reformatories	1,310,411
Hospitals, asylums, and other charities	4,754,380

It is fair to the author to state that she does not declare in so many words that the shutting up of the saloons would obviate all the arrests and all the hospital, jail, and charity bills. Instead of *wipe out* she says *shrivel*. No truth would have been lost by avoiding all misrepresentation.

[345]The author probably felt as I did when I took my total abstainer's protest to a celebrated scientist who had exposed certain misstatements regarding the effect of small quantities of alcohol: "Is not the untruth of these exaggerated statements less dangerous than the untruth of dispassionate, scientific statement? So long as the child mind takes in only an impression, is it not better to write this impression indelibly?" He sadly but indulgently replied, "And in what other studies would you substitute exaggeration for truth?"

The reaction has already begun against exaggeration in hygiene text-books, against drawing lessons from accidental or exceptional cases of excessive use of alcohol, against classing moderate drinking and smoking with drunkenness as sins of equal magnitude, and against overlooking grave social and industrial evils that threaten children far earlier and more frequently than do tobacco and alcohol. Instead of adding an ell to the truth, text-book writers are now adding only an inch or two at a time. No longer do we favor highly colored charts that picture in purple, green, and black the effect of stimulants and narcotics upon the heart and brain, the stomach, the liver, the knee, and the eardrum, *assuming that all resultant evils are concentrated in one organ.* Menacing habits, such as overeating and indulgence in self-pity, are beginning to receive attention. It is also true that physiology and anatomy are progressively made more interesting. Publishers are looking for the utmost originality compatible with the purpose of the present laws and with the only effective public sentiment that has hitherto been interested in the interpretation of those laws.

A score of improvements in the method of carrying out a small ideal will not take the place of enlarging that ideal. If existing laws stand in the way of broadening the purpose of school hygiene, let the laws be changed. If text-book publishers stand in the way, let us induce or compel them to get out of the way. If we fear rumsellers, their money, [346]and the insidious political methods that they might employ to bring in undertruth if overtruth is once sacrificed, let us go to our communities and locate the rumseller's guns, draw their fire, tell the truth about their opposition, and educate the public to overcome it. If, on the other hand, misguided teetotalism stands in the way, then, as one teetotaler, I suggest that we prove, as we can, in our respective communities that there is a better way of inculcating habits of temperance and self-restraint than by telling untruths, overtruths, or half truths about alcohol and tobacco. Let us prove, as we can, that a subject vital to every individual, to every industry, and to every government is now prevented from fulfilling its mission not by its enemies but by its friends. We can learn the character of hygiene instruction in our schools and the interest taken in it by teachers, principals, and superintendents. We can learn how teachers practice hygiene at school, and how the children of our communities are affected by the hygiene instruction now given. Finally, we can compel a public discussion of the facts, and action in accordance with facts. Without questioning anybody's avowed motive, we can learn how big that motive is and how adequate or inadequate is the method of executing it.

Alcohol and tobacco really occupy but a very small share of the interest and attention of even those men and women by whom they are habitually used. Hygiene, on the other hand, is of constant, uninterrupted concern. Why, therefore, should it be planned to have alcohol and tobacco displace the broader subject of personal and public hygiene in the attention and interest of children throughout the school life? Beyond the text-book and schoolroom a thousand influences are at work to teach the social evils, the waste of energy, and the unhappiness that always accompany the excessive use — and frequently result from a moderate use — of stimulants and narcotics. Of the many reasons for not drinking and smoking, physiology gives those that least [347]interest and impress the child. The secondary effects, rather than the immediate effects, are those that determine a child's action. Most of the direct physiological effects are, in the majority of instances, less serious in themselves than the effects of overeating, of combining milk with acids, of eating irregularly, of neglecting constipation. Were it not for the social and industrial consequences of drunkenness and nicotinism, it is doubtful if the most lurid picture of fatty degeneration, alcoholic consumption, hardened liver, inactive stomach lining, would outweigh the pleasing — and deceiving — sensations of alcoholic beverages and cigarettes.

The strong appeal to the child or man is the effect these habits have upon his mother, his employer, his wife, his children. The vast majority of us will avoid or stop using anything that makes us offensive to those with whom we are most intimately associated, and to those upon whom our professional and industrial promotion depends. Children will profit from drill in and out of school in the science of avoiding offense and of giving happiness, but unless the categories — *acts that give offense* and *acts that give happiness* — are wide enough to include the main acts committed in the normal relations of son, companion, employer, husband, father, and citizen, those who set out to avoid alcohol and tobacco find themselves ill equipped to carry the obligations of a temperate, law-abiding citizen.

Things do not happen as described in the early text-book. Other things not mentioned hinder progress and happiness. The child at work resents the mis-education received at school and suspects that he has been following false gods. The enemies that cause him trouble come from unexpected sources. He finds it infinitely easier to eschew alcohol and tobacco than to avoid living conditions that insidiously undermine his aversion to stimulants and narcotics. The reasons for avoiding stimulants in the interest of others are more [348]numerous and more cogent than the reasons for avoiding stimulants and narcotics for one's own sake. The altruistic reasons for shunning stimulants and narcotics cannot be implanted in the child unless he sees the evil of excess *per se* in anything and everything, and unless he becomes thoroughly grounded in the life relations and health relations to which he must adapt himself.

Unclean streets, unclean milk, congested tenements, can do more harm than alcohol and tobacco, because they breed a physique that craves stimulants and drugs. Adenoids and defective vision will injure a larger proportion of the afflicted than will alcohol and tobacco, because they earlier and more certainly substitute discouragement for hope, handicap for equal chance. Failure to enforce health laws is a more serious menace to health and morals than drunkenness or tobacco cancer.

If it is true that we must attack the problem of alcohol from the standpoint of its social and industrial effects, we are forced at once to consider the machinery by which cities and governments control the manufacture and sale of alcohol. It is not an exaggeration to say that courses in regulating the traffic in alcohol are more necessary than courses in the effects of alcohol upon digestion and respiration.

If Sunday closing of saloons, local option, high license, and prohibition have failed, there is no evidence that the failure is due to the principles underlying any one of these methods. Until more earnest effort is made to study the effects of these methods, the results of their enforcement and the causes of their nonenforcement, no one is justified in declaring that either policy is successful or unsuccessful. It is very easy to select from the meager facts now available convincing proofs both that prohibition does not prohibit and that high license leads to increased drunkenness. The consequence is that the movements to control, restrict, or prohibit the use of alcohol are emotional, not rational.

[349]It is impossible to keep emotion, sensation, sentiment, at white heat. Most extremists worship legislation and do not try to keep interest alive by telling every week or every month new facts about the week or the month before. No new fuel is added to the anti-saloon fire, which gradually cools and dies down. Not so, however, with those who make money by the sale of intoxicants. The greater the opposition, the more brains, the more effort, the more money they put into overcoming or circumventing that opposition. Fuel is piled on and the bonfire is fed freely. Every day the anti-restriction bonfire becomes larger and larger, and the anti-saloon bonfire becomes smaller and smaller. By carefully selecting their facts, by counting the number of arrests for drunkenness and the number of saloons open on Sunday, by reiteration of their story the pro-saloonists gradually win recruits from the opposition, and, when the next election comes, their friends outnumber their enemies and the "dry" policy of a city, county, or state is reversed.

The failures attributed to prohibitive or restrictive measures are probably no more numerous than the failures of government in other respects. The present ambassador from England, James Bryce, writing his *American Commonwealth*, declared that municipal government was America's "most conspicuous failure." The mayor of Toledo, writing in 1907, says, "There has been a pessimism, almost enthusiastic, about the city." These failures are due not to any lack of desire for good government, not to any fundamental evils of cities, but to the fact that municipal reform, like the crusade against alcohol, has been based upon emotionalism, not upon definite proof. Reformers have been unable to lead in the right direction, because they have looked at their lantern instead of their road. Not having cumulative information as to government acts, they have been unable to keep their fires burning. To illustrate: in November, 1907, the governor of New York state, the [350]mayor of New York City, and reformers of national reputation eulogized the tenement-house department; yet this department, whose founding was regarded as a national benefaction, was the only department of the city government that did not receive an increase for 1908. It is in the position of temperance legislation, the facts of whose enforcement or nonenforcement are not promptly and continuously made public.

Fear of the negro victim of alcoholism, social evils of intemperance, whether among white or black, industrial uncertainty and waste due to alcoholism, are the three chief motives that have swept alcohol traffic out of the greater part of the South. Knowledge of physiological evils has had little influence, except as it may have rendered more acceptable the claim that alcoholism is a disease against which there is no insurance except abolition of alcohol as a beverage. Religious revivals, street parades by day and by night, illustrated banners, personal intercession, lines of women and children at the polls, made it necessary for voters to make known their intention, and made it extremely difficult for respectable men, engaged in respectable business, to vote for saloons. Some states have gone so far as to prohibit the manufacture of alcoholic stimulants, even though not offered for sale within state limits. In Georgia wine cannot be used at the communion service, nor can druggists sell any form of liquor except pure alcohol. In Louisiana it is illegal for representatives of "wet districts" to solicit orders for liquor in any of the "dry districts." In Texas the sale of liquor in dining cars is forbidden, and the traveler may not even drink from his own flask. Congress is being urged by senators and congressmen, as well as by anti-saloon advocates, to pass laws prohibiting common carriers from delivering alcoholics to any "dry" community. The more optimistic anti-saloon workers believe it is but a matter of a short time when Congress will pass laws prohibiting [351]the manufacture or sale of alcoholic beverages within any limits protected by the United States Constitution.

Southern states have been warned that they could not afford the depreciation of real estate values, of rents, and of business that would surely follow the "confiscation of capital" and "interference with personal liberty." This warning has been met by plausible arguments that the buyers of legitimate and nonpoisonous commodities could pay better rents, better profits on business and on real estate, if freed from the uneven fight against temptation to drink. The argument that schools and streets and health must suffer if the license money was withdrawn, has been met by the plausible argument that the ultimate taxpayer — the family that wants clothing, food, and shelter — will save enough money to be able to spend still larger sums than heretofore upon education, health, and public safety.

For the first time dealers in alcohol recognize the possibility of a great national movement and of national prohibition. Both the defects in methods hitherto used to oppose saloon legislation and the reasons for meeting the present situation by new methods are presented in the May issue (1907) of the *Transactions of the American Brewing Institute*. Under the title, "Social Order and the Saloon — the Measure of the Brewer's Responsibility," Mr. Hugh F. Fox, known throughout the Union as a defender of child rights, advocate of probation and children's courts, promoter of health and education, outlined a plan for research that is indispensable to the proper settling of this great question. Whether brewer or anti-saloon leaguist, total abstainer or moderate drinker, employer or trade unionist, it is necessary to the intelligent control of alcohol that each of us approach this momentous question of control or abolition of the saloon in the spirit expressed in this paper, whose thoroughness and whose social point of view would do credit to a church conference. The address is [352]quoted and its questions copied because both show how much depends upon knowing whether laws are enforced and how much greater is the difficulty of coping with a conciliatory antagonist who professes willingness to submit to tests of evidence.

The regulation of the liquor business involves fundamental questions of the function and scope of government, and there is hardly any department of organized human activity that has been the subject of so much experiment and futile tinkering.... The only people who are perfectly consistent are the prohibitionists, whose policy is abolition. Let us, however, try to detach ourselves from any personal interest that we may have in the subject, and consider it impartially as a matter of public concern.

What the brewer as an individual cannot do, the brewers as an organization have done successfully in many places in spite sometimes of official negligence, corruption, or incapacity. The Texas Brewers' Association is reported as having successfully prosecuted two thousand cases against keepers of disreputable resorts during the past three years. The object of their campaign was to purify the retail liquor trade from unclean and law-defying elements.

The greatest gain that has come to society, as distinguished from the individual, through the temperance movement is its effect in unconsciously informing the public that the regulation and administration of licensing is in itself a great and vital problem; and as a secondary result of such agitation, I should cite the growing sensitiveness of all persons in the business to the power of public opinion.

The recognition by brewers of the force of public opinion is a recent affair. In former years they were totally indifferent to it, if indeed they did not openly flout it. Even now their appeal to public sentiment is mainly a special plea for defensive purposes, and has little or no educational value. Brewers have opposed practically every effort to effect a change in excise laws, often without any convincing reason, but simply because the proposed change involved temporary inconvenience and uncertainty, and perhaps a temporary loss. The brewing trade has utterly failed to develop a constructive programme in connection with the public [353]regulation of its affairs. It does not seem to have any fixed principles or positive convictions as to excise methods and liquor laws. Its policy has been that of an opportunist, at the best,—or an obstructionist, at the worst. As in all other industries which affect the welfare of the people, reforms have been forced from the outside, with no help from within. Of course this is equally true of insurance and railroad corporations, of food purveyors, mine owners, cotton merchants, and a score of other interests. It is due not merely to human selfishness but to shortsightedness; in other words, to a lack of statesmanship.

To call your opponents hypocrites, cranks, fakirs, and fanatics may relieve your feelings, but it doesn't convince anybody, and only hurts a just cause. It is foolish to question the motives of men who, without thought of personal gain, are trying to remedy the evils of inebriety.

The church is perfectly right in urging total abstinence upon the individual. The only path of safety lies in abstinence for some individuals....

The recognition of the right of a community to establish its own licensing conditions carries with it the right of the community to determine whether there shall be any licenses at all!

To make the discussion of this subject as fruitful as possible, I venture to submit the following questions for your consideration. None of them involve any direct moral issue, but there is an honest difference of opinion about each one of them, and they are certainly of vital importance in determining the course of wise and just administration.

What has been the effect of high license?

How much public revenue should the traffic yield?

Does high license stimulate unlawful trade?

How much license tax should be imposed upon local bottlers and grocers? Should they be allowed to peddle beer or to sell it in single bottles?

Should the place or the individual be licensed?

Should the licensing authorities be appointive or elective? By whom should they be appointed, and for what term of office?

Have the courts made good or bad licensing authorities? Where the courts issue licenses, what has been the effect on the court?

[354]Should the licensing authority alone have the power to revoke a license, and discretion to withhold a license?

How can the licensing authority enforce the law? Should it not be independent of the police?

What should be the penalty for breach of the law? Do not severe penalties miscarry?

On what plea, and under what conditions, should licenses be transferred?

What has been the effect of limiting the number of saloons?

Should limitation be according to area or to population?

Is there any relation between the number of saloons and the volume of consumption?

What should be the limit to the hours of selling?

Should saloons be allowed to become places of entertainment?

How can the sale of liquor by druggists be controlled?

How can spurious drinking clubs be prevented or controlled?

How can the operation of disreputable hotels be prevented? What should be the definition of a hotel? Who should define it? By whom should it be licensed? What special privileges should be given to it?

How can the "back-room" evil be stopped? Is it legal (i.e. constitutional) to prohibit the sale or serving of liquor to women?

Has the removal of screens reduced the volume of consumption? Has it improved the character of saloons? Has it solved the problem of Sunday prohibition for any length of time? What has been the general effect of it in the tenement districts?

Should the state undertake to regulate the liquor business or to enforce liquor laws?

Is it possible to devise any working plan which will apply with equal effectiveness and equity in communities of compact and of scattered population?

Should, or should not, the principle of self-government be carefully preserved in the whole scheme of legislation to regulate the liquor business?

Whether the present prohibition wave shall wash away the legalized saloon, as ocean waves have from time to time engulfed peninsulas, islands, and whole continents, [355]depends upon the power of American educators and American officials to answer right such questions as the foregoing. The great danger is that we shall, as usual, over-emphasize lawmaking, underemphasize lawbreaking, and go to sleep during the next two or three years when we should be wide-awake and constantly active in seeing that the law is enforced. Unless exactly the same principles of law enforcement are applied in "dry districts" as we have urged for eradication of smallpox, typhoid, scarlet fever, and adenoids, local and city prohibition are doomed to failure. There must be:

1. Inspection to discover disease centers — "blind pigs," "blind tigers," etc.

2. Compulsory notification by parents and landlords, and by police and other officials.

3. Prompt investigation upon complaint from private citizens.

4. Prompt removal of the disease and disinfection of the center.

5. Segregation of individual units that disseminate disease, whether bartender, saloon keeper, owner of premises, or respectable wholesaler, none of whom should be permitted to shift to another the responsibility for violating liquor laws.

6. Persistent publicity as to the facts regarding enforcement and violation, so that no one, whether saloon leaguist or anti-saloon leaguist, shall be uninformed as to the current results of "dry" laws.

It is perfectly safe to assume that none of these things will be done consistently unless funds are provided to pay one or more persons in each populous locality to give their entire time to the enforcement of laws, just as the improvement of other ills of municipal government require the constant attention of trained investigators. Cogent arguments for such funds have recently appeared in the *New York Evening Post's* symposium on "How to Give Wisely," by Mrs. Emma Garrett Boyd, of Atlanta, and Miss Salmon, of Vassar College.

[356]If the saloon is here to stay, we must all agree that it is a frightful waste of human energy and of educational momentum to be appealing for its abolition when we might be hastening its proper control. On the other hand, if the saloon is destined to be abolished as a public nuisance and a private wrong, as a menace to industry and social order, is it not a frightful, unforgivable waste of energy to permit prohibition laws to fail, and thus to discredit the principle of prohibition? Philanthropists have provided millions for scientific research, for medical research, for the study of tuberculosis, and for the study of living conditions. It is to be hoped that a large benefaction, or that an aggregation of small benefactions, will apply to governmental attempts to regulate the sale of alcohol those methods of scientific research which have released men from the

thraldom of ignorance and diseases less easily preventable than alcoholism.

[357]

IS IT PRACTICABLE IN PRESENTING TO CHILDREN THE EVILS OF ALCOHOLISM TO TELL THE TRUTH, THE WHOLE TRUTH, AND NOTHING BUT THE TRUTH?

If children are taught that the most effective way of combating alcoholism is to insure the enforcement of existing laws and to profit from lessons taught by such enforcement; if children are taught that the strongest reasons for total abstinence are social, economic, and industrial rather than individual and physiological,—there is much to be gained and little to lose from telling them the truth, the whole truth, and nothing but the truth about alcohol. To stimulate a child's imagination by untruths about alcohol is as vicious as to stimulate his body with alcohol. Whisky drinking does not always lead to drunkenness, to physical incapacity, to short life, or to obvious loss of vitality. Beer drinking is not always objected to by employers. Neither crime, poverty, immorality, lack of ambition, nor ignorance can always be traced to alcohol. On the contrary, it is unquestionably true that the majority of the nation's heroes have used alcoholics moderately or excessively for the greater part of their lives. It is probably true that among the hundred most eminent officials, pastors, merchants, professors, and scientists of to-day, the great majority of each class are moderate users of one or more forms of alcoholics. Overeating of potatoes or cake or meat, sleeping or working in ill-ventilated rooms, neglect of constipation, may occasion physiological and industrial [358]injuries that are not only as grave in themselves as the evils of moderate drinking, but, in addition, actually tempt to moderate drinking.

All of this can be safely admitted, because whether parents and teachers admit it or deny it, children by observation and by reading will become convinced that up to the year 1908 the noblest and the most successful men of America, as well as the most depraved and least successful, have used alcoholics. To be candid enough to admit this enables us to gain a hold upon the confidence and the intelligence of children and youth that will strengthen our arguments, based upon social and industrial as well as physiological grounds, against running the risks that are inevitably incurred by even the moderate use of alcohol.

Other things being equal, the same man will do better work without alcohol than with alcohol; the same athlete will be stronger and more alert without alcohol than with alcohol; the clerk or lawyer or teacher will win promotion earlier without alcohol than with alcohol; man or woman will grow old quicker with than without alcohol. Other things being equal, a man of fifty will have greater confidence in a total abstainer than in a man of identical capacity who uses alcohol moderately; a mother will give better vitality and better care to her children without than with alcohol; a policeman or fireman or stenographer is more apt to win promotion without than with alcohol. Whatever the physical ailment, there is in every instance a better remedy for an acute trouble, and infinitely better remedies for deep-seated troubles, than alcoholics.

The percentage of failure to use alcoholics moderately is so high, the uncertainty as to a particular individual's ability to drink moderately is so great, as to lead certain insurance companies, first, to give preference to men who never use alcoholics, and later, to refuse to insure moderate drinkers. Life insurance companies have the general rule [359]that habitual drinkers are bad risks, as the alcohol habit is prejudicial to health and longevity; but they have no means of studying the risk of moderate drinkers, because, except where alcohol has already left a permanent impression upon the system, the indications are by no means such as to enable the medical examiner to trace its existence with certainty. For this reason the life insurance companies have little effect in *preventing* alcoholism. Though they are agreed that habitual drinkers ought to be declined altogether, only a few companies have taken the decided stand of declining them. "Habitual drinkers, if not too excessive, are admitted into the general class where the expected mortality, according to the experience of the Pennsylvania Mutual Life Insurance Company, is 80 per cent, as against 56 per cent for the temperate class.

Though it is only necessary to look over the death losses presented each day to see that intemperance in the use of liquors, as shown by cirrhosis of the liver, Bright's disease, diseases of the heart, brain, and nervous system, is the cause of a large proportion of the deaths, these companies prefer to grade the premiums accordingly rather than to decline habitual drinkers altogether. While this is partly due to the difficulty and expense of diagnosis, it is more probably due to an objection to take a definite stand on the temperance question."

Thus the insurance companies' rules touch only the confirmed drinker, whose physique is often irreparably injured. One company writes: "Men who have been intemperate and taken the Keeley or other cures are never accepted until five years have elapsed from the date of taking the cure, and only when it can be conclusively shown that during the whole period they have refrained entirely from the use of alcoholic liquor, and that their former excesses have not in any way impaired the physical risk."

Thus far American insurance companies are doing little preventive and educational work on the alcohol question, [360]though they have the very best means at their command for so doing. According to the Metropolitan Life Insurance Company nine tenths of the school children in New York City are insured by them, and an even greater proportion of workingmen. Even though this is done "at twice the normal cost," the most cursory medical examination is given and no attempt is made to instruct them in the relation of their physical condition to their working power, or in the evils of the alcohol and the smoking habits.

Naturally the moderate drinker is first rejected for positions where an occasional overindulgence would be most noticeable and most serious. The manager of a large factory tells his men: "You cannot work here unless you are sober. If you must drink at parties, stay at home if necessary until 12 o'clock the next day and sleep it off, but don't come here till you are straight. We cannot afford it." Occasionally his men stay at home and not a word is said, but the minute they are found at work in an unsteady condition they are summarily discharged. From this position it is but a step to that of an upholsterer in New York City, who prints on his order blanks, "No drinking man employed." His company recently discharged a man after twenty years of service because a customer for whom this man was working detected a whisky breath. Men reported to trade unions for frequent intoxication are blacklisted. A certain financial corporation permits no liquor on its grounds or in its lunch rooms. The head of one of its large branches was heard to say recently that he would discharge on the spot a man who showed evidences of drinking, even though he had previously worked faithfully for years.

Rejection of moderate drinkers by business houses is not done on moral grounds alone, but because experience has proved the danger of employing men who have not their faculties fully under control *all* the time they are at work. The rules are especially strict for men working for a railroad [361]or street railway company. The Pennsylvania Railroad Company replied to my inquiry as to their custom of discriminating against drinking men in these words: "We have no printed rules in regard to this except in a general way,—that no employee is allowed to go into a saloon during his hours of work or wearing the company's uniform. Of course the men are promptly discharged or disciplined if they show the effects of liquor while on duty, and the whole tendency of the administration of the rules is to get rid of any men who are habitual drinkers, but the administration of the rules and discipline is left to the superintendent of each division." The Interborough Rapid Transit Company of New York has these printed rules for the physical standard required for applicants for employment:

1. *Examination of heart and arteries.* Rejection of candidates showing excessive or long-continued use of tobacco and alcohol, with explanation of condition, causes, and dangers of continued use. Warning to chiefs of departments regarding those accepted who show tendency to drink at times, but whose physical examination does not disclose sufficient evidence to warrant their disqualifications. Foremen and chiefs of departments to be notified and to carry out the policy of employing only men who are at all times sober and not under the influence of alcohol at all.

2. *On reëxamination of employees.* Warning to or rejection of those showing, on physical examination, indulgence to excess of alcohol, tobacco, or drugs. Warning to chief of department of evidence of

such habits on part of any employee examined for any reason, but retained in service of the company with injunction to chief of department to speak with such employee and have him under proper supervision.

The blacklisting of habitual drinkers by their union, and the growing tendency on the part of large corporations, factories, and business houses to take a decided stand against drinking, are having a marked effect in reducing drunkenness where it does most harm. This practice has been declared by John Bach McMasters, the noted American historian, to have exerted a stronger influence in promoting temperance and total abstinence than all the temperance crusades from Hartley's time to the prohibition wave of [362]1907. The school, by instructing children how the alcohol habit will affect their chances of business success, future usefulness as citizens, and enjoyment of life, will inevitably reduce the evils of alcohol. By teaching based on facts that intimately concern the life of the child, as well as by caring for his health and his environment, the schools can help supplant the desire for alcohol with other more healthy desires.

No truth about alcohol is more important than that the craving for alcohol or something just as bad will exist side by side with imperfect sanitation, too long hours of work, food that fails to nourish, lack of exercise, rest, and fresh air. Conditions that produce bounding vitality and offer freedom for its expression at work and at play will supplant the craving for stimulants. Finally, the great truth contained in the last chapter must be taught, that success in coping with alcoholism is a community task requiring efficient government above all else.

[363]

CHAPTER XXXVIToC

FIGHTING TOBACCO EVILS

"It is not necessarily vicious or harmful to soothe excited nerves." This editorial comment explains, even if it condemns while trying to justify, the tobacco habit. To soothe excited nerves by lying to them about their condition and by weakening where we promise to nourish, is vicious and harmful just as other lying and robbery are vicious and harmful. Yet two essential facts in dealing with tobacco evils must be considered: tobacco does soothe excited nerves, and the harm done to the majority of smokers seems to them to be negligible. For these two reasons the tobacco user, unless frightened by effects already visible, refuses to listen to physiological arguments against his amiable self-indulgence. Cheerfully he admits the theoretical possibility that by its method of soothing nerves tobacco kills nerve energy. But in all sincerity he points to men who have found the right stopping point up to which tobacco hurts less perhaps than coffee or tea, candy or lobster, overeating or undersleeping. Therefore the physician, the bishop, the school superintendent, candidly run the necessary risk for the sake of nerve soothing and sociability.

Less harm would be done by tobacco if it were more harmful. Like so many other food poisons, its use in small quantities does not produce the prompt, vivid, unequivocal results that remove all doubt as to the user's injuries and intemperance. As inability to see the physiological effect upon himself encourages the tobacco user to continue smoking or chewing, so failure to identify evil physiological effects upon the smoker encourages the nonuser to begin [364]smoking or chewing. A very few smokers give up the habit because they fear its results, but too often the man who can see the evil results would rather give up almost anything else. The one motive that most frequently stops inveterate smoking—fear—is the least effective motive in dissuading those who have not yet acquired the habit; every young man, unless already suffering from known heart trouble, thinks he will smoke moderately and without harm. Unfortunately, every boy who begins to smoke succeeds in picturing to himself the adult who shows no surface sign of injury from tobacco, rather than some other boy who has been stunted physically, mentally, and morally by cigarettes.

For adult and child, therefore, it behooves us to find some other weapons against tobacco evils in addition to fear of physiological injuries. Among these weapons are:

1. Enforcement of existing laws that make it an offense against society for dealer, parent, or other person to furnish children under sixteen with tobacco in any form; and raising the age limit to twenty-one, or at least to eighteen.

2. Enforcement of restrictions as to place and time when smoking is permitted.

3. Agitation against tobacco as a private and public nuisance.

4. Explanation of commercial advantages of abstinence.

Because the childish body quickly shows the injurious effects of what in adults would be called moderate smoking, the proper physical examination of school children will reveal injuries which in turn will show where and to what extent the cigarette evil exists among the children of a community. Even the scientists who claim that "in some cases tobacco aids digestion," or that "tobacco may be used without bad effects when used moderately by people who are in condition to use it," declare emphatically that tobacco "must not be used in any form by growing children or youths." Prohibitive laws can be rigidly enforced if a small [365]amount of attention is given to organizing the strong public sentiment that exists against demoralizing children by tobacco. Thus children and youths will not need to make a decision regarding their own use of tobacco until after other arguments than physiological fear have been used for many years by parent, teacher, and society.

One effective weapon is the sign on a ferryboat or street car: "No smoking allowed on this side," or "Smoking allowed on three rear seats only." Public halls and vehicles in increasing numbers either prohibit smoking altogether or put smokers to some considerable inconvenience. The trouble involved in going to places where smoking is permitted tends gradually to irritate the nerves beyond the power of tobacco to soothe. Again, many men would rather not soothe their excited nerves after five, than have their nerves excited all day waiting for freedom to smoke. Restrictions as to time or place make possible and expedite still further restrictions. Thus gradually the army of occasional smokers or nonsmokers is being recruited from the army of regular smokers.

The anti-nuisance motive follows closely upon the drawing of sharp lines of time and place for the use of tobacco. Like treason, smoking in the presence of nonsmokers can be considered respectable only when the numbers who profess and practice it are numerous. If the two first-mentioned weapons are effectively used, there will be an increasing proportion of nonsmokers and not-yet-smokers who will give attentive ear to proof that nicotinism is a nuisance. The physical evidences of the cigarette habit can easily be made distasteful to all nonsmokers if frankly pointed out,—the yellow fingers, the yellow teeth, the nasty breath, the offensive excretions from the pores that saturate the garments of all who cannot afford a daily change of underwear. The anti-nuisance argument is always insidious and abiding. In the presence of nonsmokers accustomed to [366]regard tobacco using as a nuisance, smokers become self-conscious and sensitive. Men and women alike would prefer a reputation for cleanliness to the pleasures of tobacco. The educational possibility of fighting tobacco with the name "nuisance" was recognized the other day by an editorial that protested against a law to prevent women from using cigarettes in restaurants. "The way for any man who has the desire to reform some woman addicted to the cigarette habit is insidiously and gently to point out the injurious effects on her appearance. Cigarette smoking stains a woman's fingers and discolors her teeth. It also tends to make her complexion sallow and to detract from the rubiness of her lips. It bedims the sparkle of her eyes. It makes her less attractive mornings." Chewing has practically disappeared, not because it ceased to soothe excited nerves but because it was seen to be a nasty nuisance.

Finally, the selfishness of the smoker is a nuisance that continues only because it has not been called by its right name. "Do you mind if I smoke?" was a polite question two hundred years ago when tobacco was rare enough to make smoking a distinction, or fifty years ago when everybody smoked at home and in public. But it is effrontery to-day when people do mind, when smoking pollutes the air of drawing room and office, and while soothing the excited nerves of the smoker lowers the vitality of nonsmokers compelled to breathe smoke-laden air. It is selfish to intrude upon others a personal weakness or a personal appetite. It is selfish to divert from family purposes to "soothing excited nerves" even the small amounts necessary to maintain the cigar or cigarette habit. It is selfish to run the risk of shortening one's life, of reducing one's earning capacity. Because the tobacco habit is selfish it is anti-social and a nuisance, and should be fought by social as well as personal weapons, as are other recognized nuisances, such as spitting in public or offensive manners.

[367]The economic motive for avoiding and for eliminating tobacco is gaining in strength. The soothing qualities of all drugs are found to be expensive to physical and business energy if enjoyed during business hours. Strangely enough, employers who smoke are quite as apt as are nonsmokers, to forbid the use of tobacco by employees at work. Some of this seeming inconsistency is due to a dislike for cheaper tobacco or for mixed brands in one atmosphere; some of it is due to the smoker's knowledge that "soothing nerves" and sustained attention do not go hand in hand, while "pipe dreams" and unproductive meditation are fast companions; finally no little of the opposition to tobacco in business is due to fear of fire. These various motives, combining with the anti-nuisance motive among nonsmokers, have led many business enterprises to prohibit the use of tobacco in any form on their premises or during business hours, even when on the premises of others. Notable examples are railroads that permit no passenger trainman to use tobacco while on duty. (Freight trainmen are restricted more tardily because the risk of damages is less and the anti-nuisance objection is wanting.)

From penalizing excessive use and prohibiting moderate use in business hours, it is a short cut to choosing men who never use tobacco and thus never suffer any of its effects and never exhibit any of its offensive evidences. No young man expects to obtain a favorable hearing if he offers himself for employment while smoking or chewing tobacco. Business men dislike to receive tobacco-scented messengers. Cars and elevators contain signs prohibiting lighted cigars or cigarettes. Insurance companies reject men who show signs of excessive use of tobacco. Why? Because they are apt to die before their time. The Interborough Rapid Transit Company of New York City rejects applicants for motormen and conductors "for excessive or long-continued use of tobacco." Why? Because, other things being equal, [368]such men are more apt to lose their nerve in an emergency and to fail to read signals or instructions correctly.

Armed with these weapons against tobacco, parents and teachers can effectively introduce physiological arguments against excessive use, against use by those who suffer from nervous or heart trouble, and against any use whatever by those who have not reached physical maturity. By avoiding physiological arguments that children will not—cannot—believe contrary to their own eyes, parents and teachers are able to speak dogmatically of that which children will believe,—injuries to children, evils of excess, restrictions as to time and place, and offensiveness to nonsmokers. But even here it is wrong, as it is inexpedient, to leave the physical strength of the next generation to the persuasive power of parents and teachers or to the faith and knowledge of minors. Society should protect all minors against their own ignorance, their own desires, the ignorance of parents and associates, and against the economic motive of tobacco sellers by machinery that enforces the law.

[369]

THE PATENT-MEDICINE EVIL

"Dhrugs," says Dock O'Leary, "are a little iv a pizen that a little more iv wud kill ye. Ye can't stop people fr'm takin' dhrugs, an' ye might as well give thim somethin' that will look important enough to be inthrojuced to their important and fatal cold in th' head. If ye don't, they'll leap f'r th' patent medicines. Mind ye, I haven't got annything to say agin' patent medicines. If a man wud rather take them thin dhrink at a bar or go down to Hop Lung's f'r a long dhraw, he's within his rights. Manny a man have I known who was a victim iv th' tortures iv a cigareet cough who is now livin' comfortable an' happy as an opeem fiend be takin' Dr. Wheezo's Consumption Cure." The Dock says th' more he practices medicine th' more he becomes a janitor with a knowledge iv cookin'. He says if people wud on'y call him in befure they got sick he'd abolish ivry disease in th' ward except old age and pollyticks.

Thus Mr. Dooley with his usual wit and insight tells the American people why they spend over two hundred million dollars annually on patent medicines. Americans consume more drugs and use more patent medicines than the people of any other country on the civilized globe. Self-medication has grown to tremendous proportions. Everywhere — in cars, on transfers, on billboards, in magazines, in newspapers, in the mails — are advertised medicines to cure disease and devices to promote health. When we consider that electric cars contain from thirty-two to fifty-two advertisements each, three fourths of which are directly or indirectly concerned with health; when we multiply these by the number of cars actually in use in American cities; when we consider the number of advertisements in magazines and daily papers, and the enormous circulation of these papers and magazines; [370]when we consider that an increasingly large proportion of advertising space is devoted to health,—we begin to realize the cumulative power for good or for evil that health advertisements must have.

To illustrate advertisements devoted to health to-day, I have kept clippings for one week of news items, editorials, and advertisements in a penny and a three-cent paper, and had them classified according to the subjects treated:

	Penny Paper			Three-Cent Paper		
	News Item	Editorial	Advertisement	News Item	Editorial	Advertisement
Milk	3	—	2	3	—	2
Teeth	—	1	2	—	—	1
Shoes	—	—	4	—	—	1
Food	1	—	—	1	—	4
Alcohol	1	—	5	3	—	7
Tuberculosis	—	—	1	1	—	—
Patent medicine	—	—	17	—	—	—
Constipation cures	—	—	4	—	—	5
Eyes	3	—	5	1	—	—
Beauty	2	5	8	—	—	6
General	8	3	3	5	—	—
Total	18	9	51	14	—	26

The following list of health topics was treated in the advertisements, editorials, and articles of a popular monthly periodical devoted to women:

	Article	Editorial	Advertisement
Babies	1	—	11

Soaps and powders	–	–	5
Beauty	3	–	6
Quack cures	–	2	–
Tooth powders	–	–	4
Household	1	–	5
Food and cooking	1	–	14
Clothes	13	–	5
Teaching sex laws	1	2	–
Medicine	4	1	–
Total	24	5	50

[371]Besides the classic patent medicines, such as Lydia Pinkham's Vegetable Compound, Castoria, Cod Liver Oil, etc., there are "Colds Cured in One Day," "Appendixine," health foods, massage vibrators, violet rays, Porosknit underwear, sanitary tooth washes, soaps, vitopathic, naturopathic, and faith cures. New ones appear every day,—enough to make a really sick person dizzy, let alone a person suffering from imaginary ailments. All seem to outline my particular symptoms. After they have flamed at me in red letters in the surface cars, pursued me in the elevated and underground, accompanied me out into the country and back again to the city, greeted me each morning in the daily paper and in my daily mail, each week or each month in the periodical, the coincidence of a familiar package on a drug-store counter seems to be providential and therefore irresistible. I know that I ought to be examined by a physician, but I am busy and not unwilling to gamble for my health; it cannot kill me and there is a chance that it will cure me. If there is nothing the matter with us, we may be cured by our faith. If we are taking a cure for consumption, the morphine in it may lull us into thinking we feel better. If we are taking a tonic for spring fever, the cheap alcohol may excite us into thinking our vitality has been heightened. Soothing sirup soothes the baby, often doping its spirit for life, or soothing it into a sleep from which it never wakes.

In spite of the fact that the "Great American Fraud" has been exposed repeatedly in newspapers and magazines of wide circulation, the appeal of the quack still catches men and women of intelligence. The other night a friend went out to a dinner and conference with a lawyer in the employ of the national government. Annoyed by a nagging headache, he made for the nearest drug store and ordered a "headache powder." He admitted that it was an awful dose, but he had been told that it always "did the business." [372]He knew the principle was bad, confessed to a scorn for friends of his whom he knew to be bromo-seltzer fiends, but he had the headache and the work to do—a sure cure and a quick one seemed imperative. The headache was due to overwork, indigestion, constipation. Plain food and quiet sleep was what he needed most. But the dinner conference plus the headache was the unanswerable argument for a dose with an immediate result.

Last winter an Irish maid slowly lost her rosy cheeks and grew hollow-eyed and thin. She was taken to a specialist who discovered a rapidly advancing case of consumption. He said that owing to the girl's ignorance, stupidity, and homesickness, her only chance of recovery was to return to the "auld countrie" at once. The girl agreed to go, but insisted on a few days "to talk it over with her cousins in New York." After two weeks had elapsed she was found in a stuffy, overcrowded New York tenement. She had found a doctor who had given her a little bottle of medicine for two dollars, which would cure her in the city. It was futile to protest. Days in the unventilated tenement and nights in a "dark room" meant that she would never live to finish the bottle.

For a year Miss H. took a patent preparation for chronic catarrh. It seemed to "set her up"; but it so undermined her strength, through its artificial nerve spur, that chronic catarrh was followed by consumption. It later transpired that the cure's chief ingredient was whisky, and cheap whisky. A good grandmother, herself a vigorous temperance agitator and teetotaler, offered to pay for it as long as my friend would take it faithfully. The irony of it makes one wonder how many earnest advocates of total abstinence are in reality addicted to the liquor habit.

Last summer a district nurse of the summer corps who visited city babies under two years of age encountered in the hallway of a tenement a bevy of frenzied women. A [373]baby lay on the bed gasping and "rolling its eyes up into the top of its head." The nurse asked the frightened mother what she had been giving it. "Nothing at all," said the woman. But a telltale bottle of soothing sirup showed that the child was dying from morphine poisoning. Happily the nurse came in time to save it.

Is it not pitiful, this grasping for a poison in an extremity; this seizing of a defective rope to escape the fire?

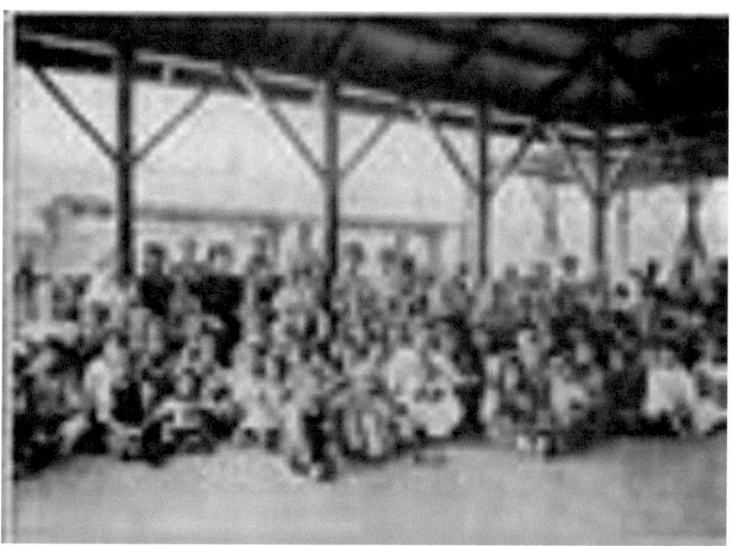

LEARNING HOW TO KEEP BABY WELL WITHOUT PATENT MEDICINES
Recreation Pier, New York City, Summer, 1908

The patent-medicine evil cannot be cured by occasional exposure or by overexposure. Nor can it be cured by legislation, legislation, legislation, unless laws are rigidly enforced.

Occasional exposure is no better than occasional advertising of good things. The patent-medicine business thrives on constant, not occasional, advertising. Leading advertisers expect so little from the first notice that they would not take the trouble to write out a single advertisement. That is the reason merchants charge advertising in [374]the programmes of church, festival, and glee-club concert to charity, not to business. Warning people once does no more lasting good than sending a child to school once a month. The exposure of patent-medicine evils must be as constant as efforts to sell the medicines.

Overexposure is ineffective. It is the evils of patent medicines that do harm, not their name and not their patents. The medical profession has in vain protested against proprietary medicines. Ethical barriers cannot be erected by resolution. Calling things unethical does not make them unethical. The mere patenting of medicines for profit does not make the medicine injurious any more than the mere mixing of unpatented drugs makes a physician safe. Physicians who would not themselves patent a drug will use certain patented drugs whose ingredients are known to be safe and uniform. True exposure of patent-medicine evils will enable the average physician and the average layman to distinguish the dangerous from the safe, the fraud from the genuine, lies from truths.

Legislation is needed to crystallize modern knowledge and to establish in courts the right to protection against the evils of patent medicines. The national Pure Food Law, passed January 1, 1907, and now in force throughout the country, requires on the "labels of all proprietary medicines entering into interstate commerce, a statement of the quantity or proportion of any alcohol, morphine, opium, heroin, chloroform, cannabis indica, chloral hydrate, or acetanilid, or any derivative or preparation of any such substance contained therein; this information must be in type not smaller than eight-point capital letters; also *the label shall embody no statement which shall be false or misleading in any particular.*" This law does not forbid patent medicines nor the use of alcohol and narcotics in patent medicines; it merely says, "Let the label tell, that all who *buy* may read." It does not require that all [375]who *run* may read, for *it does not say that advertisements of a patent medicine shall tell the truth about its ingredients or its action on the human body*; only that the label on the bottle shall tell. The object of this law is to explain to the consumer the exact nature of the medicine. But to the majority of people the word "acetphenitidin" on the label of a headache medicine does not explain. The new order that requires manufacturers to substitute acetanilid for acetphenitidin does no more than replace fog with mist. Protection requires legislation that cannot be evaded by technical terms. The present law requires that packages must be properly labeled *on entering the state*. To carry out the national law, state laws should make it an offense for dealers to have in their possession proprietary medicines without explanatory labels that explain. Where state laws to this effect do not exist, the packages once in the state may be deprived of their labels and sold as secret remedies, thus nullifying the whole effect of the national law.

Enforcement must be insured. Impure drugs may do as much harm as patent medicines containing harmful drugs. In New York a vigorous campaign was recently inaugurated by the department of health to drive out impure drugs. Drugs are dangerous enough at their best. When they are not what they pretend to be, whether patented or not, they may take life. One extreme case where a patient's heart was weakened when it ought to have been strengthened, led to the discovery that practically all of one particular drug offered for sale in New York City was unfit to use and calculated to kill in the emergency where alone it would be used. Yesterday four lives and several million dollars were lost in a New York fire because the hose was rotten or weak. As inspection and testing were needed to insure hose equal to emergency pressure, so inspection and testing of patent medicines and drugs are needed to make legislation effectual.

[376]Legislation and enforcement should reach the newspaper, magazine, billboard, street car, that advertises a falsehood or less than the essential truth regarding drugs, foods, and patent medicines. Public sentiment condemns the advertising of many opportunities to commit crime or to be disorderly or indecent or to injure one's neighbor. The facts about hundreds of nostrums can be absolutely determined. The advertising agency, whether secular or religious, that carries misrepresentation of drugs and foods should be forbidden circulation through the mails. The existence of such advertisements should be made evidence of complicity in a public offense and punished accordingly. Treat them as we treated the Louisiana lottery. Boards of health, instead of furnishing names to druggists and manufacturers who want to sell patent foods and medicines, should print circulars exposing frauds, and punish so far as the law permits.

While trying to secure adequate legislation and efficient administration of the above-mentioned standards, there is much that can be done by individuals and clubs. We can give preference to those journals that refuse drug and food advertisements unless evidence is produced that the truth is told and that the goods are not harmful. We can refuse to have in the house a paper or journal which prints notices that lie or that conceal the truth. If this drastic measure would cut us off entirely from daily papers, we could choose the least offensive and petition it to exclude specific lying methods. When it preaches health, honesty, and philanthropy, we can cut out of one issue the noble editorial and the exploiting advertisements and send them to the editor with our protest. Knowledge of the ingredients and dangers of patent medicines should be a prerequisite for the practice of medicine or pharmacy. We can help bring about such conditions, and we can patronize physicians who send patients to drug stores that cater to intelligence rather than to ignorance.

[377]Fighting patent-medicine evils is a civic duty to be accomplished by civic coöperation, not private effort. It is impossible to organize unofficial educational agencies that can offset the cumulative, lying advertisement. Personal opposition is but the beginning. Official machinery must be set running and kept running so as to protect the public health against the commercial motive that preys upon ignorance and easily inspired faith.

[378]

CHAPTER XXXVIIIToC

HEALTH ADVERTISEMENTS THAT PROMOTE HEALTH

It is usually considered futile to attempt to defeat the devil with his own methods, because he knows so much better how to use them. But abuse does not do away with use, and the success of quacks in reaching the people demands our respect. There is no reason why their methods, based on a knowledge of human nature and human psychology, should not be employed to appeal to needs rather than to weaknesses. A good thing may lie unused because of lack of advertisement. Vitality is coming to be the passion of the American people. It is on this sincere passion that fakirs have so long traded.

There can be no doubt that advertisements of health-promoting goods are quite as profitable as health advertisements that injure health, when equally effective methods are used to make them reach the public. The tradition has been repeatedly mentioned in this book that the better the doctor, the less he advertises himself, except in medical and scientific journals that notoriously fail to reach the people. The same is too often true of reputable remedies and goods. The theory that these things stand or fall on their merits is not borne out by practical experience, — conspicuously in the case of "fake" remedies. Purely philanthropic undertakings for the advancement of health fail, if not placed before the people whom they aim to help in an attractive, convincing form. Failure to advertise a worthy cause limits its usefulness, and is therefore unjustifiable, whether we speak of medicine, legal aid, or dental clinics.

[379]An intensive study of the methods used to advertise patent medicines will suggest means of extending the usefulness of health-promoting goods. Aside from clever methods of suggestion that lead many people to take medicine for imaginary ailments, especially seasonal ailments, patent-remedy advertisers have employed (as

an argument for the efficiency of their cures) scientific theory, bacterial origin of diseases, recent medical or physiological discoveries, and state and national movements for promoting health. In fact, they have turned to their own uses the very law that seeks to control them and the exposures that seek to exterminate them. Whatever may be the merits of Castoria, the "Don't Poison Baby" advertisement on the following page, printed just after the accompanying "Babies Killed by Patent Medicines," which appeared in a home journal, was surely a clever bit of advertising. Upon an editorial in a daily paper on the relation of eyeglasses to headache and indigestion, an optician based a promise of immediate relief for these ailments if he himself were patronized. The recent investigations of the Department of Agriculture, and of Professors Chittenden and Fisher, in regard to foodstuffs, are proving helpful to food quacks and advertisers of pills for constipation and indigestion. Since the passage of the Pure Food Law one health food is advertised in a column headed "Pure Food."

When the season for pneumonia comes around numerous medicines are "sure cures" for grippe and pneumonia. "Rosy teachers look better in the schoolroom than the sallow sort," is surely a good introduction to a new food. Woman's vanity sells many a remedy advertised to counteract the "vandal hand of disease, which robs her of her beauty, yellows and muddies her complexion, lines her face, pales cheek and lip, dulls the brilliancy of her eye, which it disfigures with dark circles, aging her before her time." Who in your town is as good a friend to "owners of bad breath" as the advertiser who tells them that they "whiff out odor which makes [380]those standing near them turn their heads away in disgust"? The climax of effective educational advertising as well as of consummate presumption and villainy is reached in the notice of an alcoholic concoction that uses the headline, "Medical Supervision Needed to Prevent the Spread of Consumption in the Schools." Thus grafting itself on the successful results of the medical examination in the Massachusetts schools, it enlists the aid of teachers, trades on the fear of tuberculosis, even indorses the fresh-air treatment. So convincing was this appeal that it was reprinted in the [381]news columns of a daily paper in New York as official advice to school children.

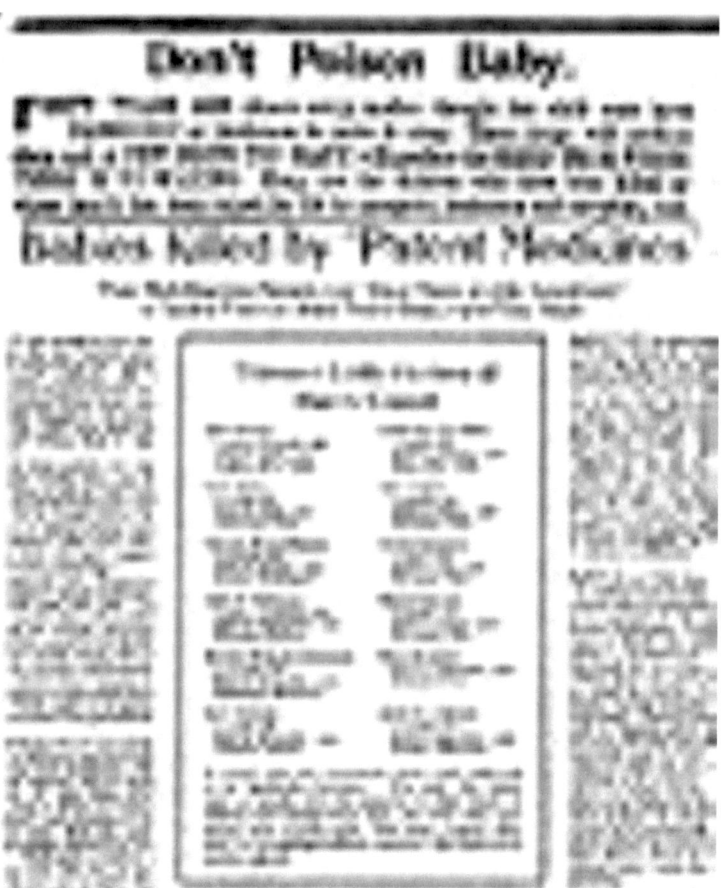

So clever are these methods of advertising and so successful are they in reaching great numbers of people, that if reputable physicians would take lessons of them, they might conduct a health crusade that would exterminate tuberculosis, diminish the use of alcohol and tobacco, and save thousands of babies that die unnecessarily. The theory of patent-medicine advertising is sound. It emphasizes the joys of health, the beauty of health, the earning power of health. It adapts its message to season, event, and need. It offers testimonials of real persons cured. It is all-appealing, promising, convincing, — a fearful menace to health when the remedies offered are dishonest, a universal opportunity for promoting health if the cure is genuine.

A classic example of health advertising that promotes health is Sapolio. The various hygiene lessons that have promoted Sapolio have done much to raise the standard of living in the United States. Few eminent physicians have done so much for public health as the "Poor M.D. of Spotless Town who scoured the country for miles around, but the only case he could find was a case of Sapolio."

Recent press discussions about furnishing free eyeglasses to the children in the public schools have so enlightened people as to the need for expert examination of their eyes that opticians will be forced to employ competent oculists to make the preliminary examination and to see that the glasses are properly adjusted. In spite of the long mis-education by makers of corsets, the persistent advertising of "good health" and "common-sense" waists has gained an increasing number of recruits from the ranks of the self-persecuting. It is only a matter of time when the term "stylish" will be transferred to the advocates of health, because advertisers who tell the truth will, if persistent, gain a larger patronage than advertisers of falsehoods; there [382]is profit in retaining old customers. The advertisement of a window device for "Fresh air while you sleep" will make prevention of tuberculosis more profitable than "sure cures" that lie and kill.

A man deserves profit who sends this message to millions of readers:

There are three kinds of cleanliness:

First, the ordinary soap-and-water cleanliness.
Second, the so-called "beauty" cleanliness.
Third, prophylactic cleanliness, or the cleanliness that "guards against disease."

But the man who sells soap ought to be the one to use this advertisement, not a man who sells toothwash that, when pure, is little better than water, that is seldom pure, and that always hurts the teeth. Many children and adults are being cured of flat foot by men who make money by selling shoes designed to strengthen the arch of the foot. Millions would never know how to discover the evil effects upon themselves of coffee and alcohol except for money-making advertisements. Little Jo's Smile taught a nation that the majority of crippled children are victims of neglect on the part of adult consumptives.

Certain it is that advertising is an art promoted by the severest competition of the cleverest brains. It is a force which we cannot afford to ignore. If we can harness it to the promotion of aids to health, it will do more good than all the hygiene books ever written. To this end we must educate ourselves to distinguish between goods which do what they profess to do and those which do not. A good eye opener would be to keep for a week clippings from a high-priced daily paper, a penny daily paper, and one or two representative magazines, including a religious paper. Teachers and parents can very easily interest children in such clippings. Moreover, they can use the bulletin method, [383]the stereopticon exhibit, the *cumulative illustration* of a fact, which is the essence of successful advertising. Boards of health can use all the typographical aids to clear understanding, — cuts, diagrams, interesting anecdotes. In New York both the health board and the school board have issued circulars and given illustrated lectures, some of them being in school and some on public squares. Medical and sanitary societies and other educators can be induced to follow what a successful business man has called the three cardinal rules of advertising:

First, put your advertisement where it will be seen. (Tell your story where it will be heard.)

Second, write it so that people will read it. (Tell it so that people will understand it.)

Third, tell the truth, so that people will believe it.

[384]

416

IS CLASS INSTRUCTION IN SEX HYGIENE PRACTICABLE?

Among remedies for preventable disease and preventable poverty, the following was urged at a national conference for the betterment of social conditions: "We have been too prudish. Because we have been unwilling to teach school children the evils of violating sex hygiene, we have been unsuccessful in combating evils justly attributable to ignorance on the part of girls as to the duties and dangers of motherhood." This point of view is shared by so many men and women that a national body was organized in 1905 to promote the teaching of sex hygiene, — the Society for Sanitary and Moral Prophylaxis. This society has its headquarters in New York, and distributes at cost lectures and essays. The second of its educational pamphlets is addressed to teachers, and is entitled "Instruction in the Physiology and Hygiene of Sex." The introduction asks eleven questions of the teachers as follows:

1. Do you wish a pamphlet on sex subjects to hand to your pupils? Why?

2. Do you wish separate pamphlets for boys and girls?

3. For what age limits and social conditions do you wish them?

4. What topics do you wish the pamphlets for boys to "handle"?

5. What topic do you wish the pamphlet for girls to "handle"?

6. If you think one pamphlet sufficient for both sexes, what should it consider?

7. How far do you go in teaching sexual hygiene or reproduction? By what method?

[385]8. What special difficulties do you find in teaching it?

9. What special need of teaching it have you found?

417

10. What special benefits (or otherwise) have you noticed from teaching it?

11. What criticisms (favorable or otherwise) do you encounter?

The difficulty of introducing formal instruction in sex hygiene, even in the upper grades of public and private schools, is hinted at in the pamphlet. The purpose of the publishing society as given in its constitution is "to eliminate the spread of diseases which have their origin in the social evil." Although sex hygiene does not begin with sex immorality, almost every text-book on sex hygiene, and almost every pamphlet urging class instruction in sex hygiene, begins with sex immorality. Yet only the exceptional school child is in danger of violating sex morals, while every school child needs instruction in sex hygiene.

Instruction in sex hygiene, whether at school or at home, should deal with sex normality, sex health, sex temperance. Instruction in sex immorality is objectionable, not merely because it offends prudists, not because it is difficult, but because it can be shown by experience to be less efficacious than training in sex health.

To expect fear to prompt sex hygiene is to make a mistake that has retarded the development of sound measures in the treatment of offenders against criminal law. For centuries man failed in attempts to fit the punishment to the crime. To deter men from committing crime by holding up a threat of prolonged and dreadful punishment has been found futile. Individuals take the risk because they think they will escape detection. It is an axiom of criminal procedure that a would-be offender is deterred by the certainty, not by the severity, of punishment. The modern theory of probation is, that children and adults may be best led away from evil practices by crowding out old influences with newer and stronger interests. Occupations [386]that are wholesome are made to rival diversions or occupations that are harmful and criminal.

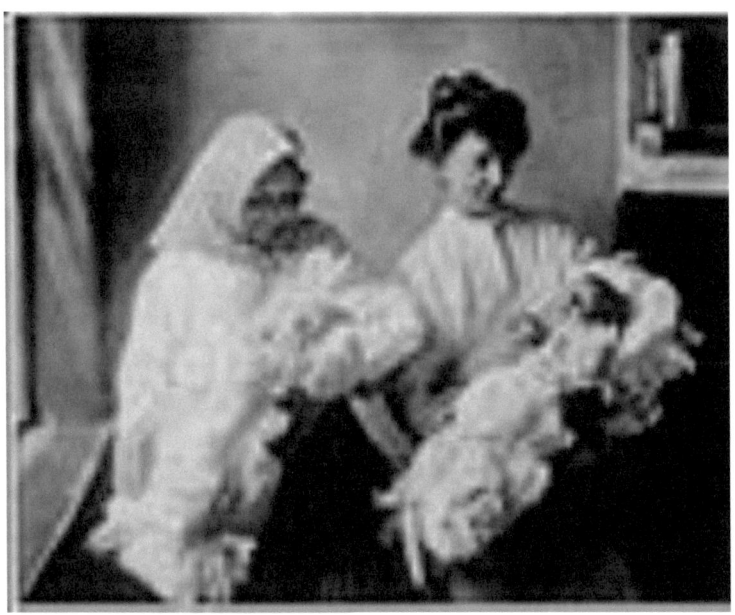

OBJECT LESSONS FOR INSTRUCTION IN SEX HEALTH
Note the uncomfortable, unhealthy overdressing

Abnormal conditions of mind and body in regard to sex can almost always be traced to general physical ill health or to an unhealthy moral environment. Cure and prevention require two kinds of treatment within reach of parents and teachers: (1) build up the child's physical condition; and (2) give him other interests. Proper physical care, and work adjusted to body and mind, may be relied upon to do infinitely more to promote sex hygiene than instruction, either at home or at school, in immoral sex diseases. That sex morality is weak and untrustworthy which is based upon fear of sex diseases. Like alcoholism and nicotinism, the saddest results of sex diseases are social and economic. The strongest reasons against such diseases are economic and social, not physiological.

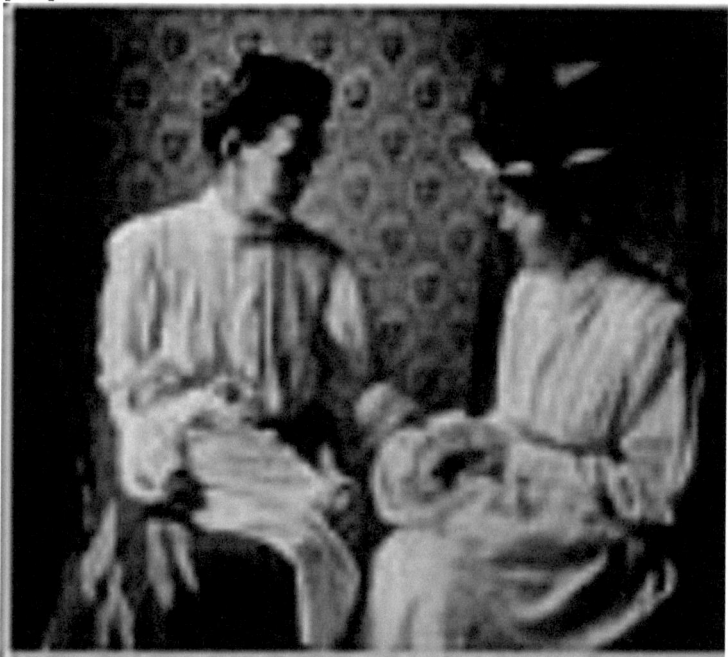

THE STUDY OF INFANT HEALTH IS CONDUCIVE TO PURE-
MINDEDNESS
Note the simple, comfortable, hygienic dress

Once having made up our minds to concentrate the teaching of
sex hygiene upon sex health rather than upon sex immorality, upon
sex functions rather than upon sex diseases, the chief objection to
school instruction and to instruction in class will disappear. Our
school text-books in history, literature, and biology abound in references to sex distinctions, sex functions, and sex health. In enumerat-
ing the daily routine of health habits I mentioned daily bathing of
the armpits and crotch. There is nothing in this injunction to offend
or injure a boy or girl. If studies and physical training are to be
adapted to physiological age, and if children are to know why they
are graded according to physiological age as well as mental brightness, we shall soon be talking of mature, maturing and not-yet-
maturing [388]girls and boys, so that everybody will be instructed

in sex hygiene without offense. Any teacher who can explain the family troubles of King Henry VIII without becoming self-conscious can easily learn to look a class of girls and boys in the face and explain how a mother's health will injure her baby before its birth, why breast-fed babies are more apt to live than bottle-fed babies, why it is as important for the mother to keep a nursing breast absolutely clean as to clean the nipple of a nursing bottle. Words whispered by children, or marked in dictionaries, to be stealthily and repeatedly looked upon and talked over with other children, lose all their glamour when pronounced by a teacher.

In these days of state subsidy of school libraries the child is hard to find who has not free access to books of fiction full of voluptuous allusions that make undesirable impressions which only blunt, candid discussion of sex facts can make harmless. Children now learn, whether in fashionable private schools or crowded slums, practically all that is lascivious and unwholesome about sex. For teachers to explain that which is wholesome and pure will disinfect the minds of most children and protect them against miseducation.

Class instruction in hygiene is practicable for all matters pertaining to normal sex health. Girls of thirteen should be taught in classes the fact and meaning of menstruation, and its grave importance to the health, in order that they may care for themselves not only before, during, and immediately after the menstrual period, but throughout the month, in order that menstruation itself shall not be unnecessarily painful, enervating, and harmful to efficiency. It is not yet advisable to discuss dangers peculiar to girls or dangers peculiar to boys in mixed classes. Generally speaking, it is undesirable that men teachers discuss girls' troubles with girl pupils. But why should it not become possible for women teachers to explain health dangers peculiar to girls to classes of boys?

[389]Individual instruction in sex matters should be reserved for the diseased mind, for the boy or girl who has already been morbidly instructed. Discussion of immoral sex diseases should be confined to individual talk. This field teachers have already entered. Repeated physical examination of children will detect symptoms of sex abnormality. When detected, the fact and the meaning should be explained to the individual by school physician, school nurse, or

school-teacher. While much can be done through mothers' meetings and through individual instruction of parents, the most effective means of improving the general attitude towards sex health is to give the simple truth to the millions of children who have not yet left school. Armed with the A B C's of sex hygiene at school, boys and girls will be prepared to select employment, associates, and newspapers that will permit normal, healthy sex development. Men and women who are leading normal lives, who have plenty of work, sleep, fresh air, nourishing food, amusement, and exercise are unlikely to be sexually abnormal.

After all, the question of instruction in sex hygiene will quickly settle itself when it is made a condition of a teacher's certificate that the applicant shall himself or herself know the personal and social reasons for sex health. The woman who does not know how to take care of her own sex health, the man who is ignorant of a woman's special needs, cannot do justice to the requirements of arithmetic, language, and discipline. Whether men and women teachers are mentally, physically, and morally equipped to be sexually normal and to teach the law of sex health will be disclosed as soon as trustees and superintendent dare to ask the necessary questions. Whether an instructor's personality will enable him to fill the minds of children with interests more wholesome, more absorbing than obscene stories or morbid sex curiosity can also be learned. When school-teachers are prepared to teach the [390]social and economic aspects of general health they will quickly solve the problem of instruction in sex health.

Just one word about country morality. It is customary to deplore the influence of large cities on the young. Of late, however, there has been a tendency to question whether, after all, sex morality is apt to be higher in the country than in the city. Parents and teachers in small towns and in rural districts will do well to take an inventory of the influences surrounding their children. It will always be impossible to give country children city diversions. One great disadvantage of country children frequently counter-acts the beneficial influence of out-of-door living; namely, isolation. The city child is practically always in or about to be in the sight of, if not in the presence of, other people. Numbers and close contact with people, though they be strangers, mean restraint and pervading social conscience. City children find it difficult to have good times in pairs. No amount of instruction of rural pupils in sex hygiene will take the place of amusements and entertainments for groups of children, forming thus a special antidote for "two's company, three's a crowd." Liberating and standardizing normal intersex relations and discouraging cramped social intersex relations are more urgent needs than instruction in sex diseases. A working environment that permits pure-mindedness will do more to inculcate a reverence for sex cleanliness and for parenthood than lectures and essays on moral prophylaxis.

[391]

THE ELEMENT OF TRUTH IN QUACKERY; HYGIENE OF THE MIND

Patent medicines and other forms of quackery could not pay such enormous dividends unless there was some truth in their claims; unless their victim found some beneficial return for his money. They win confidence because they raise hopes and combat fear. They do cure thousands of people of fear and of "ingrowing thoughts." In so doing they remove the sole cause of much disability.[17] In so doing they are merely applying by wholesale principles of mental hygiene that are legitimately used by physicians, tradesmen, teachers, and parents who deal successfully with nervousness.

Quackery makes cures and makes money because of the undoubted influence of mind in causing and in removing those ailments that originate in fear, imagination, or morbid introspection. A few years ago a little out-of-the-way town in southern Minnesota was visited by train loads of the sick and crippled from miles around. Miraculous cures were heralded broadcast. Life-long cripples left wagon loads of crutches and braces to decorate the little church with the enchanted transom. People who had not walked for years returned to their homes cured. The marvels of famous shrines were fast being duplicated when the church authorities at St. Paul issued an explanation of the alleged miraculous appearance of biblical figures in the transom of the new church. The outlines of a mother carrying a baby had [392]been vaguely impressed in the transom glass when molten. When the mystery was explained the excursions and the cures stopped.

Nearly every physician and practically every medical charlatan can count scores of cures of ailments that had previously defied the skill of eminent physicians. A child's bumps actually stop aching after the mother or nurse kisses the abused spot. Invalids forget their limitations under stress of some great excitement or some intense desire for pleasures incompatible with invalidism. Many a physician of reputation owes his success in great part to the discriminating use of the *placebo*,—a bread pill designed to supplant the patient's fear with confidence. Hypnotism and "suggestion" have been successfully used to cure alcoholism and to fill patients' minds with conviction stronger than the fear that produced the sickness. A well-known writer and preacher cures insomnia by auto-suggestion, telling himself he is sleepy, is very sleepy, is going to sleep, is almost asleep, is fast asleep. Treatment by osteopathy has been followed by disappearance of diseases that cannot possibly be cured by osteopathy. Christian Science has restored to health and happy usefulness hundreds of thousands of chronic invalids. Verily is hygiene of the mind an important factor in the civics of health.

Fear can originate with mind. Fear produces fear. Fear disarranges circulation of the blood and the nourishment of muscle and nerve. Fear can produce many bodily disorders which in turn feed fear. Fear cannot last unless bodily symptoms exist or arise to justify and feed it. Fear can be cured and removed in two ways: (1) by driving away fear and releasing bodily disorders from its thraldom; (2) by removing the disorders and making fear impossible to the logical mind. An enforced sea voyage begins with the disorder; a clever, buoyant physician begins with the fear. Patent-medicine proprietors, quacks, and fakes of every [393]kind begin by displacing the fear with hope or cheer; the physical disorders frequently vanish by the same window as fear. For *fear* write *self-pity*, *morbid self-consciousness*, *hypertrophied submission*; to *hope* and *cheer* add *smile*, *relaxation*, and *zest*; and we have the chief elements of mental hygiene and the reason why intelligent as well as unintelligent men like to be swindled by medical or other quacks.

The social aspects of mental hygiene are particularly important. Once admitting the power of the mind to decrease vitality, we recognize the duty of seeming happy, buoyant, cheerful, vital, at least when with others, for the sake of others' minds and bodies. Secondly, we find the duty to refrain from commenting on others' appearance in a way that will start "ingrowing thoughts." A "grouchy" foreman can give blues and indigestion to a roomful of factory girls. A self-pitying teacher can check the heart beats of her class, cause arteries and lungs to contract, and deprive the brain of fresh blood. An oversympathetic neighbor can put a strong man to bed by discovering signs of nervous disintegration. Shall we gradually work out a code of mental hygiene rights and nuisances that will require compulsory notification of the "blues" and compulsory segregation of every person unable to "smile dull care away"? Is the time coming when boards of health will accompany infection leaflets with messages such as this from James Whitcomb Riley:

> Talk health. The dreary, never-changing tale
> Of mortal maladies is worn and stale.
> You cannot charm or interest or please
> By harping on that minor chord, disease.
> "Whatever the weather may be," says he,
> "Whatever the weather may be,
> It's the songs ye sing, and the smiles ye wear,
> That's a-making the sun shine everywhere."

[394]Mental hygiene has hitherto enjoyed an evil reputation and has been condemned to generally evil associations, because the rank and file have been ignorant of hygiene of every kind. Medical science has so long enveloped itself in mystery that it is in danger now of becoming discredited and of falling heir to the mantle of quackery.

Quacks often get social and economic results more agreeable to the patient and more helpful to society than orthodox medicine. "When traitors become numerous enough treason becomes respectable." So when mental hygiene succeeds, it becomes science for the case in question, and for that case orthodox medicine loses its respectability. For the layman there is no safety except in having intelligence enough to know whether his trouble has defied the sincere application of mental treatment, auto-suggestion, and loyalty to the health ideal.

Mental hygiene admits the existence of dental cavities, scarlet fever germs, adenoids, cross-eyes, uncleanliness, broken legs, inflamed eyes, overeating. The organic, structural defects which are to be sought by physical examination are all admitted by mental hygienists. They work for an orderly, daily routine and affirm the penalties of its violation. They would even favor going periodically to a physician, provided that we never go to him except when organic or structural disorders may safely be assumed from the fact that cheer and relaxation treatment does not give relief. Unhygienic living and mind cure cannot go together. The mind that tries to deceive itself cannot cure either mind or body. The man who violates the habits of health cannot patch his injuries or conceal the ravages of dissipation by mental hygiene. Here is the great advantage of knowing how to live hygienically, of observing habits of health, and then concerning ourselves not with ourselves, but with conditions of living for all those whose health can be affected by our health, or can affect our health and efficiency.

[395]The most recent practical application of mental hygiene for moral and physical uplifting is the "moral clinic" or "psychotherapeutic" clinic established by Emmanuel Church in Boston. This clinic represents the union of three forces,—religion, medical diagnosis, mental hygiene. As a result of this alliance it is anticipated that both religion and medicine will be humanized, socialized, vitalized, made to express more accurately and more consistently that community consciousness and that yearning for equal opportunity and equal happiness which constitute the profoundest religious impulse. No person is treated at this moral clinic whose trouble is organic or structural. In determining whether the case belongs to this clinic, expert medical diagnosis is relied upon rather than the credulity of the patient or the zeal of the clergyman. Medical scientists of highest repute can consistently coöperate, because they recognize two scientific facts: first, that many troubles are due primarily to mental disorder; and, second, the greatest asset of the human mind is that something called religion, which is no less real and potent because peculiar to each individual. Whatever may be that deepest current of thought and feeling, whatever that synthetic philosophy, that explanation of being, which guides my life, it can be of inestimable aid if enlisted in an effort to secure normal vitality of mind and body.

The controlling motive of the moral clinic has proved infectious. There is reason to believe that the alliance of medicine and religion has come to stay, and that the present excitement over psychotherapeutics will settle down into a scientific utilization of religious motive and medical knowledge to prevent mental and moral disease. Unwholesome, morbid, self-centered thought is driven out. A recognition of others' claims takes its place. Hypnotism, suggestion, and group enthusiasm are used to their utmost possibilities. The success of the Boston moral clinic is due to establishing [396]in the mind of the neurasthenic, the alcoholic, the world-weary, and the purposeless a truer conception of the pleasures that result from vitality and from altruistic effort.

It is too early to classify by kind of functional disorder the patients treated. Results from one patient have been described in newspapers as follows:

A school-teacher, as a result of nervous collapse, had lost control, began to fear the children under her care, and thought of relinquishing her profession. She was instructed in the art of self-control and the control of others; the notion of fear was dislodged and a sentiment of love for her little charges took its place. In the course of a few weeks this conscientious and experienced teacher regained her poise and found herself performing her duties better than ever before.

Many alcoholics have for months given evidences of complete cure. Stories almost incredible are quickening pastor and physician alike throughout the country. After individual treatments are given, after religious motive is appealed to, and the soul stirred to heed the lessons of religion, medicine, and sociology, patients are given the work cure. Thus a branch of social service is established, where after-treatment is given to the patient whose thoughts have been turned from himself to others. All of a sudden the church finds itself in need of definite knowledge as to opportunities for altruistic work, as to definite community needs not met, as to people in distress who can be relieved by volunteers, as to agencies which can be called upon to coöperate both in treating the individual and in utilizing his energies for others' benefits.

Because a relatively small percentage of men and women are neurasthenic, melancholy, morbid, alcoholic, the lesson of the moral clinic is most serviceable when extended for the benefit of the "not yet alcoholic" and the "not quite neurasthenic." In other words, individuals in thinking of [397]themselves must learn the health value and soul value of purpose that centers in others' happiness. That thing which we have called tact in personality, and which in the past was discovered by induction, namely, the law of mental hygiene and the control it gives over others' health, must be taught in schools to children by wholesale, must be taught in medical and theological schools, to all physicians and all pastors. This alliance of medicine and religion, which is at present confined to one or two moral clinics, should be incorporated into education, into social work, into church work, becoming thus a part of civilization's normal point of view.

Mental hygiene cannot survive conscious violation of the fundamental laws of medicine and religion. The alliance of medicine and religion will prove utterly futile unless habits of living and of thinking are inculcated that conform to nature's law of self-preservation and to God's law of brotherly love. Self-centered religion, like self-centered medicine, destroys both body and soul.

FOOTNOTES:

[17] The alliance of mental hygiene, medicine, and religion is discussed in the Emmanuel Church book, *Religion and Medicine; the Moral Control of Nervous Disorders*; also in its bulletins, *Religion and Medicine*.

[398]

CHAPTER XLIToC

"A NATURAL LAW IS AS SACRED AS A MORAL PRINCIPLE"

When a grammar-school boy I learned from the game "Quotations" that Louis Agassiz, scientist, had written the sentence with which I introduce a final appeal for living that will permit physical and civic efficiency. Agassiz has been called "America's greatest educator," and again "the finest specimen yet discovered of the genus *homo*, of the species *intelligens*." The story of his long life as teacher of teachers reads like a romance. But among his gifts to education and citizenship none can be made to mean more than the simple proposition that natural law is as sacred as a moral principle. All who remember this "beatitude" will be helped to solve many perplexing problems of dress, diet, play, education, philanthropy, morals, and civics.

Reverence for the natural carries with it a distaste for the unnatural. Those who obey natural law soon come to regard its violation as a nuisance when not immoral. On the other hand, compromise with the unnatural, like compromise with vice, quickly leads first to toleration and thence to interest and practice. Therefore the importance of giving children Agassiz's conception of the sacredness of the laws that govern the human body. A passion for the natural is a strong foundation for habits of health and a priceless possession for one who wishes to know morality in its highest sense.

"Natural" is less attractive to us than it would be had Agassiz first interpreted it for us rather than Rousseau or present-day exponents of "the simple life," "back to nature," [399]and "back to the land." It is too often forgotten that no one sins against natural law more grievously than the primitive man or the isolated man in daily contact with non-human nature. Communing with nature seems not only to require communing with man but to give joys in proportion as the nature lover is concerned for the human society of which he is a part. Natural law does not become a moral principle until man is benefited or injured by man's use of nature's resources within and about him. Natural living according to natural law must be something sounder, more beautiful, and more progressive than can be read into or out of mountains, trees, brooks, and sky, or primitive society.

Natural law points to a Nature Fore as well as a Nature Back, to a Nature Up and Beyond as well as a Nature Down and Behind. The Nature that was yesterday will not do for to-morrow, any more than a man is willing to give up his nature aspirations for the careless, animal ways of romping childhood. Civilization is constantly urged at each step to repeat the prayer of Holmes's old man who dreams for the Autocrat of the Breakfast Table:

> Oh for one hour of youthful joy!
> Give back my twentieth spring!
> I'd rather laugh a bright-haired boy
> Than reign a gray-beard king!
> Off with the wrinkled spoils of age!
> Away with learning's crown!
> Tear out lifc's wisdom-written page,
> And dash its trophies down!
> One moment let my life blood stream
> From boyhood's fount of flame!
> Give me one giddy, reeling dream
> Of life all love and fame!

But every experiment in turning back exalts the present and the future. Gifts as well as problems are seen to come [400]with complexity, and civilization flatly refuses to relinquish these gifts. Sound maturity is better than youth or age:

> The smiling angel dropped his pen, —
> "Why, this will never do;
> The man would be a boy again,
> And be a father too!"

Problems of health and of civics can never be solved by appealing to Nature Back, when only the few could be healthy, when one baby in three died in infancy, when old age was toothless and childish, when infection ravished nations, when the average life was twenty years shorter than now, and when unspeakable filth was tolerated in air, street, and house. They can all be solved by appeals to Nature Fore, which holds up an ideal of mankind physically able to enjoy all the benefits and to conquer all the dangers of civilization. It is not looking back, but looking in and forward that reveals what natural law promises to those who obey it.

By using numerous tests which have been suggested in preceding chapters we can learn how far we and our communities obey natural law when working and playing. Health for health's sake has nowhere been urged. On the contrary, healthful living has been frankly valued for its aid to efficient living by individual and by community; wherefore the emphasis upon others' health and upon the civic aspects of our own health. Tests furnish us with the technic necessary to efficient living; civics, with the larger reason; natural law, with the "pillar of fire by night" to help us choose our path among habits and pleasures whose immediate results upon efficient living cannot easily be determined.

Fashions, tastes, mannerisms, personal indulgences, have been left for Agassiz to deal with. Generally speaking, we all know of numerous acts committed and numerous acts [401]omitted in our daily routine that convict us of not living up to our knowledge of physiology and hygiene,—wearing tight shoes or tight corsets, drinking strong coffee, smoking, reading while reclining, failing to insure clean air and clean bodies. Then there are other acts whose omission or commission violate no physical law so far as we can see, but whose unnaturalness we concede,—putting chalk on the eyebrows, wearing false hair or curious puffs, putting perfumery in the bath or on handkerchiefs, assuming artificial poses of body or mouth. These violations of natural law are forced upon us by "style" or "custom" or family convenience. When we come to choose between following fashions and disobeying them, we generally decide that it is better to do a foolish or slightly harmful thing than to occasion criticism, mirth, or even special notice by our dress or our abstemiousness.

Last night I went to a dinner party at eight. I ate and ate a great variety of palatable foods that Nature Back never knew. After two hours of eating I imbibed for two hours the tobacco smoke of the gentlemen who made up the party. I knew that eight o'clock was too late for me to begin eating, that two hours was too long to eat, that the tobacco of others was bad for my health and for to-day's efficiency. All this I knew when I accepted the invitation to dinner. I went with no intention of preventing others from smoking or of lecturing my host or his chef or his guests for the unhygienic practices of our day. Yet the physical ills were more than offset by certain definite gains to the school children of New York that will result from last night's meeting. Natural law was abated in part. But I declined certain dishes that would not agree with me, helped myself sparingly of many dishes, avoided tobacco and wines, and by a three-mile walk in the open air, a bath, and a good long night's sleep have almost recovered my right to talk of the sacredness of natural law.

[402]Nature Back says I should not have gone to this dinner. But I was compelled to go. I know I am going to others. I cannot do my work unless I overdraw my current health account. Nature Fore tells me that effective coöperation with others will frequently require me to eat at the dinner hour of others, to retire at others' sleeping time, to wear what others will approve, to violate natural law. But Nature Fore also tells me how to build up a health reserve so that I can meet these emergencies without endangering my health credit.

Nature Back demands "dress reform." Nature Fore tells me that I can march in step with my contemporaries without either attracting attention or discrediting and affronting natural law. Passion for the natural has effected numerous reforms in dress, diet, and social habits, until commerce provides a natural adaptation of practically every fashion. With regard to few things is it necessary to-day for any one who reads magazines to do violence to bodily health for fashion's sake. We may wear what we will, eat what we prefer, decline what is unnatural for us, without inviting censure. The debauches of those unfortunate people who live an unnatural, purposeless existence, affect such a small number that their laws need not be considered here. Natural law makes obedience to itself attractive; hence commerce is rapidly learning to cater to distaste for the unnatural. With few exceptions, only temporary concessions to unnatural living are required in order to dress and act conventionally.

Nature Back throws little light upon conditions necessary for modern labor. It can do nothing but demand the abolition of the factory, the big store, the tenement, the school. Nature Fore says we cannot abolish the means of working out the highest forms of coöperation. But we can make them compatible with natural living. We can modify conditions so that earning a livelihood will not compel workers [403]to violate natural law at any or all times. The greatest need of factory and tenement reform is for parents and teachers to make a religion of Nature Fore and to instill its principles in the minds of children. Parents and teachers must live the natural before they can make children love the natural. Parents and teachers cannot possibly be natural in this day, cannot live or love natural law unless they know the machinery by which their communities are combating conditions prejudicial to health, morals, and civic efficiency.